Glaserian Grounded Theory in Nursing Research

Dr. Barbara M. Artinian, PhD, RN is professor emeritus in the School of Nursing, Azusa Pacific University. She has taught courses in community health nursing, family theory, nursing theory, and qualitative research methodology. For about 7 years she conducted the Spiritual Care Research Institute that was held in collaboration with Azusa Pacific University and Nurses Christian Fellowship. Doctoral and master's level students attended the institute and through it Dr. Artinian became methodologist for three doctoral students who report their research in this book—Tove Giske, Pamela Cone, and Paula Vuckovich. Dr. Artinian has written a nursing model, the Intersystem Model, which is used internationally. The model was published by Sage Publications in 1997 in a book entitled *The Intersystem Model: Integrating Theory and Practice.* The model had been presented in many articles prior to the publication of the book. Dr. Artinian served on the doctoral committee of a student in Australia who used the Intersystem Model in his doctoral work (Taylor, 1977).

This book culminates the vision Dr. Artinian had in 1988 of what qualitative research could be when she wrote "Qualitative Modes of Inquiry" as published in the *Western Journal of Nursing Research.* It is very gratifying to see how the description of the modes presented in that article has been carried out in this book in a more sophisticated manner than was envisioned at that time.

Dr. Artinian grew up in Wisconsin and graduated from Wheaton College in Wheaton, Illinois. She attended Case Western Reserve University and earned a degree in nursing. She completed her graduate degree at the University of California at Los Angeles, earning an MSN degree. At the University of Southern California, she earned a PhD in sociology with a major emphasis in family theory. She had postdoctoral studies at the University of California at San Francisco in the area of chronic illness and studied with Strauss. She was introduced to the grounded theory method by reading and discussing the book *Theoretical Sensitivity* (Glaser, 1978) with the other postdoctoral students, Carole Chenitz and Janice Swanson. Her first use of the grounded theory method was with Mary Thompson (see chapter 11, "Nurturing Hope in Patients With Cancer") and she has continued to use the method with all her students. She has served as thesis chairperson for 24 students at the master's level and as methodologist for 5 doctoral dissertations.

Dr. Tove Giske, PhD, RN is currently an associate professor at Haraldsplass Diakonale Høgskole (HDH), the university college where she has taught nursing for over a decade. She holds a joint position of nursing research at HDH and Haraldsplass Diakonale Hospital, a sister institution of the nursing university college. Dr. Giske received her BSN from Betanien Diakonale Høgskole in Bergen, Norway, and both her MSN and PhD from the University of Bergen, where she conducted a Glaserian GT doctoral study with patients having diagnostic studies in a gastroenterology ward. Her dissertation, *Preparative Waiting*, examined the experiences of these patients as they tried to strategically balance their anxiety and hope during the long wait for a final diagnosis. Born and raised on the west coast of Norway, Dr. Giske has long been interested in spiritual caregiving. Currently the vice president of Nurses Christian Fellowship International, she has been an active member of KFSS, the Norwegian branch of NCF. She is also editor of the *Journal of Profession & Faith*, sponsored by KFSS. A vital part of the Spiritual Care Network of nurse scholars, she became a friend and colleague of both Dr. Artinian and Dr. Cone through the Spiritual Care Research Institute of 2001. Her continued interest in spiritual care research prompted her to join Dr. Cone as co-investigator on the spiritual care Fulbright research project in the fall of 2008. In addition, Dr. Giske is an active member of the Bergen, Norway, grounded theory (Bergen GT) group of research scholars.

Dr. Pamela H. Cone, PhD, RN, CNS received her BSN from Alderson-Broaddus College in Philippi, West Virginia, and her MSN from Azusa Pacific University (APU). Currently an assistant professor, she has been teaching nursing at APU for 17 years. Born and raised in Haiti, Dr. Cone's interest in people and cultures around the world has enabled her to successfully promote international experiences for nursing students at APU. In 2006 Dr. Cone received her PhD from the University of California, San Francisco. Her doctoral dissertation was based on a Glaserian GT study with formerly homeless mothers in the Pacific Southwest of the United States, and she continues to have an interest in vulnerable populations such as the homeless and immigrants. Her interest in spiritual care research goes back to a master's program completed in 1994. Since then she participated in an ongoing study on spiritual care for 7 years and remains an active member of an international network of nursing scholars who conduct research in this domain. In August of 2008, Dr. Cone received a Fulbright Scholar award that enabled her to conduct a six-month study requested by Norwegian nursing educators on how well their programs are preparing nurses to provide spiritual care. Her collaboration with Dr. Artinian dates from a qualitative research class in 1992. Dr. Tove Giske became a friend and colleague through the Spiritual Care Research Institutes, and together they remain actively involved in spiritual care research and part of the Bergen GT group of researchers.

Glaserian Grounded Theory in Nursing Research

Trusting Emergence

BARBARA M. ARTINIAN, PhD, RN
TOVE GISKE, PhD, RN
PAMELA H. CONE, PhD, RN, CNS

SPRINGER PUBLISHING COMPANY
New York

Springer Publishing Company, LLC
11 West 42nd Street
New York, NY 10036
www.springerpub.com

Acquisitions Editor: Allan Graubard
Project Manager: Mark Frazier
Cover design: Steve Pisano
Composition: Apex CoVantage, LLC

Ebook ISBN: 978-0-8261-0539-4

09 10 11 / 5 4 3 2 1

Library of Congress Cataloging-in-Publication Data

Glaserian grounded theory in nursing research : trusting emergence / editors, Barbara M. Artinian, Tove Giske, Pamela H. Cone.
p. ; cm.
Includes bibliographical references and index.
ISBN 978-0-8261-0538-7 (alk. paper)
1. Nursing—Research. 2. Grounded theory. I. Artinian, Barbara M. II. Giske, Tove. III. Cone, Pamela H.
[DNLM: 1. Glaser, Barney G. 2. Strauss, Anselm L. 3. Nursing Research. 4. Nursing Theory. 5. Qualitative Research. 6. Research Design. WY 20.5 G548 2009]
RT81.5.G57 2009
610.73072—dc22 2009014798

Printed in the United States of America by Hamilton Printing

We dedicate this book to Dr. Barney Glaser, who provided direction for our research through his many books.
We also dedicate this book to Dr. Rose M. Liegler, former dean of the Azusa Pacific University School of Nursing, during whose tenure most of the research reported in this book was done. Her support and encouragement made the research possible.

Contents

Contributors

Maureen Friesen, MSN, RN, CNS
Patient Flow Coordinator in Labor & Delivery
Huntington Hospital
Pasadena, CA
Adjunct Faculty, School of Nursing
Azusa Pacific University
Azusa, CA

Esther Hjälmhult, PhD, MAEd, RN, RPHN
Associate Professor, Faculty of Health and Social Sciences, Center of Evidence Based Practice/ Department of Postgraduate Studies
Bergen University College
Bergen, Norway

Judith Milligan-Hecox, MSN, RN, CNS
Former CEO of Livingston Memorial Health Agency
Ventura, CA

Pamela Sircar Osuri, MSN, RN, CNS, CCRN
Assistant Professor, Anne Arundel Community College
Arnold, MD

Lynda Pash, MSN, RN, CNS
Retired Hospice Case Manager and Admissions Nurse; ELNEC Trainer

Jane Pfeiffer, MA, MS, RN
Assistant Professor, School of Nursing, Azusa Pacific University
Azusa, CA

Milka Satinovic, PhD, MSN, RN
Associate Professor, Faculty of Health and Social Sciences, Bergen University College
Bergen, Norway

Mary Thompson, MSN, RN
Nurses Christian Fellowship Planned Giving Specialist
Former President of Nurses Christian Fellowship International, InterVarsity/ Nurses Christian Fellowship USA

Leslie Van Dover, PhD, MScN, RN, PN
Professor, School of Nursing, Azusa Pacific University
Azusa, CA

Paula Vuckovich, PhD, MSN, RN
Assistant Professor and Primary Undergraduate Advisor, California State University at Los Angeles
Los Angeles, CA

Katharine S. West, MPH, MSN, RN, CNS, PHN
Nurse Clinical Systems Project Manager, Kaiser Permanente
Pasadena, CA

Victoria Winter, MSN, RN, CNS, CCRN
Clinical Nurse IV, Children's Hospital Los Angeles
Los Angeles, CA
Adjunct Faculty, School of Nursing, Azusa Pacific University
Azusa, CA

Foreword

Grounded theory, a research method used internationally and by myriad disciplines, was developed by Barney G. Glaser and Anselm Strauss in 1967 (Glaser & Strauss, 1967) while they were studying patients dying in California hospitals (Glaser & Strauss, 1965). According to Morse (2009), grounded theory (GT) is likely the most widely used qualitative method of research. From the beginning, the method found favor with the nursing community, both because Glaser and Strauss held positions at the University of California, San Francisco, School of Nursing and because they mentored students in the then new doctoral program in nursing. The first graduate of the program, Jean Quint (later Benoliel), published the findings from her grounded theory study as the widely read book *The Nurse and the Dying Patient* (Quint, 1967), thereby giving further credence to the method for nurses. When the sociologists Glaser and Strauss (1967) wrote their first methodology book, *The Discovery of Grounded Theory*, it was natural that they used the jargon of their discipline; while nurses appreciated the findings from GT studies as true and meaningful to their work, they didn't have the sociology vocabulary to understand how it was done. It was only after Glaser wrote his follow-up book *Theoretical Sensitivity* (1978), and when students of Glaser and Strauss began writing clarifying articles that nurses were able to use the method (Stern, 1980).

Barbara Artinian was among the early interpreters of the method in her 1988 article "Qualitative Modes of Inquiry." The present book is an expansion and illustration of the ideas put forth in that article, where Artinian examined the range of GT and the possible levels of abstraction. During her 21 years as professor at Azusa Pacific University (APU), Artinian mentored masters and doctoral students through their thesis studies, teaching them the Glaserian version of GT (as opposed to the later Straussian adaptation [Strauss & Corbin, 1990; Stern, 1995]). In other ways Artinian followed the pattern set by Barney Glaser by publishing the work of her protégés in this book, as Glaser has done in his collections of studies (Glaser, 1993, 1994, 1996; Glaser & Holton, 2007).

I find the figures that illustrate the GTs developed by the authors (which they call conceptual maps) to be clear and helpful to the reader's understanding. As a rule, I admit that I tend to be dismissive of figures because beginning researchers spend so much effort depicting *everything* they found in the figure that the text suffers from a lack of explication. Perhaps *conceptual map* is a better term than figure, as for the visual learner, tracing the work as a drawing helps the GT researcher understand what is going on in the social scene.

The focus of this book is particularly clinical, to the extent that the final chapters deal with nursing interventions. In their work, Glaser and Strauss (1967) argued that the final level of abstraction would lead to formal theory. For nurses, intervention may be more useful than formal theory, even if the more professorial of us might be attracted to work that impacts the world as opposed to easing the discomfort of our charges.

During her tenure at APU from 1984 to 2005, Barbara Artinian conducted a series of Spiritual Care Research Institutes sponsored by APU and The Nurses Christian Fellowship. Azusa Pacific University was originally founded in 1899 as a Bible college, and today lists its purpose as continuing "to prepare young men and women to serve Christ throughout the world" ("Our History," 2009). It was as a result of these institutes that the authors of chapters in the present book looked to Artinian for mentorship in their research work. Therefore, it is no surprise that these authors seem particularly sensitive to the spiritual needs of patients.

Artinian's institutes attracted nurses from as far away as Norway, where one of her coeditors, Tove Giske, is an associate professor of nursing in Bergen (gateway to the fjords). Dr. Giske defended her dissertation at the University of Bergen in March 2008. Such is the popularity of her decade of teaching and leadership in the community that a whole contingent of friends and colleagues attended her graduation party. Dr. Giske has a long history of teaching nursing students about the importance of spiritual care in both clinical and didactic settings.

The second coeditor, Pamela Cone, assistant professor at APU, gained her PhD in 2006 from the University of California, San Francisco. She has long been a proponent of spiritual care and based her master's thesis in its provision. She received a Fulbright Scholarship in 2008 to respond to Norwegian nurse educators' request for a review of their programs in regard to spiritual care. She and Dr. Giske became colleagues as a result of the Spiritual Care Research Institutes; thus the institute brought scholars together, providing another avenue beside research meetings for colleagues to exchange ideas.

Barbara Artinian stands out as a mentor and colleague. With this book she provides a model for the retired academic's second career, spreading the grounded theory and spiritual care message in meaningful ways.

REFERENCES

Artinian, B. (1988). Qualitative modes of inquiry. *Western Journal of Nursing Research, 10*, 138–149.

Glaser, B. G. (1978). *Theoretical sensitivity.* Mill Valley, CA: Sociology Press.

Glaser, B. G. (1993). *Examples of grounded theory: A reader.* Mill Valley, CA: Sociology Press.

Glaser, B. G. (1994). *More grounded theory methodology: A reader.* Mill Valley, CA: Sociology Press.

Glaser, B. G. (1996). *Gerund grounded theory: The basic social process dissertation.* Mill Valley, CA: Sociology Press.

Glaser, B. G., & Holton, J. A. (2007). *The grounded theory seminar reader.* Mill Valley, CA: Sociology Press.

Glaser, B. G., & Strauss, A. (1965). *Awareness of dying.* Chicago: Norton.

Glaser, B. G., & Strauss, A. (1967). *The discovery of grounded theory.* Chicago: Norton.

Morse, J. M. (2009). The Banff symposium. In J. M. Morse, P. N. Stern, B. Bowers, K. Charmaz, & A. E. Clarke (Eds.), *Developing grounded theory* (pp. 9–11). Walnut Creek, CA: Left Coast Press.

Our history: About APU—Azusa Pacific University. Retrieved April 2, 2009, from http://www.edu/about/history

Quint, J. (1967). *The nurse and the dying patient.* New York: Macmillan.

Strauss, A., & Corbin, J. (1990). *Basics of qualitative research.* Thousand Oaks, CA: Sage.

Stern, P. N. (1980). Grounded theory: Its uses and processes. *Image: The Journal of Scholarly Nursing, 12*, 20–23.

Stern, P. N. (1995). Eroding grounded theory. In J. M. Morse (Ed.), *Critical issues in qualitative research methods* (pp. 212–223). Thousand Oaks, CA: Sage.

Phyllis Noerager Stern, DNS, LLD (Hon.), FAAN
Professor Emerita, Indiana University School of Nursing, Indianapolis, Indiana, USA

Preface

The purpose of this book is to illustrate the development of the Grounded Theory (GT) method developed by Glaser and Strauss (1967) and further described by Glaser in *Theoretical Sensitivity* (1978) and his recent publications. By staying true to the original description of the method, the researchers presenting their studies in this book have discovered grounded theories of various types and levels of abstraction. Dr. Barbara M. Artinian has either trained all of the authors, or has served as methodologist or consultant for their research projects in master's or doctoral studies. Her persistent efforts have enabled these scholars to maintain consistent use of a purist Glaserian GT method as we understand it.

This work is divided into four sections. Part I, "Theoretical Considerations," includes an overview of the GT method followed by a discussion of various experiences in developing grounded theories. It discusses the use of conceptual mapping as an assist to the analytical process, and explains how clearly medical personnel must understand the intent of Glaser's directives in order to use his method while satisfying research committee requirements. The final chapters of this section describe the process of a scholar moving from a novice state to that of an experienced researcher in the Glaserian GT method.

Part II, "Studies Using Early Modes of Grounded Theory," presents six examples of research using the early modes of Glaserian GT. The main modes are the descriptive, the gerund, and the emergent fit. The descriptive mode is the most detailed and least abstract of the GT modes. Two GT studies are presented in the descriptive mode. The gerund mode with its basic social process (BSP) is one of the most commonly reported of the GT modes, and two studies are presented in the gerund mode. Finally, part II presents two examples of the emergent fit mode. This mode starts with a theory or with variables thought to be relevant for the area under study, with the intent of clarifying or expanding the existing theory, or of clarifying the relationships among the variables.

Part III, "Studies with Emergent Theoretical Codes: Theoretical Code Mode," presents research from which a theoretical code emerged. This mode is more abstract than the modes discussed above and is more difficult to use because it requires the researcher to discover the overall organizing principle that relates the substantive codes into an integrated theory. These theoretical codes, which emerge from the data, describe in a more abstract way than in the other two modes how the main concern of the subjects is resolved. Glaser has identified many theoretical codes in his books. Ten studies depicting five specific codes are presented in this section. This level of abstraction is not often seen in GT work and is a unique focus of this book.

Part IV, "The Intervention Mode," is the final section, and it presents four research studies. In this mode, findings from fully integrated studies are used to conduct a research study in a clinical area, after which outcomes are further analyzed to improve nursing practice and to refine and extend the theories involved. These examples are presented to provide direction to other researchers who might use the intervention mode to test and extend their theories in their own practice settings.

A digital adjunct for this book, developed by Katharine S. West and Barbara M. Artinian, is available through Springer Publishing and includes the following content:

- The tables and conceptual maps presented in the book, converted into formats that can be used for PowerPoint presentations
- The watercolor paintings from which emerged the name of the theory "Preparative Waiting" (see chapter 5)
- Definitions of the modes of Grounded Theory
- Definitions of the types of theories emerging from Grounded Theory research
- An outline of how the use of the literature review as required by research committees evolved
- The Intersystem Model, which is the nursing model that uses the methodology of GT. A diagram of the model is also provided, and is illustrated by care plans based on data from studies reported in this book.

REFERENCES

Glaser, B. G. (1978). *Theoretical sensitivity.* Mill Valley, CA: Sociology Press.

Glaser, B. G., & Strauss, A. (1967). *The Discovery of grounded theory.* Chicago: Norton.

Acknowledgments

First of all, the editors thank all of the authors who contributed to this book. We appreciate your scholarly work. We all thank Dr. Barbara Artinian for her invaluable assistance with Glaserian grounded theory. Her mentoring and consulting assisted us in producing sound and rigorous research.

We also thank the university graduate programs where these studies were conducted. The leaders, colleagues, and peers from Azusa Pacific University, the University of California at San Francisco, the University of San Diego, the University of Bergen, and the University of Trondheim assisted us in numerous ways.

We cannot thank Katharine West enough. She was the graphic designer and is also a GT researcher. Without her knowledge of nursing, GT methodology, and graphic design, we would not have been able to prepare all the conceptual maps, figures, and tables presented in this work. We also thank Kathie Speck, who prepared the first version of this manuscript, and Katharine West, who integrated all the edited changes into the final manuscript.

Last, but not least, we wish to express our appreciation to God and to all our families and friends who helped us in countless ways, great and small, to accomplish this project.

Theoretical Considerations

PART I

INTRODUCTION: BARBARA M. ARTINIAN

The purpose of Part I is to give an introduction to the Glaserian Grounded Theory method and to discuss and give examples of learning and working with classical Grounded Theory (GT). In chapter 1, Artinian gives an overview of the GT method and discusses its historical development. The strengths and weaknesses of GT design as well as types of nursing problems for which the method is suitable are described. Issues in theory development such as sample size, data collection methods, levels of data analysis, reliability and validity, and human subject issues are presented. Practical issues such as proposal development and critiquing a GT study are also addressed.

In the 1990s, the controversy between adherents of a classic Glaserian approach and the axial coding method developed by Strauss and Corbin was the subject of many nursing journal articles. In chapter 2, Artinian discusses the relative usefulness of the two methods. Examples of theories developed using a classic Glaserian approach are contrasted with the descriptive data produced by the axial coding method.

Conceptual mapping is a strategy for graphically mapping the relationships between and among the variables in a research study. It serves as a tool to help the researcher clarify the probabilistic relationships emerging from the data. Principles for constructing conceptual maps are discussed by Artinian and West in chapter 3, and references are made to conceptual maps found in parts II and III.

In chapter 4, Cone and Artinian discuss the need to adjust a number of Glaser's directives found in *Theoretical Sensitivity* (1978) and *Doing Grounded Theory* (1998). Often the need to adapt Glaser's method for graduate committee requirements prompts some bending of the rules in GT research. Some of Glaser's directives can be followed with very slight adjustments, while others need major adaptation. The challenge is to understand the underlying principle of each directive so that the intent of the rule can be upheld while the manner of its use is adjusted. Thirteen directives are addressed in this chapter with examples from Cone's research.

Giske and Artinian describe the process of planning and carrying out a grounded theory study in chapter 5, "Learning Glaserian Grounded Theory by Doing It." The chapter contains examples of producing memos and analyzing data as well as the steps in the analysis of Giske's research. The tedious process of fitting concepts to data and further developing a parsimonious theory is explicated in well-constructed tables.

The three book editors write the final chapter in this section and address several ways to learn Glaserian GT and stay close to its original methodology. Cone discusses finding a mentor and engaging in scholarly dialogue, while Giske relates her experiences in a supportive scholarly GT group that continues to meet on a monthly basis. Artinian describes how she came to understand the grounded theory method by reading and discussing Glaser's work with other scholars who were learning the method. For all the editors, the most effective learning experiences occurred in community rather than learning the method by themselves.

REFERENCES

Glaser, B. G. (1978). *Theoretical sensitivity.* Mill Valley, CA: Sociology Press.
Glaser, B. G. (1998). *Doing grounded theory.* Mill Valley, CA: Sociology Press.

1

An Overview of Glaserian Grounded Theory

BARBARA M. ARTINIAN

The grounded theory method was developed by Glaser and Strauss during the 1960s. It was first described by them in their 1967 book, *The Discovery of Grounded Theory,* and was further explicated by Glaser in his 1978 book *Theoretical Sensitivity.* It is an inductive qualitative methodology that allows the researcher to identify the main concern of a group of subjects and the behaviors they use to resolve their main concern. The researcher then expresses this understanding in a theory named by a carefully chosen word or phrase that captures the subjects' experience. In this process, Glaser describes the main concern as the variable that motivates the behaviors that attempt to resolve the main concern. For example, in a study of elderly caregivers providing home care for their spouses, the main concern was to keep the spouse out of institutionalized care. The spouses were motivated to resolve their main concern by strategizing ways to provide care and "Making it Work" (the core category; Artinian, 2003). It is appropriate to use the grounded theory method when there is no existing theory to guide the research process. Glaser says that "grounded theory is the systematic generation of theory from data acquired by a rigorous research method" and the product is an "integrated set of hypotheses which account for much of the behavior seen in the substantive area" (1998, p. 3). Stern (1985) states that the purpose of grounded theory "is to identify problems and discover what the actors themselves see as solutions" (p. 153).

THE GLASERIAN GROUNDED THEORY DESIGN

Qualitative unstructured interviews and participant observation are the usual data collection methods for generating hypotheses. Nevertheless, other sources of data such as journals, formal documents, newspaper reports, literature from the substantive area or other areas, and personal experience can be added to the data set in the form of memos. In this methodology, the basic assumptions are that (a) the underlying main concern and core category will emerge with consistent use of the method, (b) the social organization of a group exists and is available to be discovered, and (c) the concerns of the participants rather than those of the researcher are the focus of the research (Glaser, 1998, p. 44–45).

Very early in the development of the method, Glaser and Strauss made the decision to develop theory around one aspect of a phenomenon even though the data provided many avenues of exploration. The most well-known example of this use of data centers on dying hospital patients. Glaser and Strauss divided the experience of dying in a hospital setting into two aspects: the trajectory of dying and the communication of information to the patient that dying was occurring. They used categories such as "death expectations," "nothing more to do," and "social loss" to develop hypotheses about the research area (Glaser & Strauss, 1967). They presented the subsequent theories in two separate books, *Awareness of Dying* (1965) and *A Time for Dying* (1968). Their method of targeting one core variable at a time in order to develop a theory distinguishes classic grounded theory methodology from qualitative data analysis.

Another important distinction Glaser makes is the twofold principle of (a) entering into the study of a phenomenon with no preconceived ideas of what data should be there and (b) remaining true to the data that are found. There can be no predetermined hypotheses or coding schemes to guide the analysis of data.

A third distinction in using Glaser's approach is the need to stay long enough in the setting to allow the researcher to identify the major concern of the participants so that the core category or process that depicts their answer to the problem is allowed to emerge. Glaser insists that the theory must respect and reveal the perspective of the subjects and not that of the researcher (1992, p. 17). Revealing the perspective of the subjects requires multiple interviews. The result of conducting too few interviews was exemplified in a study I reviewed, wherein the researcher claimed to have achieved saturation of her categories after three interviews, and then did two more interviews to confirm this. After carefully reading her work, I determined that she was only saturating her own preconceived categories.

The basic method of grounded theory, constant comparative analysis, is based on theoretical sampling: the concurrent collection, coding, and analysis of data, which is used to direct further data collection appropriate for developing the emerging theory. Grounded theory is developed by constant comparison of incident with incident. The comparisons are recorded in theoretical memos, which are the "theorizing write up of ideas about codes and their relationships as they strike the analyst while coding" (Glaser, 1978, p. 83). By recording the comparisons in memos using theoretical codes, the researcher develops categories and hypothesizes relationships among categories. These relationships are then tested through theoretical sampling until categories are saturated and a core category emerges that describes the behavior used by the subjects to resolve their main concern. The goal of grounded theory is to discover the core category. This goal is aided by theoretical sorting of the memos, which makes possible the integration of connections among the categories and leads to a rich, multivariate theory.

Grounded theory can be done using different modes. What the modes have in common is that they all use the constant comparative approach to identify the main concern of the subjects and how the subjects resolve the concern. The research can be initiated in the discovery mode or in the emergent fit mode. The discovery mode is used when the researcher enters the field with no preconceptions about what will be found and allows the variables to emerge. When a basic social process or a core category has been discovered by the researcher in a prior study or by some other researcher and is used as the starting point for the new research, the emergent fit mode is used. In this way, a program of research can be initiated such that each study builds on the prior study (Wuest, 2000). (For an example of this approach, see chapter 12, "Partnering With God and the Patient.")

In the past, a grounded theory study could be started with variables identified in a literature review that were thought to be relevant to the area of study. Identifying these variables was required by the research committee. An example of this type of emergent fit study (chapter 11, "Nurturing Hope in Patients With Cancer") shows how, by using the constant comparative approach, a basic social process (BSP) was identified—Nurturing Hope. This approach is not recommended now that research committees are more familiar with the grounded theory method. Glaser says that the problem with using the emergent fit mode is that the identified basic process (or variables) may not fit the new data. However, he states that this mode "has a place in grounded theory if done properly" (1978, p. 108). Although the researcher starts with a preconceived framework, early thoughts can be corrected by proceeding in the constant comparative method.

Both the discovery mode and the emergent fit mode can be used to develop theories in the descriptive mode, the gerund mode (a basic social process) (Glaser, 1996), or the theoretical code mode. All theories must begin with substantive codes, which are the categories and their properties that emerge from the data. With further analysis of the same data, either the discovery mode or the emergent mode can be moved to a higher level of abstraction by relating the substantive codes to each other with a theoretical code. Glaser says, "Without substantive codes, theoretical codes are empty abstractions" (2005, p. 11). However, if substantive codes are used without theoretical codes, the findings cannot be conceptualized in a meaningful way. The value of allowing a theoretical code to emerge from the data is illustrated by Giske, who presents the same study in the descriptive mode (see chapter 7 of this volume, "Preparative Waiting: Patients Hospitalized for Diagnostic Workups") and in the theoretical code mode (see chapter 21, "Patterns of Balancing Between Hope and Despair in the Diagnostic Phase on a Gastroenterology Ward"). Cone also illustrates the emergence of theoretical codes (chapter 17, "Mutuality: Reconnecting to Overcome Homelessness") by analyzing her BSP of reconnecting in terms of the theoretical code of cutting point and subsequently amplifying causal loops. Theories at the gerund or theoretical code mode level of abstraction can be used to conduct research in the intervention mode. The potential relationships between these modes are diagrammed in Figure 1.1. Each of these modes is discussed in later chapters, where examples of research using the modes are presented.

The Strengths and Weaknesses of the Design

The major strength of the grounded theory method is its ability to move data from the descriptive level to the conceptual level. There are no set formulas for doing this and some researchers find the progression from the descriptive to the conceptual level perplexing. However, Glaser has written several books in the past few years that describe in more detail how to conceptualize data (2001, 2003, and 2005). These books are not

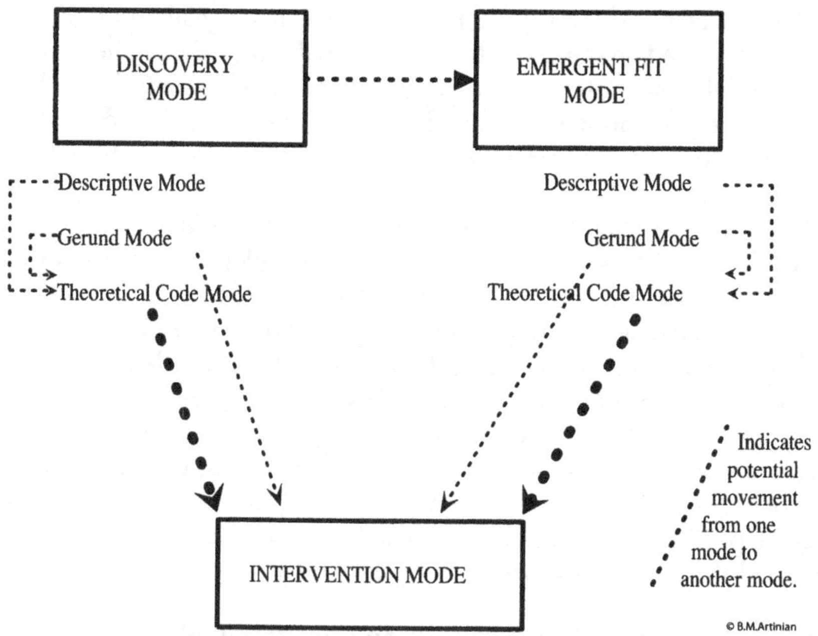

Figure 1.1 Modes of grounded theory.
Printed with permission from B. M. Artinian.

easy reading but can provide understanding of how to integrate hypotheses into a grounded theory. In addition, Glaser has developed a Web site (www.groundedtheory.com) to connect the global network of grounded theory researchers (Glaser, 1999, p. 845).

The benefit to the researcher of undertaking a grounded theory study is that he or she can progress from knowing very little about the main concern experienced by the participants to being an expert on the theory that accounts for their behavior. The moment when the core category that integrates the data is found can be truly exciting. The theory integrated by the core category works to explain relevant behavior in the substantive area, has relevance for the participants and academic community, and fits the situation because it has been developed from data that have been gathered from the participants. In addition, the theory can be modified if new data point to new categories or properties of a category.

Some of the problems that are encountered in using the design stem from the researcher rather than from the method. The most difficult problem often is the researcher's unwillingness to give up preconceived ideas of how the subjects should be responding. For example, one student initially wanted to test the hypothesis that nurses in the labor and delivery setting would interact with patients in the manner in which they had experienced their own labor. When she was willing to give up this hypothesis, she found that the development of the nurse-patient relationship was influenced by other variables that primarily had to do with patient characteristics or the environmental setting (see chapter 8, "Caregiving Behaviors of Intrapartum Nurses").

Another researcher-generated difficulty is the desire to tell the whole story in all its details. When focusing on theory development, peripheral aspects of the data that are not related to the core variable must be left out. An example of a study that includes the life stories of each subject is *Good Days, Bad Days* (Charmaz, 1991). Glaser describes this storytelling type of study as *qualitative data analysis* but not *grounded theory.* He suggests that Charmaz could have developed a grounded theory of "simplifying life styles" under a condition of impairing chronic illness that would resolve the patient concern of needing to redesign life (Glaser, 2003, p. 178). In this way, there would have been direction and organization of the data rather than merely descriptive accounts.

Kinds of Nursing Problems for Which the Grounded Theory Design Is Suitable

The grounded theory method can be used to study any type of problem that involves the discovery of a patient or nurse concern. It cannot be used to study professional problems that are preconceived from the nursing literature. For example, Glaser reported that Amy Calvin (2000) wanted to study how dialysis patients handled end-of-life directives. She could not get them to talk about directives because their main concern was not how to plan for death but how to stay alive by "beating the odds" (Glaser, 1998, p. 124). Because she was willing to explore with the patients what they were really thinking about, she identified the core category, "*personal preservation*" to describe their experience. The grounded theory method can be used to study any problem provided that the researcher is willing to let the subjects define the problem, is willing to let go of any preconceived ideas, and is willing to trust that the ways the subjects resolve their concern will emerge.

THEORY DEVELOPMENT

The grounded theory method is primarily an inductive method. Incident is compared to incident to develop categories and then to see how these categories are related. As incidents are compared in line-by-line analysis, the researcher asks the question, "What category does this incident indicate?" or "What property of what category does this incident indicate?" Lastly, the researcher asks, "What is the participant's main concern?" (Glaser, 1998, p. 140). These categories are then related in hypotheses using theoretical codes. Glaser says that selective coding "starts only after the analyst is sure that he has found a core variable" which "then becomes a guide to further data collection and theoretical sampling" (1992, p. 75). As hypotheses emerge, they are tested deductively by theoretically sampling to gather and compare more data. The researcher then generates concepts to round out the theory. Theoretical sampling is usually done within the same substantive area so that a theory that describes how the concerns of that group are resolved can be developed.

Sample

Sample size cannot be predicted at the beginning of a grounded theory study since it is not possible to know what concern will emerge as problematic and how it will be resolved. The object of study is the concern particular to a group of people experiencing the same social situation. Therefore it is important to ensure homogeneity of the sample, just as a quantitative design controls for extraneous variables. Later, when a theory is developed, theoretical sampling can direct the researcher to other groups in which the same main concern may be occurring, resulting in further development of the theory. Data collection continues until categories are saturated and a core category emerges that integrates most of the categories. For example, in a study of socialization of novice nurses to the intensive care unit, it was thought that a sample of 15 nurses would be sufficient for the study. However, by using the constant comparative approach, it was found that the male nurses resolved their main concern (to find out where they fit into the nursing profession) in a different way than did the female nurses. Therefore, in order to saturate the categories, more interviews and observations of male nurses needed to be done (Osuri; see chapter 10, "Moving On: A Study of Male Novice Nurses in the Critical Care Unit").

Data Collection Methods

Data are usually collected initially through tape-recorded interviews using an interview guide. In his work, Glaser counsels against developing interview guides. However, an interview guide may help beginning researchers to get started. The researcher must use the guide knowing most of its questions will be peripherally relevant (at best) to the particular participants being questioned. If participant responses are vague or not meaningful, the researcher then asks questions related to the experience of the subjects until their concerns are brought forth. Since the goal of the research is not to get a response from each subject to a set of questions, but to discover their main concern and patterns of behavior, any questions or observations are suitable if they help the researcher to know what is going on in the participants' world of experience. The participants do not all need to respond to the same questions, either.

Glaser makes a strong case against the taping of interviews because he believes that taping produces too much data without distilling the main ideas. Also, the need for transcription of the tapes slows down the time between data collection and analysis because often the researcher does not begin interacting with data until the transcriptions are available. Glaser recommends writing detailed notes after leaving the setting, which can be immediately analyzed for patterns. However, my students and I have found it useful to tape record interviews so that the interviews can be listened to a number of times to detect themes and nuances we may not have been aware of during the interview. To begin the process of data analysis before the tapes are transcribed, we listen to the interviews immediately until the salient ideas are embedded in memory so that our brains can be working on the process of analysis while the tapes are being transcribed.

In many settings, tape recording cannot be done because to tape record would destroy the relation-building process that occurs during participant observation. In these situations it is important to record extensive field notes that include the actual words and interactions of the participants. It is also true that data given during a formal tape-recorded interview can be qualitatively different from that given in casual conversation. During a study that I did of a drug rehabilitation program for women, I did a follow-up interview in their homes. Often the participant would engage me in a 45-minute conversation at the door of her home as I was preparing to leave. What was told to me then was often of a more intimate nature than what had been told me on tape. So as not to lose this information, as soon as I entered my car, I would turn on the tape recorder and record it (Artinian, 1975). Therefore, I find that a combination of formal tape-recorded interviews and field notes based on casual interviews and observations constitutes the best data set.

Types of Data Analysis

Data analysis is based on a three-level conceptual perspective analysis. Glaser (1998) outlines these three levels as follows:

- The first level is the data.
- The second level perspective is the conceptualization of the data into categories and their properties. There are sublevels that exist within this level.
- The third level is the overall integration of data into a theory through data sorting.
- A fourth level perspective is the formalization of a substantive theory to a more general conceptual level by constantly comparing substantive theory articles (p. 136).

Most published research in the grounded theory tradition uses only the above-named three levels of analysis, but Glaser gives further examples of formal theory development from his own work, such as the theory of status passage (Glaser & Strauss, 1971). Glaser gives more complete guidelines about how to develop formal theory in the *SAGE Handbook of Grounded Theory* (Glaser, 2007).

Substantive categories are developed into codes that name the participant actions in the substantive area. These codes can be "in vivo" codes, which mirror the conceptual talk of the participants, or they can be researcher-generated codes. During the coding of substantive categories, theoretical codes emerge that relate the categories and develop the theory. As the theory is developed using theoretical codes, coding changes from open coding (in which everything is coded) to selective coding focused only on the core category and related categories. When a theoretical code does not emerge from the data, the theory can be described as "descriptive telling of what happens." Finding a theoretical code allows the researcher to tell *how* it happens.

There are many families of theoretical codes described by Glaser in the book *Theoretical Sensitivity* (1978), and he added more in 1998 and 2005. A basic social process is one theoretical code in which the core category has two or more distinct stages. This code was commonly used in the earlier grounded theory studies (Glaser, 1996) and is still useful when a theory describes how the subjects move through a situation. However, many other theoretical codes can emerge from the data. For example, this book presents additional codes: strategizing, cutting point, amplifying causal loops, role theory, and balancing. Glaser says, "theoretical coding is the least understood aspect of generating grounded theory" (2005, p. 10). He describes theoretical codes as "abstract models of integration, based on best fit . . . which conceptualize how the substantive codes will relate to each other as a modeled, interrelated, multivariate set of hypotheses in accounting for resolving the main concern" (2005, pp. 10–11). Glaser answers the question of whether theoretical codes are necessary with the response by saying no, they are not, "but a grounded theory will appear more relevant and more enhanced when integrated and modeled by an emergent theoretical code" (2005, p. 14). In order to model how the theoretical code integrates the substantive codes, I find the technique of conceptual mapping to be useful in analyzing relationships among the variables. A conceptual map is "a diagram of the relationships among the variables" (Artinian, 1982, p. 379). The map illustrates the process subjects use to resolve their main concern.

Treatment of Reliability and Validity in Grounded Theory

Initially Glaser specified the criteria for judging the quality of a grounded theory as "fit, work, relevance, and modifiability" (1978, pp. 4–5). In an analysis of these criteria using a realist interpretation, Lomberg and Kirkevold (2003) conclude that fit "is a matter of correspondence to facts in social reality" and that work, relevance, and modifiability "are argued to support the fitness of a theory and to be useful in the broader evaluation of the quality of grounded theories" (p. 189).

More recently, Glaser has addressed the issues of reliability and validity and concludes that grounded theory does well in meeting the established criteria:

1. Credibility. A grounded theory is abstract of time, place, and people. Because the categories are constantly compared to vary them for application and to develop new properties, he states that when a theory is generalizable, fits, works, is relevant, and is highly modifiable, this method produces a product that is credible.
2. Transferability. Because a grounded theory transcends experience it moves from description of what is happening in a particular situation to an understanding of the process by which it happens. Since it is abstract of time, place, and people it can be more readily applied to a new situation with emergent fit.

3. External validity. The concept of fit means that the theory both fits the situation from which it was generated and can be generalized to other situations by constant comparison.
4. Dependability. All categories and properties are constantly verified during the process of generating theory. New data or changing conditions just require modification as categories vary and these modifications are worked into the theory.
5. Confirmability. The problems of reproducibility, replication, and objectivity are not pertinent to the grounded theory method because conceptualization is the goal, not description. The conceptual patterns, once discovered, stand on their own and new data will only extend or modify the theory (Glaser, 2001, pp. 123–124).

The best argument for the validity of a grounded theory is the affirmation of the knowledgeable person when the grounded theorist is able to explain how his or her world fits together and works. By providing categories that reveal the underlying patterns in their world of experience, the theorist helps the participants understand how to manage their world. In an article on the value of grounded theory for nursing (Artinian, 1998), many examples are given of subject responses to the theoretical explanation of their behavior. For example, after sharing the results of one study describing how patients managed their dialysis, a head nurse in a dialysis unit said to me, "We know these things, but how do you?" and also added, "I never thought of it in that way." Understanding the patients' main concern and how they resolved it, opened up the world of experience of the patient for the nurses in a way they had not understood before and provided them a sense of direction in working with the patients.

Research Proposal Issues

In their introduction to an article on writing a proposal in the naturalist paradigm, Sandelowski, Davis, and Harris (1989) capture the major problem in proposal development:

> The preparation of the research proposal for a study that involves an emergent research design compels the investigator to negotiate the paradox of planning what should not be planned in advance. (p. 77)

Their suggestion is to describe a tentative plan for sampling and data collection with the explicit statement that this plan is only to provide the initial direction for the study. Glaser makes it clear that theoretical sampling provides the impetus for directing data collection and analysis. In order not to preconceive the concepts to be studied, Glaser recommends reading in a "general area that is along side [sic] the area of research" (2001, p. 136). A more in-depth literature review is done after the core category is identified. For example, Winter (see chapter 19, "Preserving Identity in a Nursing Home Setting") did an extensive literature review on role theory after finding it to be a theoretical code of significance in understanding the behaviors of the subjects in her study.

Because it is not possible to know what direction the investigation will take, it is not possible to know what data will be needed to continue the investigation. Therefore, a research proposal must be understood as no more than a framework for getting started. Glaser says that the proposal is "designed to keep the research open to generating while keeping preconceptions to the minimum" (2001, p. 111). The researcher must retain the flexibility to allow the unanticipated to emerge, maintaining the right to modify the design and the right to flexibly change the research as emergent theory corrects it (Glaser, 2001, p. 114). For Glaser, the ideal proposal would be very simple. It would need only to describe a relevant area of interest, identify a site where it can be studied, establish that there is entry, and state that the GT method of collecting, coding, and analyzing data would be followed until the theory emerges. He realizes that this will not satisfy most research committees and so he says that the researcher must do what is necessary; but as Stern writes, the proposal "does not necessarily constitute the study that will actually be done" (Stern, 1985, p. 152). However, Glaser concludes that the researcher must do what needs to be done to get started and the grounded theory methodology will correct any preconceptions that were written into the proposal (2001, p. 114).

Human Subjects Issues

Glaser makes the argument that the privacy and identity of subjects are not revealed in the research report because "grounded theory is conceptualized patterns abstract of time, place, and people. No person or place can be recognized" (Glaser, 2001, p. 129). However, he comments that the grounded theory researcher must choose illustrations carefully for very sensitive substantive areas. Despite the safeguards to privacy built into the GT method, most institutional review boards require that the participants sign a consent form. Glaser lives in the real world of institutional review boards and devotes several chapters to the research proposal so that the researcher can develop a proposal with the required consent form that meets the requirements of the review board thus allowing research to begin (2001, pp. 111–143). Glaser's main concern is that the consent form must contain language that allows for flexibility of data collection and analysis of data. Glaser advises the researcher to keep human subjects issues and consents to a minimum (2001, p. 130). My approach is to use a consent form whenever a tape-recorded interview is done, but to secure no consent other than approval from the research site for casual conversations or observations that are recorded in field notes or memos.

Critique of a Glaserian Grounded Theory Research Report

When I review a published research report that claims to use the grounded theory methodology developed by Glaser, the most important question I ask myself is: "Would it be possible using the stated problem, the sampling strategy, and the method of analysis to develop a theory that has fit, work, relevance, and modifiability?" Specific issues to consider are:

1. Is there evidence that the problem has been preconceived by the researcher rather than emerging as a concern of the subjects?
2. Is the focus on quantity of data for full description rather than theoretical sampling of data to develop a theory?
3. Does the theory appear superficial? Is it what would be expected after a cursory analysis of the data? An example of a superficial theory might be an analysis suggesting that a basic social process is to experience an event, respond to it, and complete the event, rather than identifying the process taking place in each of these stages. This "theory" is merely reporting the developmental stages of the event, such as a parent bringing a baby to a hospital, enduring the hospital experience, and taking the baby home. It is not a true theory and has no grab and interest. In contrast, when the core category of the event is found and integrated by a theoretical code, such as "strategizing" done by prenatal patients in a rural area, a useful theory is described that has implications for prenatal practice and for other rural population groups (see chapter 13, "Strategizing Safety by Perinatal Patients in a Rural Setting").
4. Does it appear that the sample selection and data collection points are theoretically driven or preconceived? Do the subjects have an experience in common that can be understood theoretically?

5. Are the data forced into an existing theoretical framework or are the subjects' concerns and their way of resolving their concerns allowed to emerge from the data?

CONCLUSION

A grounded theory transcends the experience of a group of subjects and can provide direction for understanding the patterns of other groups of subjects experiencing a similar condition, such as a chronic illness. Using the emergent fit mode to study the new situation, a program of research can be initiated (Wuest, 2000). When a theoretical code emerges, it moves the study from a description of what is happening (descriptive mode) to an understanding of the process by which it happens by identifying and integrating patterns of behaviors that subjects use to resolve their main concern (gerund mode and theoretical code mode). When an integrated theory is used to develop interventions to improve clinical practice, and data from the study are analyzed to refine, modify, or extend the theory, the theory becomes more useful to the nursing profession (intervention mode).

REFERENCES

Artinian, B. (1975). *Identity change in a therapeutic community.* Unpublished doctoral dissertation, University of Southern California, Los Angeles.

Artinian, B. (1982). Conceptual mapping: The development of the strategy. *Western Journal of Nursing Research, 4,* 379–393.

Artinian, B. (1998). Grounded theory research: Its value for nursing. *Nursing Science Quarterly, 11*(1), 5–6.

Artinian, B. (2003, August 5–8). Making it work: Elderly spouses as caregivers. Thinking Qualitatively Workshop. University of Alberta, Edmonton, Canada.

Calvin, A. (2000). *Hemodialysis patients and end of life medical treatment decisions: A theory of personal preservation.* Unpublished doctoral dissertation, University of Texas at Austin.

Charmaz, K. (1991). *Good days, bad days: The self in chronic illness and time.* New Brunswick, NJ: Rutgers University Press.

Glaser, B. G. (1978). *Theoretical sensitivity.* Mill Valley, CA: Sociology Press.

Glaser, B. G. (1992). *Basics of grounded theory analysis: Emergence versus forcing.* Mill Valley, CA: Sociology Press.

Glaser, B. G. (1996). *Gerund grounded theory: The basic social process dissertation.* Mill Valley, CA: Sociology Press.

Glaser, B. G. (1998). *Doing grounded theory: Issues and discussions.* Mill Valley, CA: Sociology Press.

Glaser, B. G. (1999). The future of grounded theory. *Qualitative Health Research, 9*(6), 836–845.

Glaser, B. G. (2001). *The grounded theory perspective: Conceptualization contrasted with description.* Mill Valley, CA: Sociology Press.

Glaser, B. G. (2003). *The grounded theory perspective II: Description's remodeling of grounded theory methodology.* Mill Valley, CA: Sociology Press.

Glaser, B. G. (2005). *The grounded theory perspective III: Theoretical coding.* Mill Valley, CA: Sociology Press.

Glaser, B. G. (2007). Doing formal theory. In A. Bryant and K. Charmaz, *The SAGE handbook of grounded theory* (pp. 97–111). Los Angeles, CA: Sage.

Glaser, B. G., & Strauss, A. (1965). *Awareness of dying.* Chicago: Aldine Publishing.

Glaser, B. G., & Strauss, A. (1967). *The discovery of grounded theory: Strategies for qualitative research.* Chicago: Aldine Publishing.

Glaser, B. G., & Strauss, A. (1968). *Time for dying.* Chicago: Aldine Publishing.

Glaser, B. G., & Strauss, A. (1971). *Status passage.* Chicago: Aldine Publishing.

Lomberg, K., & Kirkevold, M. (2003). Truth and validity in grounded theory—a reconsidered realist interpretation of the criteria: Fit, work, relevance and modifiability. *Nursing Philosophy, 4,* 189–200.

Sandelowski, M., Davis, D. H., & Harris, B. G. (1989). Artful design: Writing the proposal for research in the naturalist paradigm. *Research in Nursing & Health, 12*(2), 77–84.

Stern, P. (1985). Using grounded theory method in nursing research. In M. Leininger (Ed.), *Qualitative research methods in nursing* (pp. 149–160). Orlando, FL: Grune & Stratton.

Wuest, J. (2000). Negotiating with helping systems: An example of grounded theory evolving through emergent fit. *Qualitative Health Research, 10*(1), 51–70.

2

Experiences in Developing Grounded Theory Through Emergence

BARBARA M. ARTINIAN

Since the publication of the book *Basics of Qualitative Research* by Strauss and Corbin in 1990, many qualitative researchers have used the axial coding methodology described in it to guide their research studies. Glaser (1992) has written a response to Strauss and Corbin in his book *Basics of Grounded Theory Analysis: Emergence Versus Forcing*, in which he asserts that the Strauss and Corbin method is not grounded theory but rather a method that develops "forced, conceptual description" (p. 5). In an issue of *Qualitative Health Research* (August, 1996) devoted to an examination of advances in grounded theory methodology, Melia (1996) states, "it still remains to be seen if other social scientists conclude that Strauss is indeed saying something different from Glaser" (p. 370). This author's chapter is a response to Melia's challenge. It is written in the hope that it will encourage other researchers to describe their experiences using the two approaches. The author provides several examples of research completed by herself, her students, or colleagues using the traditional method of emergence described by Glaser (1978) in the book *Theoretical Sensitivity*.

EXPERIENCES WITH GLASERIAN GROUNDED THEORY

"Grounded theories have grab and are interesting. People remember them; they use them." (Glaser, 1978, p. 4). Despite the fact that numerous theories with "grab" and excitement have been generated using the traditional methodology described by Glaser and Strauss (1967) and Glaser (1978), many researchers are now using the Strauss and Corbin methodology of axial coding. Glaser (1992) suggests that the novice to the grounded theory methodology may use the axial coding method because it is so easy to use. He says that if you follow the prescribed process that Strauss and Corbin describe, "you are sure of finding something" (p. 5). The axial coding method insists that the researcher look for the conditions and dimensions of any situation; these always exist, so researchers are certain to be able to describe them. The problem in Glaser's eyes is that they may not be relevant to the situation under investigation. In contrast, the painstaking Glaserian process of integrating categories into a theory is difficult and cannot always be accomplished. I myself have pondered the behaviors of certain subjects in my investigations for years before finding time to do the analysis that identified the theory guiding their actions.

For example, in my study of young adults on dialysis (Artinian, 1983), I found that their two major developmental tasks were to find a job or to find a spouse. Few of them were able to accomplish both tasks. However, two dialysis patients who were very successful businessmen had also married. After several years of marriage, they both divorced their wives. For over seven years I puzzled over why they did this when it is so difficult for a disabled person to find a spouse. Finally, by looking closely at all the examples of marital relationships discussed by all of the patients and their spouses, the category of marital role performance became pivotal to my understanding. The category was saturated by examining the indicators of the same essence. For example, a bride of six months told me, "I almost divorced my husband because he was babying me too much. But we had a long talk and now he doesn't do it anymore." This indicated to me that she expected her husband to expect her to do what a wife should do. On the other hand, the expectation could not always be fulfilled. Another young dialysis wife told me, "There are a lot of times I just don't feel good, and he has to be very understanding about that, and it's just that I can't help it. Maybe I'm tired and the laundry doesn't get done right away. He has to be a lot more understanding of me than I of him."

One of the divorcing husbands told me, "She always expects me to be up." Further insight into the essence of the process came from a conversation with a 24-year-old unmarried man. In talking about dating, he commented, "She's not old enough yet." When I asked if he had someone specific in mind, he said, "No, but in order to marry someone on dialysis she would have to be very mature. Since I think the husband should be older than the wife, she's not old enough yet."

From these comments and others, I realized that the main concern of the partners in a successful marital relationship was the acknowledgement of the role responsibilities of the disabled spouse. This was resolved by willingness to set the expectations aside if fatigue prevented carrying out the responsibility at a particular time. The wives of both the successful businessmen were unable to relax their expectations and the men found it impossible to continue the relationship. From this analysis, the theory of "bending expectations" in a marriage in which one spouse is at a disadvantage because of a chronic illness emerged from the data (Artinian, 1990). Because this theory emerged directly from the data, there was no need to "validate the theory against the data" in order to ground it as suggested by Strauss and Corbin (1990, p. 133).

When analyzing the data about the dialysis patients, I did not attempt to show the whole range of variation possible within each indicator but rather to show how each indicator was related to the main category so that a theory would emerge. It can be assumed that as variables, the indicators pointing to a concept will vary, but it is not their range of variability that is important, but their essence—in this case, the ability of spouses of dialysis patients to both hold role expectations and bend them. The emergent method of coding and writing memos about the emerging process is very different from the axial coding method described by Strauss and Corbin (1990) in which every category is fully dimensionalized. Glaser says that the axial coding method produces "forced, full, conceptual description" but not grounded theory (Glaser, 1992, p. 5), because a grounded theory emerges directly from the data rather than from fitting data into axial codes.

In order to absorb "data as data, to be able to step back or distance oneself from it, and then to abstractly conceptualize the data" (Glaser, 1992, p. 11), it is necessary to immerse oneself in the data. In working with a graduate student who was studying the experience of colostomates, we found the category of "valuing of self." This did not prove to be useful in understanding her data. As I was driving home from grocery shopping and thinking about the many instances where self-image had been enhanced in these patients, I realized that the basic social process occurring was "revaluing of self." This process integrated all the categories of experiencing loss of the normal self, acceptance of the person by significant others, and finally acceptance of self as all right even with a colostomy (Woodward, 1982). Once the basic social process was discovered, the writing that had floundered for months was completed in two weeks. Glaser (1978) talks of this mental process of reflecting on data so as to understand the essence of the indicators as "delayed action phenomena" and "preconscious processing" (p. 18).

It takes time to allow the theory to emerge from the data rather than from the experience of the analyst. It is much easier to think about situations from the experience of the researcher and to use those insights to analyze the new data, but the grounded theory method requires analysis of the data to find out if other subjects also describe their life experience in a similar way. Glaser (1992) insists that the theory must respect and reveal the perspectives of the subjects (p. 17).

In developing a grounded theory it is necessary to ask questions of the data, analyze the data line by line, and develop the theory oneself. Development of a grounded theory requires immersion in the data in order to assimilate it. I have found that the best way to foster this assimilation is to allow the brain to store the data by hearing the interviews and reading the transcriptions of the interviews. By developing categories and writing memos, the analysis process is started, but often the brain analyzes the stored data in ways we cannot understand. In one case, I was writing an abstract for a conference and had just written that what I would present would be a description of nurses' activities with cancer patients. Even as I wrote, I heard in my mind from the taped interviews the nurses saying "Never again," "I decided," and "There is no other way I could nurse." I suddenly realized that these nurses were making a decision whether or not to risk emotional involvement with patients. The basic social process of risking involvement integrated all the categories and provided a useful way to understand the experience of the nurses. The theory came to me when I least expected to discover it (Artinian, 1995; see chapter 18 "Risking Involvement With Cancer Patients").

Although axial coding is one way to "get into the data," it can result in the "overconceptualization of a single incident" (Glaser, 1992, p. 40). It is very difficult for discovery to break through the analysis and the product is usually mere thick description. In a research session at the Western Institute of Nursing conference in Portland in 1997, Dr. Judy Kendall first presented a detailed analysis of the concept *disruption* in families with attention deficit hyperactivity disorder (ADHD) children. She presented antecedent factors, mediating interactions, context, phenomena, family responses to disruption, actions, intervening conditions, and outcomes (Kendall, 1997). By doing this, she was able to identify five family responses to their experience. However, she felt that she had missed what was going on in the experience of the families. Glaser (1992) says that:

> Once this form of forced coding starts, the grounded theory is usually lost because the analyst is led far away from relevance. He is led away from an analysis that does not "work" or account for a concern of relevance. He is struck with continued forcing description of the full scene to justify his time and effort. (p. 47)

Of course, it is possible for emergence to "poke its reality" (Glaser, 1992, p. 95) through the forcing of the data into the axial paradigm, but it is difficult.

When Kendall decided to go back and reread *Theoretical Sensitivity* (1978) and begin memoing ideas as they emerged, the basic social process of Reinvesting was discovered. This is a very important theory for anyone working with these families. The identification of the stages families go through, from doing everything they can do to help the child, to letting go of the anticipated normal child, to reinvesting in their own lives again, provides a useful theory for understanding the family experience (Kendall, 1998). Since this theory of reinvesting transcends the specific disease entity, it was useful for me in understanding the experience of families with autistic children at various ages.

Anyone familiar with the richness of grounded theories knows that they capture the essence of the human process under investigation. A true grounded theory needs to show how the subjects resolve their main concern. Glaser (1992) suggests that the "need to preconceive is very strong when there is no trust in the discovery of a problem" (p. 24) and that the research problem should not be stated until it emerges from the data. The beauty of grounded theory is that statements of relationship emerge from the data rather than being preconceived if the researcher is willing to look at the total experience of the subjects.

Rafuls, a researcher who defined herself as "a newcomer to qualitative research in general, and grounded theory specifically" (Rafuls & Moon, 1996, p. 67), felt that she was obliged to use the Strauss and Corbin method because it would only be possible to implement the Glaser method if "Glaser himself, or one of his disciples, for that matter, were there to coach me all the way through . . . so that I would not wonder whether I was proceeding correctly" (p. 67). However, this is not an adequate reason for selecting a method that does not produce grounded theory. There are many books available to the novice wishing to learn the Glaser method. For example, the Chenitz and Swanson (1986) book, *From Practice to Grounded Theory*, gives much practical advice on how to do the constant comparative approach of grounded theory in addition to giving examples of research completed using this method. Glaser has also published a reader, *More Grounded Theory Methodology* (1994), which gives many examples of research illustrating his method.

In addition, a growing number of scholars who have used the Glaser method successfully are available for consultation. When a group of doctorally prepared nursing faculty members and doctoral students wanted to learn the grounded theory methodology, I implemented the week-long Spiritual Care Research Institute. This institute took place each year from 1997 to 2002. It was jointly sponsored by Nurses Christian Fellowship and Azusa Pacific University. To date, more than 30 scholars have attended the Spiritual Care Research Institute. The week focused on data analysis methods for coding and memoing using *Theoretical Sensitivity* (Glaser, 1978) as the basis of the discussions. My research associates, Pamela Cone and Katharine West, introduced the participants to computer coding and data retrieval methods using the NVivo program (Richards, 1999).

Prior to attending the institute, all participants read *From Practice to Grounded Theory* (Chenitz & Swanson, 1986) and interviewed both patients who had received spiritual care and nurses who had given spiritual care. "Office hours" were held every evening of the institute, often in a group format, to discuss individual ideas for research and formulation of research questions. By the end of the week, all participants were able to clarify either how they could develop their own studies, or how they could participate in the ongoing study, using the interviews generated for the institute. One participant made this comment: "Grounded theory is so much clearer. The assignments guided our preparation, but hands on coding and office hours clarified so much."

CONCLUSION

Axial coding may lead one into great insights about subject data because one instance is examined in great detail, such as the concept of disruption. However, it may prevent the researcher from seeing the overarching phenomenon underlying the data. Grounded theory analysis leads to hypotheses about the process emerging from the phenomenon. Whereas the pure description of the Strauss and Corbin method is situation specific, a grounded theory transcends the data by explaining the variations in the events that comprise the data. By comparing incident to incident as depicted in patient interviews, patterns revealing significant aspects of human behavior are identified that were not previously conceived. Therefore, Glaser says that patience is needed to let relevance emerge (1992, p. 47). Trust in the subjects is also needed. Through persistence in coding the responses and behaviors of the subjects, the data from the subjects will let the researcher know what the subjects' main concerns are. These insights will emerge into grounded theory for anyone willing to patiently immerse himself or herself in the experience of the subjects.

NOTE

This article was submitted to Dr. Glaser to be reviewed for publication in his online journal a number of years ago. It was never published, but he referred to it in his book *The Grounded Theory Perspective III: Theoretical Coding* (2005, p. 52). He incorrectly stated that I took a long time to develop theory because I combined grounded theory procedures with non-GT procedures. In my 20 years of using the Glaserian methodology, I have constantly advised students and colleagues not to use Strauss and Corbin's axial coding methodology. Therefore I was shocked to have Glaser attribute this method to my work. In a discussion with Dr. Glaser he understood his mistake and asked what we should do for damage control. He suggested that I write a memo that he could include in copies of his book to explain how I do grounded theory. Following is the memo that I sent to him:

> Dear Dr. Glaser,
>
> I am writing this memo at your request to correct an error that occurs on page 52 in the book *The Grounded Theory Perspective III: Theoretical Coding* (2005). From an incorrect reading of an article I submitted for consideration to www.groundedtheoryinstitute.com entitled "Experiences in Developing Grounded Theory Through Emergence," Dr. Glaser made the assumption that I combine the GT method and the method of axial coding and thus prolong the time needed to develop a GT. Nothing could be further from the truth. In the article I report (with her permission) Judy Kendall's attempt to use the Strauss and Corbin method to analyze data for her dissertation. She reported that she felt obligated to use that method because she had received funding for the proposal, which stated she would use that method. At a Western Institute of Nursing research conference (1997) she reported that after 3 years of attempting to analyze her data using the axial coding method, she concluded that her analysis did not match what she was seeing in the families she was observing. She then started her analysis over using the GT method outlined in *Theoretical*

Sensitivity and developed the GT of Reinvesting. At no time did she use both methods concurrently. My article also cites the experience of other researchers who attempted to use the Strauss and Corbin method without success. I then described my experience of developing the GT of Bending Expectations. I had written several articles from my study of young adults on dialysis, but other research and teaching responsibilities kept me from further analysis of the data. However, for over seven years I puzzled about why some dialysis patients had divorced their wives. I finally went back to the data and used the concept-indicator model and the other procedures of GT. Within a very short time, the major concern of the subjects emerged (marital role performance), which was resolved by the process of bending expectations. It was lack of time to do the analysis, not the use of the axial coding method, that prolonged the emergence of the theory.

REFERENCES

Artinian, B. (1983). Role identities of the dialysis patient. *Nephrology Nurse, 5,* 10–14.

Artinian, B. (1990). Bending expectations for marital role performance of dialysis patients. *Family and Community Health, 12,* 47–57.

Artinian, B. (1995). Risking involvement with cancer patients. *Western Journal of Nursing Research, 17,* 292–304.

Chenitz, C., & Swanson, J. (1986). *From practice to grounded theory.* Menlo Park, CA: Addison Wesley.

Glaser, B. G. (1978). *Theoretical sensitivity.* Mill Valley, CA: Sociology Press.

Glaser, B. G. (1992). *Basics of grounded theory analysis: Emergence vs. forcing.* Mill Valley, CA: Sociology Press.

Glaser, B. G. (1994). *More grounded theory methodology: A reader.* Mill Valley, CA: Sociology Press.

Glaser, B. G. (2005). *The grounded theory perspective III: Theoretical coding.* Mill Valley, CA: Sociology Press.

Glaser, B. G., & Strauss, A. (1967). *The discovery of grounded theory.* Chicago: Aldine.

Kendall, J. (1997). *Reinvesting.* Paper presented at the meeting of the Western Institute of Nursing Conference, Portland, OR.

Kendall, J. (1998). Outlasting disruption: The process of reinvestment in families with ADHD children. *Qualitative Health Research, 8,* 839–857.

Melia, K. (1996). Rediscovering Glaser. *Qualitative Health Research, 6,* 368–378.

Rafuls, S., & Moon, S. (1996). Grounded theory methodology in family therapy research. In D. Sprenkle & S. Moon (Eds.), *Research methods in family therapy* (pp. 65–82). New York: Guilford Press.

Richards, L. (1999). Data alive! The thinking behind NVivo. *Qualitative Health Research, 9,* 412–428.

Strauss, A., & Corbin, J. (1990). *Basics of qualitative research.* Newbury Park, CA: Sage.

Woodward, B. (1982). An exploratory study of the phenomenon of embarrassment in colostomates. Unpublished master's thesis, California State University, Los Angeles.

3 Conceptual Mapping as an Aid to Grounded Theory Development

BARBARA M. ARTINIAN
KATHARINE S. WEST

"Grounded Theory is the systematic generation of theory from data acquired by a rigorous research method resulting in an integrated set of conceptual hypotheses" (Glaser, 1998, p. 3). Glaser has discussed how to move from substantive data to memos to integrated hypotheses in many of his books. Although Glaser (1978) says that categories emerge from the data, behind that emergence is a thought process that makes it possible to see the relationships that exist among the categories. One useful method for developing theory from integrative memos, which describe the categories emerging from the data, is conceptual mapping.

DESCRIPTION OF CONCEPTUAL MAPPING

Conceptual mapping is a strategy first developed by Artinian in 1977 and published in 1982a. A conceptual map "is a diagram of the relationships among the variables" (Artinian, 1982a, p. 379). A conceptual map is useful in displaying the theoretical relationships identified in qualitative studies, as when a basic social process has been discovered in grounded theory research, such as the theory of Letting Go in chapter 9.

Just as Glaser (1998) used his background in quantitative research and the "explication of the text" (p. 24) to conceptualize the grounded theory method, so I used my understanding of quantitative research, especially path analysis (Duncan, 1966), and qualitative research (Lofland, 1971) to develop the technique of conceptual mapping. Glaser states, "Much of grounded theory uses qualitative math. That is, it uses probability statements assessing patterns of properties" (1998, p. 22). The conceptual map organizes data into a probabilistic schema of how variables are related to each other to resolve the main concern. It is a theoretical model that shows a tentative diagram of reality as understood by the investigator. For example, the theory of Reconnecting (see chapter 17 "Mutuality: Reconnecting to Overcome Homelessness") illustrates the steps a homeless mother goes through in reintegrating into society.

I (Artinian) had already developed the technique of conceptual mapping before I was introduced to grounded theory, and it has been very useful in identifying and clarifying basic social processes and research with emergent theoretical codes. The technique can be used for presenting any type of completed research. The first time I presented the conceptual mapping technique at a research conference (Artinian, 1982b), a doctoral student told me, "Now I know what to do with my data."

Conceptual maps have three purposes:

1. To aid in theory development by illustrating how a theory is being conceived at a particular time. They are a graphic representation of the thought process as the theory evolves. Maps reduce the integrative memos to a diagrammatic representation. This aids the researcher in identifying inconsistencies or gaps in the emerging theory.
2. To provide a structure for organizing and presenting data. Burns and Grove (1997) suggest that a map that is well developed will be easily understood by colleagues and by the subjects.
3. To visually present the theory to the reader.

Principles for Constructing Conceptual Maps

Because maps are visual rather than verbal, they have a different and possibly greater impact on understanding of a theory than verbal descriptions. Therefore they must very accurately and graphically display the theory. The ways in which we construct conceptual maps have expanded and improved since West began using computer programs in 1996 to generate conceptual maps. Since she is trained in both grounded theory and in graphic design, she has been able to work with many of the authors who present their research in this book to help them visually express their theories. Mapping technique has progressed from lines and arrows as originally done (see chapter 11, "Nurturing Hope in Patients With Cancer," Figure 11.1) to a graphic representation of the theory of bending expectations as a balancing scale (see chapter 22, "Bending Expectations by Spouses of Dialysis Patients: Balancing Between Alternatives," Figure 22.2). Because electronic graphic files can overwhelm typical e-mail services, West uses the Internet file transfer protocol (FTP) feature of her Web site to share a newly rendered map with its authors for review and collaboration. Subsequent versions can incorporate the author's desired changes.

Some of the most important principles that are used in constructing maps have been described by Artinian (1982a). These principles have been expanded as we have used computer programs to generate maps. Each principle will be discussed and a map in the book will be referenced that illustrates the principle.

1. Every arrow must indicate that a variable leads to the next variable or several variables that collectively lead to another variable in the model (see Figure 16.2).
2. When the process is iterative, the arrow may have two heads or a feedback loop can be indicated by an arc (see Figure 18.1).
3. The map must visually represent the theory (see Figure 19.1).
4. When a particular outcome occurs under a particular condition, that condition can be written within the arrow (see Figure 18.1).
5. Revise the map to better express the relationships of the phenomenon under investigation in an ongoing process until the map is consistent with the experience of the subjects and communicates that experience to the readers (see chapter 5, "Learning Glaserian Grounded Theory by Doing It").
6. The more descriptive the study, the more words are used to describe the theory and the conditions under which it occurs (see Figure 8.1). However, when a theoretical code emerges that integrates all the categories, fewer words are needed. By reducing the number of words, a clearer view of the process is achieved (see Figure 21.1).
7. Maps do not need to quantify a particular process because quantities may change yet the theory remains consistent.
8. Maps can be presented in their entirety and then a stage can be taken out for presentation or for further analysis (see Figure 12.2; see Figure 14.1, which shows one phase of a four-phase theory).

DISCUSSION

An advantage of constructing a conceptual map is that it reduces integrative memos to a diagrammatic representation and clearly shows the relationships of the variables emerging from the data. This helps the researcher make sense out of seemingly unrelated variables by providing a structure for organizing ideas. By mapping the theory, the researcher is provided with an outline for presentation of the data in the final report.

The complexity and accuracy of the conceptual map that is constructed depends on the state of knowledge for the particular phenomenon under investigation. A descriptive study may be done from which data can be collected to identify the relationships that can form the structure of the conceptual map. If some theory is thought to explain the phenomenon of interest, a research design can be developed in the emergent fit mode (Artinian, 1986; Glaser, 1978).

When using the emergent fit mode, one must be willing to correct earlier thoughts based on preconceived theoretical notions, which are diagrammed in the conceptual map, and instead follow the theory that develops through theoretical sampling of comparison groups. Blumer (1969) also supports the use of the emergent fit mode if opportunity is given for the empirical world to "talk back" to our representation of it (p. 22). The conceptual map that is drawn at the conclusion of the study may or may not be similar to the original map depending on how closely the original map fits the data that emerged from the study.

Conceptual maps are also very useful in generating grounded theory using the theoretical code mode. After integrative memos have been written describing categories of the phenomenon under investigation, the memos can be sorted to show the relationships among the variables. A preliminary map can be constructed to display the theory. As more is learned about the process through rereading and further analyzing the data, the map evolves to include more relationships or becomes more parsimonious. For example, early conceptual maps developed by Giske contained more concepts than the final one (see chapter 5, "Learning Glaserian Grounded Theory By Doing It"). In this way the integrated theory can emerge from the successive maps.

Graphical Design and Conceptual Map Construction

Nurse researchers can render conceptual maps in a variety of ways. Sketching maps with pencil and paper is one way to represent data within reach of every researcher. Also available are the mapping features within qualitative research software, niche software designed expressly for creating conceptual maps, and standard presentation or drawing and illustration software. More sophisticated maps or rendering of final maps may lead a researcher to collaborate with a graphic designer. Additionally, scanners or fax machines connected to a computer can be used to digitize manually drawn maps. Although it is not necessary to use software during the data analysis and theory development stage, the final conceptual map will need to be replicated if the research is ever presented or published.

Graphic illustration software has become easier in the last few years for the average computer user. No longer does the user have to know complicated high-end digital illustration techniques to create a digital image. In fact, the digital process now incorporated within most qualitative research software applications very closely mimics the original grounded theory process, which consisted of writing each code on an index card, and then sorting and rearranging the cards until a map of the process emerged. All that needed to be added to the paper cards were arrows showing movement from one concept to the next. The computer does this in a click of the mouse and records the final product at the end of each research session, creating a visual memo trail of the conceptual process.

Conceptual mapping software is designed to encourage a similar type of sorting and movement on screen. The number of concepts can easily expand or contract as needed for clarification. Each concept has its own shape that can be changed from a rectangle to a circle or other form with a few clicks of the mouse. Concept shapes can be enlarged or diminished to show relative importance, colored or shaded to match color-coded memos or color-coded concepts, and made bold or thin. Labels can be easily added, moved, edited, or removed. Interconnective arrows or lines can be unconnected or reconnected to shapes at will. Freedom to play with the organization of the visual tools taps into the researcher's unconscious knowledge and experience about the research data. The shapes themselves and their orientation in space on the page engage the right brain in the research process, whereas reading the code words engages the left brain. Conceptual mapping supports whole-brain research analysis. Selected conceptual mapping software resources are provided in Table 3.1.

A very gratifying activity in the development of conceptual mapping has been the collaboration of nurse researchers and graphic designers. The graphic designer brings to the collaboration a marriage of artistic

Table 3.1

SELECTED CONCEPTUAL MAPPING RESOURCES

SOFTWARE APPLICATION	COMPANY	WEB SITE
The Graphic Organizer	Graphic.org	http://www.graphic.org/concept.html
Graphic Organizers	North Central Regional Educational Laboratory	http://www.ncrel.org/sdrs/areas/issues/students/learning/lr1grorg.htm
Graphic Organizers	Schools of California Online Resource for Education	http://www.sdcoe.k12.ca.us/SCORE/actbank/torganiz.htm
Inspiration	Inspiration Software, Inc.	http://www.inspiration.com/Inspiration
MyWebspiration	Inspiration Software, Inc.	http://www.mywebspiration.com/index.php
SmartDraw	Smartdraw.com	http://www.smartdraw.com/
Xsight	QSR International	http://www.qsrinternational.com/default.aspx

ability, technical skill, and concept. Ultimately, the designer is a problem solver who uses the resources of typesetting, reiteration or contrast of design and words, color theory, proportional beauty, accuracy of shape and size, or whatever illustrative tool is needed to deliver a suitable product for the researcher.

When I (West) work with nurse researchers to render their conceptual maps digitally, I bring my training in art and illustration design as well as my expertise as a nurse and grounded theorist to the collaboration. As the researcher explains what depiction is intended, I help the researcher problem solve: "Is this section a process (sequential) or a filter (through)?" "Does this cause that (loop)?" "Is this more/less (larger/smaller, darker/lighter) important than that?" In providing answers for me, the researchers are compelled to clarify the concepts, which in turn help them conceptualize their research.

When I work with a nurse researcher, my intention is simply to render, or illustrate, what he or she has conceptualized. I design visual patterns and arrange the research elements to convey in the best way possible the message of the research itself. I make it a point not to read the research in progress, because the conceptual map must stand alone and still make sense to me. One interesting issue I have encountered is that the researcher's brain can fill in gaps in the conceptual map because of his or her intimate relationship with the data. Bringing the map to a neutral third party demands that a certain knowable logic prevails at all steps of mapping.

When grounded theory codes and conceptual ideas can be visually communicated to a viewer so that the viewer understands, the map works. If there are only shapes connected with arrows with no "thinking" or objective behind them, the map may merely be a design, and open to interpretation. After all, which is stronger: a rectangle containing two concepts opposite each other to show that the ideas must be balanced, or a depiction of a familiar balance scale figuratively weighing the choices (see chapter 22, "Bending Expectations by Spouses of Dialysis Patients: Balancing Between Alternatives")? The point is visual communication: to depict the research findings, and ultimately a basic social process or an integrated theory, in a visually accurate way that conveys information quickly and succinctly, because the map has succeeded in engaging both sides of the brain of the viewer.

CONCLUSION

In summary it has been shown that there are many advantages in diagramming the relationships that are identified in a research study. By abstracting and conceptualizing the phenomenon in a graphic manner, we can come to a better understanding of the relationships in the data than would be possible solely from a narrative description of the categories. Tracing the effects of the variables on the outcome variable through the map serves to clarify thinking. It also "makes it possible for someone exposed to the theory for the first time to grasp the central variables of the study" (Artinian, 1982a, p. 392). The conceptual map further serves as an organizing structure for the final report since each step of the process is depicted in the map. Glaser (1978) has said that by diagramming the theory, the reader has "a succinct, interesting, and easy way to remember the data and a transcending way to view it" (p. 3).

REFERENCES

Artinian, B. (1982a). Conceptual mapping: Development of the strategy. *Western Journal of Nursing Research, 4,* 379–393.

Artinian, B. (1982b, April). *Conceptual mapping: A strategy for theory development.* Fifth Biennial Eastern Research Conference on Nursing Research, Baltimore, MD.

Artinian, B. (1986). The research process in grounded theory. In C. Chenitz & J. Swanson (Eds.), *From practice to grounded theory* (pp. 16–23). Menlo Park, CA: Addison-Wesley.

Blumer, H. (1969). *Symbolic interactionism.* Englewood Cliffs, NJ: Prentice-Hall.

Burns, N., & Grove, S. (1997). *The practice of nursing research.* Philadelphia: W. B. Saunders.

Duncan, O. (1966). Path analysis: Sociological examples. *American Journal of Sociology,* 72, 1–16.

Glaser, B. G. (1978). *Theoretical sensitivity.* Mill Valley, CA: Sociology Press.

Glaser, B. G. (1998). *Doing grounded theory: Issues and discussions.* Mill Valley, CA: Sociology Press.

Lofland, J. (1971). *Analyzing social settings.* Belmont, CA: Wadsworth Publishing.

4

Bending the Directives of Glaserian Grounded Theory in Nursing Research

PAMELA H. CONE
BARBARA M. ARTINIAN

The stringent requirements of graduate research often slow the progress of theses and dissertations, and adherence to particular methodologies can be extremely challenging. Many graduate students struggle to balance the demands of master's or doctoral committees against their chosen method of inquiry. The following discussion addresses the primary author's efforts to remain true to Glaser's grounded theory (GT) method while meeting the requirements of some dissertation committee members at the University of California at San Francisco who were not familiar with the method. Glaserian grounded theory is a useful approach to qualitative inquiry (Glaser, 2003), and the results of my study conducted among formerly homeless mothers confirmed that theory development is possible when using Glaser's method of GT research. Through all phases of the research process, careful attention was given to classical GT methodological issues and Glaser's reasoning behind each. Sometimes his directives were clear and were followed closely; others were not so clear and needed careful exploration of the thinking that led to the rules in order to follow them accurately.

Often, it was not possible to strictly follow the directives, and I found it necessary to bend them in order to meet my dissertation committee requirements. Through my doctoral research (Cone, 2006a), I came to understand the background and intent of each directive addressed in this chapter. Solutions to problems with Glaserian directives are described here and the rationale for each is explained. Glaser's recent publications (2001, 2005) on GT make it quite clear that his approach is unique and most appropriately called grounded theory. This chapter does not refute or support Glaser's assertion; it simply explores rules that are particularly Glaserian in approach and addresses the need, in some instances, to adjust certain of Glaser's directives during my doctoral research. In the following pages, my methodologist and I will address 13 directives, or "don'ts," of Glaser.

THIRTEEN DIRECTIVES

1. Don't Have a Predetermined Theoretical Framework in Mind

Glaserian GT requires approaching data with an open mind rather than coming to the project with a preconceived framework (Glaser, 1978, 1998). While the researcher who has read widely knows many theories and theoretical frameworks, those should not guide the developing theory unless the emergent fit mode is being used (see chapter 12, "Partnering With God and the Patient"). Symbolic interactionism (SI), often considered foundational for a study where meanings are being explored, should not guide the analysis along the path of the propositions of SI (Denzin & Lincoln, 2005). In addition, while feminist theory might seem an appropriate approach in light of the nature of the participants, it can guide the choice of formerly homeless mothers as the informants, but it cannot guide the analysis of their stories.

Of the other approaches often associated with GT, axial coding requires that codes drawn from data bits be placed into a structural grid that addresses preconceived codes and categories (Strauss & Corbin, 1997), dimensional analysis requires that all dimensions be addressed, and qualitative data analysis (QDA) requires details to flesh out any coding grid (Denzin & Lincoln, 2005). All of these use predetermined theoretical frameworks that assist the researcher in being thorough and extremely detailed during analysis (Glaser, 2001). Glaserian GT seeks to find themes and patterns that answer the main concern of the participants, so theory development can be done more effectively using the GT method. Based on our study among formerly homeless mothers, the theory of reconnecting was enhanced using the emergent theoretical codes of cutting point and amplifying causal loops (see chapter 17, "Mutuality: Reconnecting to Overcome Homelessness"). This theory is being tested in an intervention study (see chapter 26, "Implementing Reconnecting Theory in Community Practice").

2. Don't Do a Review of Literature

This is a classic statement of Glaser (1978, 1998), and it certainly has merit. Glaser says that a bias may be introduced by your reading, you can be misdirected onto a tangent, and you might be tempted to force your findings into a pattern rather than allowing the patterns to emerge. Glaser does agree that a theoretical background in general literature is helpful during the researcher's planning of the research project as well as during the discussion (Glaser & Strauss, 1967). Glaser is very concerned that the researcher avoid being led down the wrong analytical path or, more commonly, trying to force the findings into a preconceived theoretical framework.

The problem with Glaser's directive that arises in doctoral research is that literature reviews are required by most committees, whose desire is to ensure that students understand the state of the science in that area of study. Supervisors want doctoral students to determine where a gap in research literature exists and to avoid senseless duplication of previously conducted studies. A statistical review of what has been published is acceptable to many committees. The dilemma is to find a gap in research literature while not tainting researcher thinking. One effective approach is to conduct an Internet search of databases that cover the topic. In our recent study of homeless mothering, such a search through literature (see Table 4.1) on homelessness revealed extremely limited research on homeless mothers, particularly from their own perspective. The Psychinfo database was found to include most of that final group of studies from the other databases, but of those, only 75 focused on the mothers themselves rather than on the children or the whole family.

For my doctorate, a brief overview of literature in the broad substantive area of homelessness was first done, which was then narrowed to homeless women. The next step was to look for literature on homeless mothers, and finally, to identify research focused on homeless mothers. After a thorough exploration of extant research among homeless mothers, 75 studies were found that dealt specifically with homeless mothers. A review of the abstracts on these studies revealed what questions had been addressed among that population and confirmed the paucity of research on homelessness

Table 4.1

USING A TABLE FORMAT FOR IDENTIFYING GAPS IN THE LITERATURE

DATABASES	YEARS COVERED	HOME-LESSNESS	HOMELESS WOMEN	HOMELESS MOTHERS	RESEARCH ON HOMELESS MOTHERS
ATLA	1985–2005	207	14	3	1
CINAHL	1985–2005	1,381	238	83	31
Cochrane	1800–2005	3,925	116	31	3
SSA	1985–2005	236	73	10	5
HAPI	1985–2005	102	31	27	20
Med-Line	1985–2005	1,110	173	48	23
PAIS	1985–2005	149	10	4	3
Psych-Info	1985–2005	3,690	625	195	145
SIRS	1985–2005	61	14	2	2
Wilson Web	1985–2005	1,393	206	56	41

from the perspective of homeless mothers, a definite gap in the literature. A lengthy and detailed table identifying the specific elements of each study (design, sample, research question, etc.) satisfied the doctoral committee's desire for me to determine the gap in the literature while avoiding the actual reading of the studies until after analysis was completed. This satisfied the intent of Glaser as well as the doctoral committee.

3. Don't Get Consent Forms From Participants

Glaser objects to consent forms (Glaser, 1978, 1998), but their use is actually a situational issue. Glaser's reasoning is that the findings should be abstract of time, place, and people, and that obtaining consent will jeopardize the rapport needed during data collection. In most cases in the United States, university research programs require formal consents to be obtained from the participants in order to gain approval from institutional review boards, as well as the site where the research is being conducted. Other countries, such as Norway, have a national ethics board that reviews and approves all research before it can be conducted. Recorded interviews usually need signed consent forms, and individuals participating in such a study need to have a clear understanding of the study in order to give informed consent. Some studies can be done without consent if the review board determines that no infringement of personal confidentiality will occur, such as when attendance at a focus group interview provides implied consent and no names are used.

Occasionally, gatekeepers may give consent for a study on their grounds or in their facility, particularly when the researcher is simply gathering observational data. Participants in my study were asked to give their consent, and all indicated a willingness to sign once they had read the document, discussed it, and been given a copy to keep. I believe this willingness was inspired by my efforts to build rapport and by the participants' eagerness to share their stories. Researchers must check with the appropriate review board to determine whether or not a consent form is needed.

4. Don't Use Demographic Data

Glaser says data are abstract of time, place, and people so it is not important to gather such information (1978, 1998). His point is that the theory will be abstracted through data analysis, so demographic data are not necessary and often distract from the theory development. However, demographic data are often a requirement of review boards/committees. One can report these data in charts giving statistics while keeping separate all participant interview data, making it possible to meet doctoral committee requirements and still adhere to Glaser's directive to avoid the use of demographic data in the analysis of participant responses. This keeps to the intent of Glaser's rule while enabling the researcher to adhere to university protocols. In addition, researchers who have a program of research may use demographic data to help determine future directions in ongoing research studies.

In the homeless mothers study, demographic data answered questions relating to length of time in homelessness. We noted those who had repeat homelessness prior to connecting with a care provider who helped them reconnect with society, and we identified questions for future studies relating to the trajectory out of homelessness. In GT, demographic data are unrelated to data analysis unless something emerges as relevant to the developing theory (Glaser, 1992).

5. Don't Tape Record Interviews

The big concern that Glaser (1978) had about tape recording interviews was the obtrusiveness of tape machines and the danger of interrupting the interview process or distracting and constraining the participants, a problem that is of limited concern in this modern day of miniaturized technology. It is true that tape recording is not always appropriate or necessary. When extremely vulnerable populations or sensitive issues are being addressed, for participant observations or for some seasoned GT researchers it is possible to conduct research simply using field notes at or after the time of the interaction.

However, tape recording is very important at times. The novice GT researcher needs help to record the pertinent data rather than trying to write down everything as it is being said. Even a seasoned researcher usually needs to tape record the initial interviews on a new study. With one-on-one interviews or focus groups, audiotapes allow for listening again to make sure all the nuances are understood. In addition, taping is a good form of accurate record keeping so that the words of participants are intact and themes are in vivo. In my study among formerly homeless mothers, we found that once rapport was established, it was relatively easy to ignore the tape recorder. To minimize distraction potential, we used digital recorders that required no manipulation once the recording had begun.

6. Don't Use Computer Programs or Software for GT Studies

This Glaserian rule relates primarily to computer use in data analysis. Glaser (1978, 1998) wants to make it clear that computer programs cannot replace the researcher's analytical processes. It is true that technology cannot replace researcher thinking, nor can it create codes, answer questions, or do theorizing. Technology can, however, manage, sort, and retrieve data at the researcher's direction. Qualitative software can assist the researcher with managing data by storing the interviews for data retrieval, by keeping track of all types of data (memos, field notes, etc.), by making it possible to retrieve data and connect them to codes, and by providing an audit trail of conceptual thinking and theorizing.

In our study, all the interviews were stored in the database on NVivo 7, as well as field notes from participant observations, reflections on interviews, memos, firsthand stories from literature, and conceptual maps. In addition, the lists of open, substantive codes, as well as selective and theoretical codes, were connected to each theme in the data. The ability to retrieve data relating to particular themes in order to insert participant comments that highlighted the meaning of the theme or code was a tremendous bonus for me during the writing process. See Table 4.2 for a list of selected software programs.

7. Don't Analyze One Incident Without Comparing It to Others

Constant comparative analysis is the foundational principle of GT (Glaser & Strauss, 1967). The concern is to avoid going off onto a tangent that is not meaningful and does not truly fit in the study. During early analysis,

Table 4.2

SELECTED QUALITATIVE RESEARCH SOFTWARE

RESOURCE	VENDOR	WEB SITE
AnSWR: Analysis Software for Word-based Records	Centers for Disease Control	http://www.cdc.gov/hiv/topics/surveillance/resources/software/answr/index.htm
Atlas.ti	Atlas.ti	http://www.atlasti.com/index.php
CDC EZ-Text.	Centers for Disease Control	http://www.cdc.gov/hiv/software/ez-text.htm
Choosing Qualitative Data Analysis Software. Atlas/ti and Nudist Compared. Sociological Research Online, 3(3)	Barry, C. A. (1998)	Retrieved from: http://www.socresonline.org.uk/socresonline/3/3/4.html
Ethnograph	Qualis Research	http://www.qualisresearch.com/
NVivo	QSR International	http://www.qsrinternational.com/default.aspx
QDA Miner 3.1	Provalis Research	http://www.provalisresearch.com/QDAMiner/QDAMinerDesc.html
Qualrus	Idea Works	http://www.ideaworks.com/qualrus/index.html
Reviews of Qualitative Software	Wilk, Richard	http://www.indiana.edu/~wanthro/softrev.htm

themes are occasionally found that do not occur in the next interview or two. In addition, reification of data is not helpful in GT (Glaser, 1998); instead, the researcher should analyze multiple data to understand the main concern that needs to be resolved and how the participants resolve it. Always stay with the data at this early stage, and avoid bringing into the analysis any thinking from other researchers or studies. Make comparisons constantly to keep on track, and be willing to let go of interesting themes if they do not fit with the rest of the data.

Memo writing is a tool that helps when discerning if the theme belongs in the picture or not. In this way, the researcher reflects on a theme found in a unique incident and then compares it to the overall findings rather than to a similar incident. During this memo writing process, it is important to avoid the "what ifs" of a participant's experience or a particular incident, that is, to avoid dwelling too much on one example or pattern. Dwelling on one element leads to qualitative data analysis rather than true GT. In our study, it was memo writing that helped with effective comparisons and ensuring the fit of codes and categories. Memos can best assist the researcher when only one theme is addressed per memo and when researcher thinking is being recorded about that theme in comparison to other data where the theme occurs.

8. Don't Answer the Researcher's Question if It Is Not the Main Concern of the Participants

Discovering and adhering to the main concern of the participants is another of Glaser's foundational principles (Glaser, 1978, 1998). While the research question guides the study, understanding participants' motives to work through their main concern is the focus of the research. This main concern is something that must be discovered over the course of data collection and analysis. It may or may not be the answer to the researcher's question.

We found this to be a very important principle when in-depth analysis of the homeless mothers' stories clearly revealed that getting off the streets into stable housing was their main concern. The process of *reconnecting* emerged, which helped them resolve this concern. Many times a supervising committee requires students to answer the original research question in the final report. This can be done in creative ways that keep to Glaser's principle while meeting committee mandates. In my dissertation, I addressed this issue in the methodology section, pointing out that analysis addressed part of the research question in identifying a process that resolved the participants' main concern.

9. Don't Make Conceptual Maps

Glaser (1978, 1998) is adamant against the use of conceptual maps in GT analysis, believing that they are counterproductive and will interfere with the analytical process. This is an area where we differ completely from Glaser. Perhaps Glaser is not a visual learner; but for those who are, these maps can be extremely helpful. The concern that Glaser seems to have is that the researcher not resort to forcing data into an interesting-looking map. Conceptual maps are not meant to and do not replace verbal explication of the core category and subcategories; they simply illustrate researcher analysis. Conceptual maps are not necessarily final; rather, they are modifiable diagrams of the researcher's thinking processes. They often reveal flaws in the researcher's thinking processes (Figure 4.1), and the clear inaccuracy of the map can be very helpful in redirecting researcher thinking.

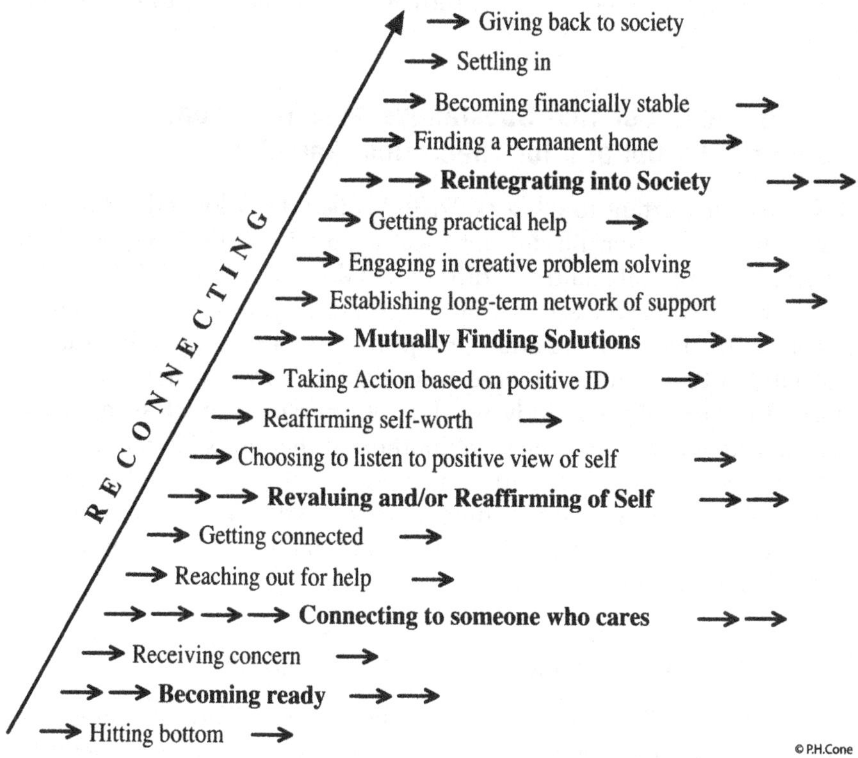
Giving back to society
Settling in
Becoming financially stable
Finding a permanent home
Reintegrating into Society
Getting practical help
Engaging in creative problem solving
Establishing long-term network of support
Mutually Finding Solutions
Taking Action based on positive ID
Reaffirming self-worth
Choosing to listen to positive view of self
Revaluing and/or Reaffirming of Self
Getting connected
Reaching out for help
Connecting to someone who cares
Receiving concern
Becoming ready
Hitting bottom
RECONNECTING
© P.H.Cone

Figure 4.1 Model 3: Reconnecting to get out of homelessness.
Printed with permission from P. H. Cone.

We found that maps were useful to visually demonstrate the emerging concepts and processes. They can clarify a pattern, path, or process (see chapter 3, "Conceptual Mapping as an Aid to Grounded Theory Development"). Our conceptual maps clarified and presented an understandable picture of a process after constant comparative analysis had revealed the themes and categories, and they helped the primary researcher avoid some pitfalls in selective coding and collapsing of categories. Our series of conceptual maps helped identify Reconnecting as the core category that answered the participants' main concern. The use of conceptual maps clarified when the cutting point occurred in the basic social process of reconnecting. Another map provided a way to depict the theoretical code of amplifying causal loops by showing the progressive acts of mutuality that took place in the reconnecting process (see chapter 17, "Mutuality: Reconnecting to Overcome Homelessness"). Their use clarified the cutting point of the basic social process and identified the theoretical code, mutuality, in the substantive grounded theory of Reconnecting (see chapter 17, "Mutuality: Reconnecting to Overcome Homelessness").

10. Don't Go Out of Your Substantive Area Too Soon, and Do Not Go Out of It for Theoretical Sampling

This is very important to Glaser (1978). While Glaser looked at families with a dying member, he did not look at families with dying children because that was substantively different (Glaser & Strauss, 1967). The main point is to have clarity about the group in your own study rather than allowing themes from other groups to enter and muddy the waters. A grounded theory must emerge from data, not from other studies or substantive areas. In our study, we did not interview homeless men. We interviewed only women who were mothers at the time of homelessness. Instead of going out of the substantive area, try going to another group experiencing the same type of thing, perhaps a similar site in a different area. We explored a group of homeless mothers in another large city to see if the patterns were the same.

11. Don't Sample to Make the Picture Complete

Glaser (1978, 1998) encourages researchers to avoid any sampling procedure that would alter the sample population. Instead, use theoretical sampling to clarify a pattern, concept, or hypothesis. Sampling to complete the picture places the researcher at risk of forcing data into preconceived themes or ideas. It is important to analyze and compare data already gathered until the picture is clear and the categories are defined. This process will avoid the "selective sampling" that Schatzman and Strauss (1973) discuss as a calculated decision based on preconceived dimensions that may seem reasonable but are worked out ahead of time. The use of selective sampling will actually move you away from your data and cloud the emerging categories or patterns.

Theoretical sampling, on the other hand, can be used to verify category saturation. Glaser (1978) writes that this process is "controlled by the emerging theory" (p. 36) rather than by a need to flesh out description. In our study, we found that many of the formerly homeless mothers in our first series of interviews had some type of mental illness and/or substance abuse issue. In order to discover if women without these problems expressed similar themes, we interviewed more mothers who had neither been mentally ill nor abused substances. We then found that the patterns were similar and no new concepts emerged.

12. Don't Try to Fully Describe Everything

According to Glaser (1998, 2001), detailed description moves you toward qualitative data analysis (QDA), situational analysis (SA), dimensional analysis (DA), or axial coding (AC). Glaser strongly opposes all of these methods. Researchers often feel compelled to tell the whole story; but in GT, the emergent pattern or process that identifies the main concern of the participants is what is important, not the extensive detail found in QDA (Glaser, 1992; Stern, 1994). Discovering what resolves that main concern is the critical element in GT, rather than a detailed description of the participants' personal experiences in a particular situation (SA), a thorough discussion of all the dimensions of a particular phenomenon (DA), or comprehensive coverage of researcher-devised codes (AC) (Glaser, 1998, 2001).

In our study among formerly homeless mothers, we found that the participants all described the overall phenomenon of experiencing homelessness. To use all of that description would not be true to Glaserian GT. Resolving the participants' concern about how to get off the streets became the focus of in-depth analysis. Only categories related to Reconnecting to Overcome Homelessness were included: *becoming ready, connecting with someone, revaluing self, mutually finding solutions,* and *reintegrating into society*. These were carried out through the process of mutuality (see chapter 17, "Mutuality: Reconnecting to Overcome Homelessness").

13. Don't Discuss the Study With Others

Glaser makes the point that discussing ideas often results in the diffusion of thoughts (Glaser, 1978). This is a concern but the real issue is knowing who should hear the researcher's thoughts and ideas. In his more recent writings, Glaser (1998) actually encourages collaboration in research as well as the frequent discussion of findings to flesh out the emerging process. Do discuss it with research colleagues; be careful, however, that you do not share it with nonresearchers because they often want to share new examples that are not relevant to the study. Some researchers have discovered that group or team analysis is a fruitful strategy for GT research (see chapter 6, "Learning Glaserian Grounded Theory Through Mentoring and Scholarly Dialogue"). In our study of homeless mothering, verbal memos, that is, memos from mentoring discussions, were very helpful to our understanding the process of reconnecting to overcome homelessness. It was important for us to record these memos for later sorting; some gems were uncovered in this way that would not have been seen if analysis had been done without communal discussion.

CONCLUSION

Glaser had his own comments to offer on following and bending his directives. First, take courage and trust your data; they will give you results if you are patient and stay true to the process. As you work with the data, be aware of the potential to stray from Glaserian GT either during analysis or during the writing phase. Most qualitative methods use similar data collection techniques that ground the findings in the data, but that does not make them grounded theory, writes Glaser (2001). If you realize you have used a different qualitative method, all is not lost; you simply need to call it what it is based on the method of analysis and continue with the work. Second, engage in dialogue with other scholars. Scholars who sincerely want to pursue grounded theory research must dialogue with each other to understand the emerging concepts. When you dialogue with other researchers, be sure to credit their contribution. The scholars presenting research in this volume agree that Glaser's method is most effective for theory development, so Glaserian GT is worth the effort.

Finally, we know there are problems and pitfalls related to the GT method. No matter where you do your doctoral studies, there will be differing opinions about grounded theory. It is important to develop a deeper understanding of Glaser's terminology in order to stay true to Glaserian GT methodology. Mentoring is helpful, so look for GT researchers who have expertise in Glaser's method to help you. Identify the areas where you can adhere strictly to Glaser's approach and those where you will need to adjust the directives to meet doctoral committee requirements at your university. Bending the "don'ts" of Glaser while adhering to Glaserian GT is a balancing act, but it can be done.

REFERENCES

Cone, P. (2006a). *Reconnecting: A grounded theory study among formerly homeless mothers.* Unpublished doctoral dissertation, University of California at San Francisco.

Cone, P. (2006b). *Model 3: Reconnecting to get out of homelessness* [Conceptual map]. Unpublished.

Denzin, N. K., & Lincoln, Y. S. (Eds.). (2005). *Handbook of qualitative research* (3rd ed.). Thousand Oaks, CA: Sage.

Glaser, B. G. (1978). *Theoretical sensitivity: Advances in the methodology of grounded theory*. Mill Valley, CA: Sociology Press.

Glaser, B. G. (1992). *Basics of grounded theory: Emergence vs. forcing.* Mill Valley, CA: Sociology Press.

Glaser, B. G. (1998). *Doing grounded theory: Issues and discussions.* Mill Valley, CA: Sociology Press.

Glaser, B. G. (2001). *The grounded theory perspective: Conceptualization contrasted with description*. Mill Valley, CA: Sociology Press.

Glaser, B. G. (2003). *The grounded theory perspective II: Description's remodeling of grounded theory methodology*. Mill Valley, CA: Sociology Press.

Glaser, B. G. (2005). *The grounded theory perspective III: Theoretical coding*. Mill Valley, CA: Sociology Press.

Glaser, B. G., & Strauss, A. L. (1967). *The discovery of grounded theory: Strategies for qualitative research*. Chicago: Aldine.

Schatzman, L., & Strauss, A. L. (1973). *Field research: Strategies for a natural sociology.* Englewood Cliffs, NJ: Prentice-Hall.

Stern, P. N. (1994). Eroding grounded theory. In J. M. Morse (Ed.), *Critical issues in qualitative research methods.* Thousand Oaks, CA: Sage.

Strauss, A. L., & Corbin, J. M. (Eds.). (1997). *Grounded theory in practice.* Thousand Oaks, CA: Sage.

5 Learning Glaserian Grounded Theory by Doing It

TOVE GISKE
BARBARA M. ARTINIAN

This chapter is a personal account of the journey from being new to the method of grounded theory (GT) to becoming experienced in developing a substantive grounded theory. Our aim is to illustrate the thinking and working processes involved in generating a substantive grounded theory by making explicit a seemingly chaotic process. We used the classical method developed by Glaser and Strauss (1967) and the later writings of Glaser (1978, 1998, 2001, 2005), which offer the principles of how to conduct a GT study. Many researchers have discussed how to follow these principles (Baker, Wuest, & Stern, 1992; Cutcliffe, 2000, 2005; Duchscher & Morgan, 2004; McCallin, 2003); however, few examples are given that illustrate the actual research process (Backmann & Kyngäs, 1999). In this chapter we discuss key areas related to data collection, analysis, and development of a conceptual theory, which are central to GT research.

GT is a general inductive method based on a concept-indicator model where the aim is to generate new theory that is grounded in ongoing data collection (Glaser, 1999, 2005). Meaning, action, and interaction are central to GT research; however, a GT is conceptual, not interactional.

Used by permission, this chapter is a further development of the article: Giske, T., & Artinian, B. (2007). A personal experience of working with classical grounded theory: From beginner to experienced grounded theorist. *International Journal of Qualitative Methods, 6*(4), 68–80.

A GT gives a conceptual account of how the participants resolve their main concern. The main concern is the prime mover of participant action in the area of study, and the core category and its variables explain how participants work to solve their main concern (Glaser, 2001). A *core category* is the highest-level concept of the theory, relating to the other categories and properties of a GT; however, it does not indicate how the different categories are related to each other (Glaser, 1978, 1998).

The substantive area in which this study took place was a gastric ward at a university hospital in Norway. The purpose was to learn more about how patients going through the diagnostic phase experience and handle their situation. The study was approved by the regional ethical board. The inclusion criteria for the participants were that they should be 35 years or older, be hospitalized because of symptoms in the stomach-intestine area, and be physically and mentally able to take part in an interview. Data came from 18 in-depth interviews with 8 women and 7 men, aged 35–84 in 2002–2003. A descriptive mode of the theory is presented in chapter 7 and a theoretical code mode is presented in chapter 21.

The substantive GT in this study was called "Preparative Waiting." Preparative Waiting showed how the participants resolved their main concern, which emerged in relation to how patients could prepare themselves for the concluding interview and life after receiving a diagnosis. Preparative Waiting emerged as the core category, and all the concepts of the theory were connected and could appear at any time. *Seeking and giving information* and *interpreting clues* moved the participants forward in trying to make more and more sense of their situation. *Handling existential threat* and *seeking respite* were more focused on dealing with the threat they experienced to self. *Balancing between hope and despair* was the filter through which everything flowed and described the way in which the participants tried to keep themselves on an even keel. The final model of Preparative Waiting is presented at the end of the chapter.

The first author conducted interviews and data analyses under the supervision of the second author, who is an expert in grounded theory methodology.

CRITERIA FOR EVALUATION OF A GT

The credibility of a GT rests on the four criteria of fit, work, relevance, and modifiability (Glaser, 1978, 1998). In analyzing data, it is important that categories not be forced or selected out of preconceived understandings of the phenomena studied. It is essential that they be generated systematically from data and constantly validated by the hard work of fitting and refitting the categories to data. Later in the analysis, categories are fitted together into a dense and parsimonious theory that fits the substantive area (Glaser, 1978, 2001). Lomborg and Kirkevold (2003) have pointed to the criterion fit as most important for evaluating validity and truth of the grounded theory. Therefore, fit is more fundamental to a theory than the other three criteria of work, relevance, and modifiability.

The second criterion is work, which means that a grounded theory must be able to explain what happens in the data, predict what will happen, and interpret what is happening in the area studied. Workability is related to how well a theory accounts for the way in which participants solve their main concern (Glaser, 1998). The third criterion concerns relevance. A theory is relevant and has good grab for participants and practitioners in the substantive field when it allows the core problems and processes in the area to emerge. The fourth criterion is modifiability. A substantive GT has only partial closure because new ideas and more data can modify the theory. Modifiability is therefore a continuous process, and all GTs have potential for further development (Glaser, 1978).

PREPARATION FOR A GROUNDED THEORY STUDY

In search of a final problem, a suitable method, and a supervisor for my doctoral dissertation, I (the first author) was introduced to a one-week grounded theory research course in 2001. The openness required in searching for the participants' problems and perspectives in GT and the way of analyzing data so that it should result in a dense and parsimonious conceptual theory sounded like a challenge full of meaningful work.

According to GT methodology, the researcher, independent of how much knowledge and experience he or she has at the outset, enters the field of study with an attitude that he or she does not know the participants' main concern (Glaser, 1998). The researcher must take a "no preconceived interest" approach and not ask questions that might be on his mind (p. 122). Such initial openness, which might require letting go of pet ideas, can be hard to obtain, but is nonetheless a principal attitude in GT. Initial openness in early data collection and analysis will best allow the participants' main concern to emerge as appropriately and quickly as possible (Glaser, 1992).

I approached the doctoral study with an interest in learning more about how patients existentially experienced uncertainty and life-threatening situations. To be able to use GT, I had to be willing to enter the field with the attitude of not knowing the main concern of the participants, acknowledging that patients do not necessarily share professionals' view of problems. When I had accepted this initial openness in the planning process, we could move on to discuss what could be a suitable area for data collection. We searched for a field with multiple outcomes of diagnostic examinations and decided on a gastric ward because patients there could be diagnosed with either malignant or benign diseases, and each case could significantly influence their lives.

To accord with the principle of seeking the participants' perspective, the aim of the research had to be formulated in a way sufficiently open to encompass the entirety of the participants' problems and how they worked to solve them. The main purpose of this study, therefore, was set to gain knowledge on how patients going through diagnostic workups in a gastroenterological ward experienced and handled their situation, and how health care professionals could help them in the best way. Qualitative interviews were chosen for data collection (Fog, 2004) because our study's aim was to learn the participants' perspective, experience, meaning, and reason for action.

In planning the study, we worked on phrasing possible questions to make sure that our own ideas, interests, or theoretical understandings were not imposed on the participants (Glaser, 1992). We especially worked on the opening of the interviews. The opening question used was some variation on, "Can you tell me what it is like for you to be here in the hospital?" The ethical guidelines in Norway demand that participants receive oral and written information about the study. An information sheet was prepared, describing the aim of the study, and participants were invited to speak openly about their experience of being in the hospital as well as to share their thoughts, resources, and what they thought might make their situation more tolerable. The contact nurse at the unit provided this information to potential participants.

WORKING FOR QUALITY IN DATA COLLECTION

The credibility of a grounded theory study depends on how data are collected, analyzed, and developed into a conceptual theory. In GT, data collection and analysis are done jointly, guided by the constant comparative method and theoretical sampling. Constant comparison means to constantly code new data and compare them with already developed codes to generate concepts in order. These concepts are the basis on which to generate a conceptual and saturated theory (Glaser, 2001).

Most of the interviews were conducted in the ward of the hospital bath area, examination room, head nurse's office, or patient room, depending on what was convenient for the ward and the patient. To meet with the participants in their environment facilitated an understanding of what they discussed in the interviews. In all contact with patients in qualitative research, ethical discernment is needed to avoid violation of personal integrity (Johnson & Long, 2006; World Medical Association, 2004).

Because quality and content of interviews depend to a great extent on the rapport developed between researcher and participant, the researcher must commit to high levels of sensitivity in asking questions and to intent focus on the dynamics in the interaction between them. To provide a relaxed beginning to the taped interviews, we started with a brief personal introduction, signed the consent form, and talked about facts to facilitate the filling in of biographies and background variables. Then participants were invited to share how they experienced being in the hospital and going through diagnostic workups. During the interviews, it was important to establish an open atmosphere of trust so that the participants would feel free to share their experiences, thoughts, and feelings. As the researcher, I sought to balance the openness with the participants' need for emotional protection by not dwelling too deeply on the possibility of a threatening future. I had to trust my judgment and be sensitive to gestures, silence, facial expressions, weeping, and change in the atmosphere between us.

Theoretical Sensitivity

Theoretical sensitivity is the ability the researcher increasingly develops to conceptualize and formulate a theory by constant comparison of data. It is about thinking in theoretical terms about what he or she knows (Glaser & Strauss, 1967). To quote Glaser: "The researcher does not go blank or give up his knowledge. He goes sensitive with his learning which makes him alert to [the] possibility of emergence and how to formulate it conceptually" (Glaser, 1998, p. 123). Different researchers, therefore, bring different theoretical sensitivities to a study (Glaser, 2002). Openness and sensitivity toward data in this study were stimulated by our reading literature in related fields (Glaser, 1978, 2005), such as suffering, grieving, ambiguous loss, and philosophy of science. As more data were collected and analyzed, my theoretical sensitivity increased, leading to more focused interviews. Then I used a variety of interview styles depending on the conceptual level of the different categories in focus during data collection. Open questions promoted the participants' thoughts about their experiences, and more specific questions were asked in relation to certain events, behaviors, or experiences, such as relationships with staff, fellow patients, and medical examinations. These were helpful in saturating concepts and their properties.

My background as a nurse and nursing teacher had given me considerable experience in meeting patients in the diagnostic phase, which influenced my theoretical sensitivity, as did my interest in spiritual care (Giske, 1993, 1995). It is generally known that uncertainty about one's health condition and consequences for the future can bring into focus the existential and spiritual aspects of life. Relying on clinical experience, research, and knowledge, I knew that most Norwegian patients would not easily speak about such concerns (Mjølnerød, 1997; Thoresen, 1993; Tønnessen, 1999; Ueland, 1997). In fact, none of the participants in our study talked explicitly about their spiritual concerns before they were asked, but once prompted, all of them had something to share about it. The question chosen to investigate possible existential concerns was formulated openly enough to give room for their total experience: "Where do you draw your strength from?" This is an example of how preunderstanding and theoretical sensitivity could influence data collection. By constant comparison of data from interviews, I knew that my ideas would either fade out as irrelevant or earn their way into the theory. In this study we found that *handling existential threat* was an important concept of the theory.

Theoretical Sampling

My growing understanding of data, concepts, and their properties also guided further data sampling in relation to selecting participants and choosing areas to sample (theoretical sampling). As the participants' main concern and their ways of resolving it became clearer, variations were sought in the participants' age, time spent waiting, medical history, and whether they stayed in the hospital or patient hotel or slept at home. Questions such as what it meant to them to receive a diagnosis and what information they wanted are examples of asking more specifically about aspects and processes so that I could saturate categories and establish the relationship between them (Glaser, 1978; Glaser & Strauss, 1967).

Taping instead of writing notes during interviews gave much better qualitative data because taping preserves the wording, the tone of the voice, the silence, laughter, sighs, crying, and so on. This provided rich data with considerable variety for coding. The transcribed interviews contained data for which we did not see the relevance at the time of the interview but which emerged as important later in the analyses. In this way, early and rich interviews became a source of theoretical sampling in the selective coding process.

WORKING FOR QUALITY IN CODING AND ANALYZING

In this section we describe steps and processes we went through in the analyzing process. The phases overlapped each other; they moved back and forth and were not as clear-cut as this presentation implies.

Open Coding

As soon as interviews were transcribed (by the first author), they were coded by hand in the right-hand margin, with keywords summing up what the participants were sharing. In open coding everything is coded so as to find as many codes as possible without considerations of relevance (Glaser, 1978) (see Table 5.1).

Memos were written along the way, recording thoughts, questions, relationships between interviews, specific themes that emerged, and references to concepts and themes in the literature. Memos were organized so that only one idea, hypothesis, or question was written for each memo, and every memo was given a heading and a date; for example, "Ambivalence and balancing, 19.08.03" and "Properties of making sense, 18.03.04." This made it possible to track the process and make the upcoming sorting easier (Glaser, 1978). An example of a memo is in Table 5.2.

Searching for Participants' Main Concern

After open coding of the first interview, we sought to identify the participants' main concern and to name the core category that resolved it. To search consciously for their main concern was very important as well as creating a practical way to ask the question, "What is this data a study of?" (Glaser, 1978, p. 57). After seven interviews we tried *knowing what is wrong with me;* later we used *balancing fear until they get to know* and *how to manage life/self while waiting for a diagnosis.* The analysis continued with validation of the participants' main concern until in April 2004 when we reached the formulation *how to prepare for the concluding*

Table 5.1

EXAMPLES OF HOW DATA WERE CODED

DATA	OPEN CODING	SELECTIVE CODING	FINAL CONCEPTS
Sometimes you **think about the worst,** you know, but they have informed me that they have taken so many tests; I have been to gynecological examinations, they have taken **lots** of blood **samples,** and my liver is okay, and they **find nothing.** But still it lies there **smoldering.** (Interview 3)	**Thinks about the worst** Uncertain despite **many samples** and **no findings** **Smolders**	Ambivalence Uncertainty	**Balancing between hope and despair**
It is important for me to get **to know,** to be able **to move on,** either with treatment or not, that I am well, or that I have **to live with this.** If they can tell me okay, this is nothing dangerous, you can gain some control, then I can manage to live with the pain. But I **have to know** the reason **why** it is so. (Interview 9)	Wants **to know to move on** **Can live with it** If **he knows why**	To receive information	**Seeking and giving information**
I read a book I brought and I listen to music **to possess another world** while I am here. I need to overcome a threshold to get rid of what fills my head. (Interview 11)	Try to **think of other things**	Create a room of rest	***Seeking respite***

Printed with permission from T. Giske.

Table 5.2

AN EXAMPLE OF MEMO WRITING

THE WAITING PROCESS, MARCH 17, 2003

The participants wait to get the result, the diagnosis, and it seems to be two processes at the same time—at least.

1. **They seek information about the investigations and the results of them.** For some, the time at the medical investigation unit is a good opportunity to discuss their case and get information from the doctor. The doctor can tell the patient what the doctors investigated and what they see and think. Most patients are active in this process.

2. **They also prepare themselves for the future** and what that will bring. This preparation occurs on two levels. This process is not so easily perceived by a researcher. It is as though the participants hold their breath as they wait for diagnosis, but underneath they work.

The first level is preparing themselves for the information about the results, which hopefully will bring them over to a new phase of life, that is, knowing what is going on in their bodies.

Some are looking forward to knowing the diagnosis with fear. They may fear a diagnosis of cancer or another disease with a prognosis that will mean they face death or big changes in life.

Those who have waited long for a diagnosis prepare themselves for the possibility that they cannot be helped this time either, and consider how to handle the situation once they receive that information.

They also are working on preparing themselves for different scenarios after they get the final results of the investigations. This facing of possible futures is a process difficult for others to see. It seems like since the participants do not know the final outcome, it's not worth taking the whole burden of what they fear into their full consciousness yet. They are "tasting" what the future might be, and then leaving the matter there.

Printed with permission from T. Giske.

interview and life afterwards (Table 5.3). Going back to memos written at an early stage (fall 2002), we see that we were well on our way to understanding the main concern and the core category as we were reflecting on how the participants could prepare themselves and make a plan for handling uncertainty. It took 1.5 years of analysis and comparative work before we were able to verbalize this as exactly as required by the rigor of GT.

Table 5.3

THE PROCESS OF DATA COLLECTION, ANALYZING, AND DEVELOPING THE GROUNDED THEORY OF PREPARATIVE WAITING

DATE	INTERVIEWS	CODING: 0 = OPEN S = SELECTIVE T = THEORETICAL	EXAMPLES OF VALIDATION OF MAIN CONCERN	EXAMPLES OF VALIDATION OF CORE CATEGORY	DEVELOPMENT OF PICTURES AND MODELS	EXAMPLES OF READING LITERATURE
May 2002	1 2 3 4	O O O O				GT Method
June 2002	5 6	O O				GT Method Uncertainty
July 2002		O				GT Method
August 2002	7 8 9	O O O	Knowing what is wrong with me			GT Method
September 2002	10 11	O O	Knowing what is going on in my body			Suffering, endurance
October 2002				Living on hold		
November 2002				Striving to get to know		Philosophy
December 2002						Existential grief Ambiguous loss

March 2003			S		Contingency planning & preparation		
April 2003	12	O	S			Working on the pictures to be made	Qualitative method
May 2003	13 14 15 16 17 18	O O O O O O	S S S S S S	Understanding what is going on in my body	– Giving and receiving information – Enduring uncertainty – Becoming certain	Working on the pictures to be made	GT Method Existential grief Fellow patients To investigate what cannot be expressed
June 2003			S		– Struggling with uncertainty – Challenging uncertainty – Struggling with ambivalence – Enduring uncertainty and promoting an outcome	Working on the pictures to be made	Løgstrup: Life utterances, untouchable zone
August 2003			S				Illness & disease Ambiguous loss

(*continued*)

Table 5.3

THE PROCESS OF DATA COLLECTION, ANALYZING, AND DEVELOPING THE GROUNDED THEORY OF PREPARATIVE WAITING (*Continued*)

DATE	INTERVIEWS	CODING: O = OPEN S = SELECTIVE T = THEORETICAL	EXAMPLES OF VALIDATION OF MAIN CONCERN	EXAMPLES OF VALIDATION OF CORE CATEGORY	DEVELOPMENT OF PICTURES AND MODELS	EXAMPLES OF READING LITERATURE
September 2003		S	Balancing fear until they get to know			GT Method Philosophy of Science
October 2003		S T	How to manage life/self while waiting for a diagnosis?	– Preparing self for getting the diagnosis/ concluding talk – Becoming prepared		GT Method Philosophy of Science Symbolic Interactionism
March 2004		S T			Model 1	Endurance, suffering Hope
April 2004		S T	How to prepare themselves for the concluding interview—and life after	– Preparing for alternatives – Preparative waiting		Symbolic Interactionism
May 2004		S T				
June 2004		S T			Models 2–4	
August 2004		T			Model 5	

September 2004	T	Model 6	
October 2004	T		GT Method
November 2004	T	Models 7–9	
April 2005	T	Model 10	Suffering and life utterances
May 2005	T	Model 11	Intensive searching and reading of relevant research findings Method Nursing care
October 2005	T	Model 12	Method Philosophy of Science Coping Uncertainty theory Narratives and communication
Spring 2006			Stress and coping theory Intensive searching and reading of relevant research findings
February 2007		Model 13	GT Method

Printed with permission from T. Giske.

Creating Paintings Assisted the Conceptualization Process

Our inability to conceptualize the theory gave birth to a creative idea of expressing our current understanding of waiting for a diagnosis as a picture. It was obvious that being in the diagnostic phase meant experiencing many feelings simultaneously. We also found that the participants were preparing themselves for different possible outcomes by tasting a small portion of emotions in these scenarios. Memos concerning the waiting process written at that time (Table 5.1) stated that the participants prepared themselves for the future in two ways: first, to face the information about their results; and, second, for different scenarios after they had received the final result of examinations. I invited Gunhild Øverli, a student nurse and a painter, to work with me. She discussed my analysis with me and was able to paint pictures that caught the whole process.

In the first painting, the patient is alone in the hallway, waiting to pass through the door at the end; the door was a symbol of the concluding interview. The doors along the corridor symbolize the patient's hopes and fears. Some of the doors are ajar; others are shut. The patient does not walk into these rooms; he or she just knows what is inside them and what might become a reality when he or she gets to know the results from the medical team at the concluding interview. The second painting depicts patients who have had their health problems for only a brief time when admitted to the hospital. The hallway is short with few doors on either side before the end door to the concluding interview. In the last painting, patients have been waiting for a long time and have gone through former examinations and hospitalizations before they were admitted to the hospital this time. Pathways traveling up and down multiple hills lead in different ways to the largest hill with the last building where the concluding interview awaits. The way they have come is long, and their troubles have increased over time.

Naming the Core Category

As our understanding of data developed, we tried to fit different concepts to the core category. The first attempt, in November 2002, was *living on hold,* but that was too passive and did not describe the process well enough. *Striving to get to know* was more active but still not broad enough to cover all of our data. We moved on to *contingency prepara-*

tion, which touched on an important aspect but was still not satisfactory. Then we tested different combinations of uncertainty, which was a very important theme in our data, but it did not fit as the core category. In October 2003, we considered *preparing self for the concluding talk,* but rejected it because it was too weak and had no grab. *Preparing for alternatives* was closer but was still missing grab along with being too ordinary for the painful process the participants experienced.

After hard work fitting concepts together to a theory, we discussed the pictures. My mentor stated that when we would at last find the name of the process, it would come out of these pictures. When we came up with Preparative Waiting, we immediately knew that we had fit the core category with our data, that this concept covered the whole process, and that it had grab (see Table 5.3). In this way, the pictures facilitated our process of conceptualizing what was happening in our study. Having done so, we later could explain the pictures to others.

Selective Coding

Simultaneously with validating participants' main concern and the core category, we went on to selective coding, which meant limiting coding to those variables that were related to the core category (Glaser, 1978). For selective coding, I used the software NVivo 2.0. A memo from March 2003 discussed balancing, creating meaning, and creating a room of rest, which were key categories in our data, and these concepts are examples of what was coded for. The coding reports for every concept, which NVivo 2.0 offered, were helpful as I could go back to data, compare incidents to incidents, and see more easily how concepts and patterns emerged from data (Glaser, 1978). Table 5.1 gives examples of how we coded data.

At this stage (spring 2003) we had many concepts at different abstraction levels, such as uncertainty, patient putdowns, giving information, and contact qualities of staff; however, it was hard to find the right way to organize them. Living with this chaos is important when doing grounded theory, and it is necessary to go through it so that the participants' main concern and how they resolve it can emerge from data and not be forced. This unforced emergence is crucial to the relevance of the theory. Perhaps the conceptualization of what was going on in this study was particularly difficult because it was a partially hidden process for the participants themselves, living as they were under the threatening uncertainty of diagnostic workups.

Along with creating the paintings and conceptual maps (Artinian, 1982), selective coding continued, and we coded for 14 aspects of being in the hospital and waiting for a diagnosis. Examples of codes were examination, information (getting, giving, and information to family), diagnosis, uncertainty, ambivalence, staff qualifications, room, and clues about seriousness. The limited application of NVivo 2.0 made data classification and entry time consuming, but the software still offered a good overview of codes and their properties. In the final stage of selective coding, theoretical sampling and theoretical memo writing assisted in saturating categories and their properties (Glaser, 1978; Glaser & Strauss, 1967). As an example of saturation of properties (dimensions or aspects of the category) for the category of *interpreting clues*, we identified the properties to be *one's own bodily symptoms, former experiences with one's own and others' illness, nonverbal expressions of the staff, hospital environment, examinations conducted,* and *schedule patterns.* Theoretical saturation of the theory was reached when no new properties of the categories were found in data and the integration and density of the theory was at a high level. In GT theoretical coverage is partial because a substantive theory always can be modified as more data are compared (Glaser, 1978).

THEORETICAL CODING

After open and selective coding, which had fragmented the data but had provided us with dimensions and variations within the concepts, it was time to move on to theoretical coding. Theoretical coding relates the concepts of a theory to each other in a clear and distinct way. In this work, sorting memos was important because it assisted us in developing categories that covered all the concepts related to the core category, preparative waiting. A lot of work was put into fitting and refitting the codes and in trying out different ways of relating concepts to each other. We found that conceptual mapping and experimenting with different models were helpful tools (Artinian, 1982; Glaser, 1978).

Different models were discussed with members of the Bergen Grounded Theory Research Group, at doctoral seminars at the university, and at several international conferences. Questions and critical feedback from various people were essential in driving the theoretical coding forward. In the next paragraphs we will comment on some models as they occurred over time. Only the models representing major changes are presented here.

Conceptual Mapping and Models

Figure 5.1 shows the first attempt to express key concepts of the theory and how they were related to each other. The main concern was put in the middle to illustrate what was driving the participants to action. The concepts of *balancing, trying to make sense,* and *creating a room of rest* were seen as closely related to each other and were important aspects of how the participants resolved their problem. We were aware that the process the participants went through was more complicated and had more concepts, but at that time we were not able to fit them into the model.

A later model (Figure 5.2) had many more categories, and tried to picture the process whereby patients worked to find meaning in their situation and at the same time take care of themselves. *Balancing* was recognized to be a more appropriate guide for the whole process than

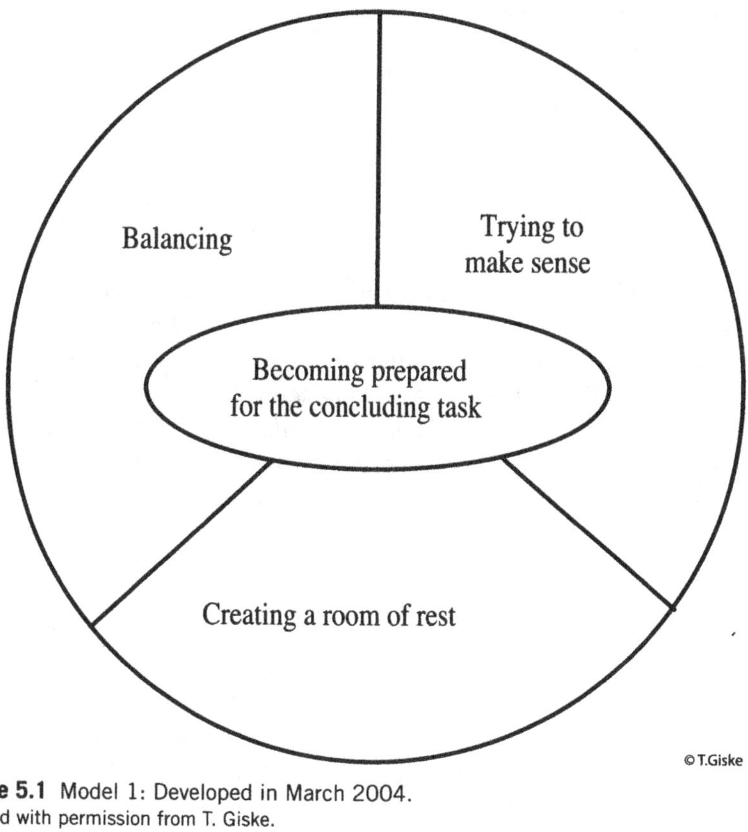

Figure 5.1 Model 1: Developed in March 2004.
Printed with permission from T. Giske.

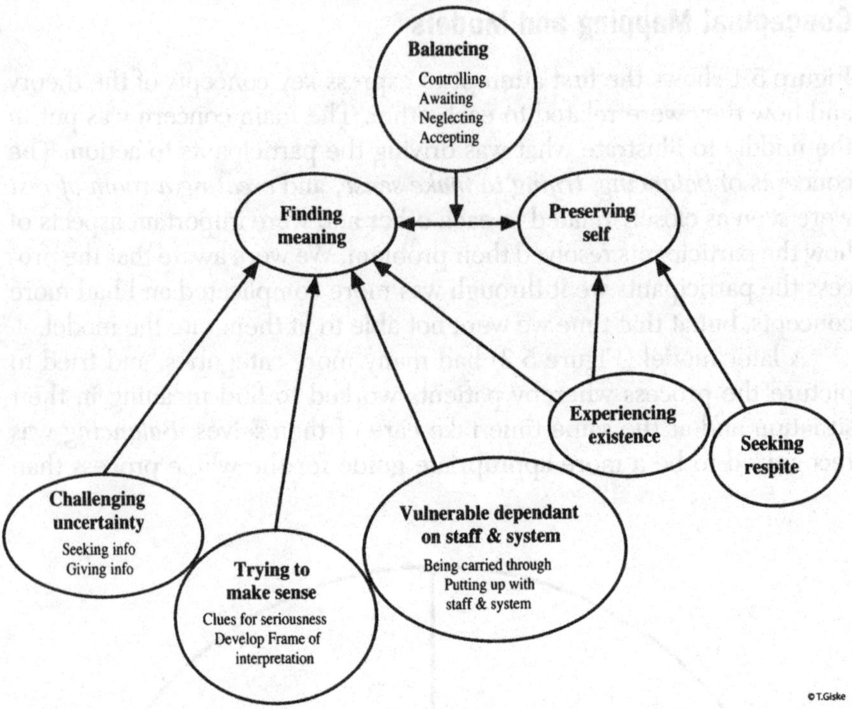

Figure 5.2 Model 3: Developed in early June 2004.
Printed with permission from T. Giske.

the other concepts and therefore was placed on top of the figure. Already at this stage we saw four patterns of *balancing between hope and despair,* which later on turned out to be another way to theoretically code our theory. The category of *making sense* from Model 1 was split into *challenging uncertainty* and *trying to make sense,* and the categories *vulnerable: dependent on staff and system* and *experiencing existence* were added to the model. Placing the arrows turned out to be difficult as the process of the theory was not clear. When presenting this model to other researchers they found it confusing and not helpful in understanding how patients prepared for getting a diagnosis.

The fourth model (Figure 5.3) tried to grasp that *balancing* was very important and guided how the other strategies were conducted. Therefore, *balancing* was placed in the middle of the model. Having the arrows passing through it was intended to indicate that the other categories were dependent on how *balancing* was conducted. Further analysis made it clear that this model mixed conditions *(vulnerable: dependant*

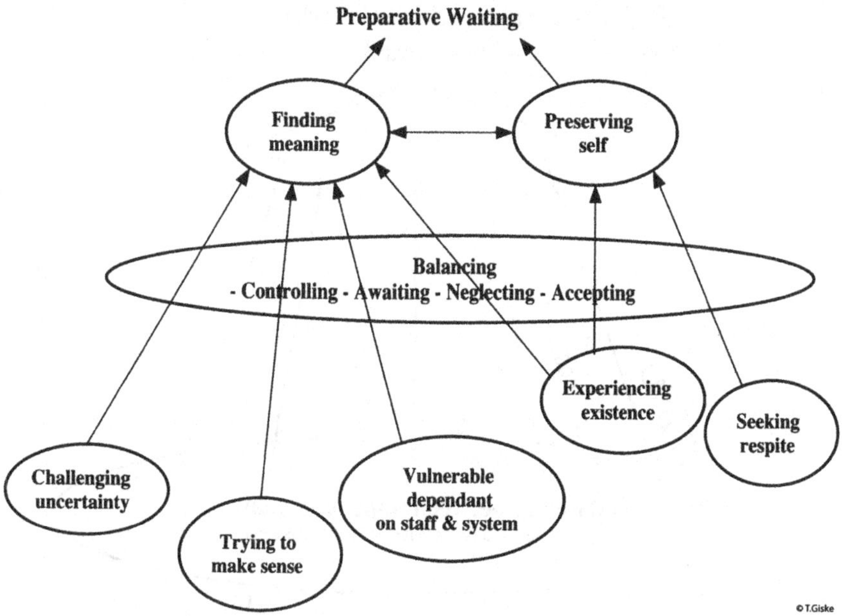

Figure 5.3 Model 4: Developed in late June 2004.
Printed with permission from T. Giske.

on staff and system) with strategies patients used. The conceptual fit was improved, but the theory did not work well to explain what was happening in the area, and the relevance and grab of the theory were still low.

Balancing as the Theoretical Code

Theoretical coding continued until *balancing between hope and despair* was identified as the theoretical code that integrates the substantive GT of Preparative Waiting (see chapter 21, "Patterns of Balancing Between Hope and Despair in the Diagnostic Phase on a Gastroenterology Ward"). Theoretical codes are difficult to understand and therefore are often missed by novice researchers. They are not necessary, but a GT becomes more integrated and relevant when theoretical coding is used because it raises the theory to a higher level (Glaser, 2005). Model 13 (Figure 5.4) is more dense and parsimonious, and contains fewer concepts. The core category of preparative waiting integrates the whole process of preparing for the concluding interview and life afterward, and the theory is more solidified, with interrelated categories reduced to a smaller set of higher-level concepts. *Challenging uncertainty* was reformulated to *seeking and giving*

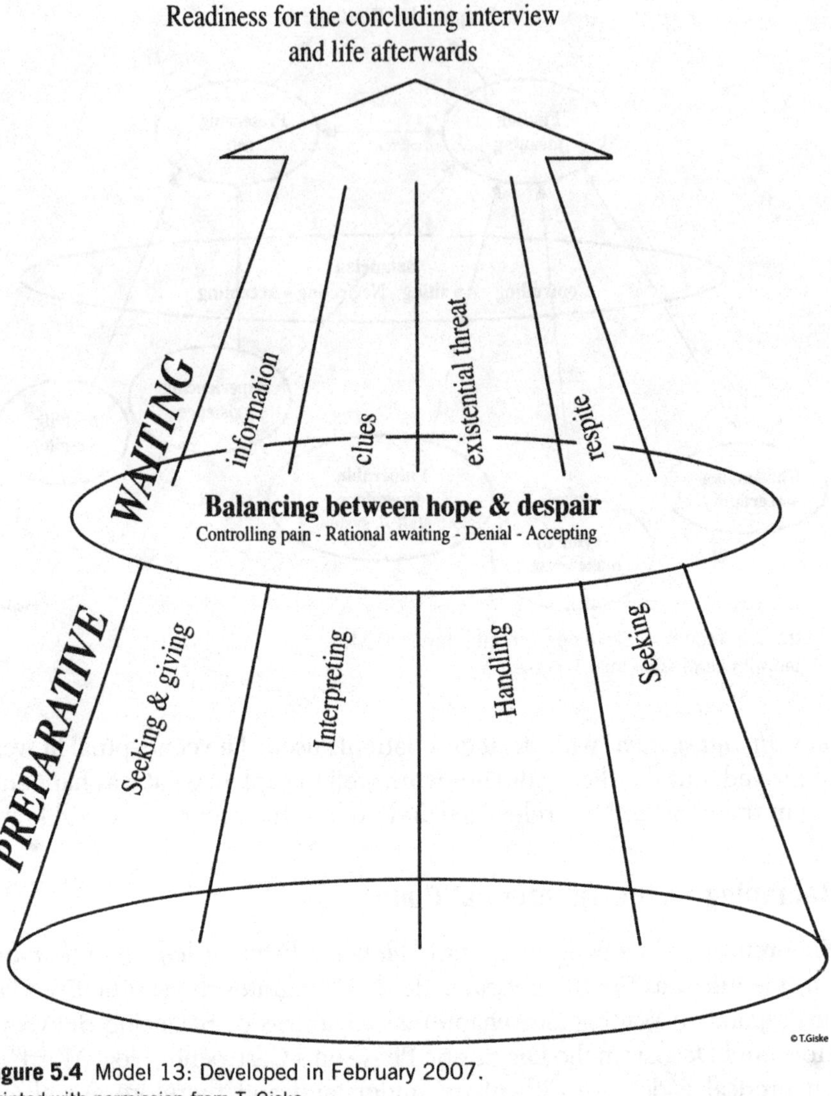

Figure 5.4 Model 13: Developed in February 2007.
Printed with permission from T. Giske.

information, a concept that is easier to understand. *Trying to make sense* was changed to *interpreting clues. Dependent on staff and system* (Figure 5.4), which had a considerable number of codes in our data, was a condition participants acted in relation to. In Model 13 this is built into all the other categories. The theoretical code of balancing between hope and despair, with its four patterns, is put in the middle of the figure to demonstrate that it is the guiding principle of how preparative waiting is carried out by patients. In analyzing more closely how the different patterns of balancing were carried out, we realized that the best fit to the full data set of the category covering the existential threat was *handling existential threat* rather than the former *struggling with existential threat.* The whole process of preparative waiting was formed as an arrow, indicating that it led to readiness for the concluding interview and life afterward. When this final model was presented, people listened, accepted it, and said they understood. The fit, relevance, and workability had improved.

LITERATURE REVIEW

The last key area to address is how a grounded theorist relates his or her substantive theory to other theories and previously developed bodies of knowledge (Table 5.3). According to classical grounded theory, searching and reading literature is done differently in different stages of a study. In the planning stage literature is searched in an attempt to identify gaps in knowledge. In our study we were aware that women with breast disorders had been studied, but we could not identify any study of patients with gastroenterological problems going through the diagnostic phase. During data collection, coding, and writing of memos, literature related to grounded theory methodology, symbolic interactionism, and other areas were read to improve openness to our actual study (Glaser, 1998). When our substantive theory of preparative waiting was grounded and developed enough to stand on its own feet, we reviewed the literature to compare and contrast our findings with the knowledge base of the field. Even at this stage, however, the attitude of a GT researcher is to read research and theories as ideas and not as truths and to compare other concepts and ideas with the concepts of our theory. This can be fruitful work where the theory can be extended further and transcended.

To contribute to the field, we wanted to show how our work fitted into the area by weaving our findings into the body of already existing knowledge. Thus, in spring 2005 we undertook a systematic literature review. A GT is abstract of time, place, and people because it conceptualizes processes (Glaser, 1978), and the concept of preparative waiting applies to many fields, which challenged our ability to judge the relevant reading of research and other theories. In the systematic review we did not find research conducted with patients where the outcome of the diagnostic examination was as open as it was with our participants. We found numerous research studies conducted on breast disorders, and these studies were evaluated as important because the diagnostic phase was crucial to our research. The drawback of comparing our findings with this body of knowledge was that it covered only women and that the examination process was much more defined and organized than for our participants.

We also looked for theories that were relevant to our GT of preparative waiting, such as uncertainty in illness, motivated information management, and stress and coping; and we have discussed the vulnerability that patients experience in relation to health care professionals (Giske, Gjengedal, & Artinian, 2009). Theories in other areas, such as system theory and authority structure, highlighted other aspects of the theory of preparative waiting that traditionally are less focused on in health care professions. Pursuing these aspects is a future challenge for us.

Summing Up the Process

We have shown how we developed a conceptual grounded theory from our rich data. Table 5.3 illustrates the whole process of data collection, coding, and development of the substantive grounded theory of preparative waiting. It shows the time schedule of interviews, when the different kinds of coding took place, how we worked on validating the participants' main concern, and the core category. The table demonstrates how we worked to improve the fit and relevance of the emergent theory by testing many terms (Glaser, 1998), illustrates our process of conceptualizing data and our work in theoretical coding of the theory by developing pictures and models to meet the criteria of *work* in order to constitute a credible GT, and also gives examples of theory and research that we read during the different stages of the analyzing process.

CONCLUSION

To be able to carry out a GT study, one must be willing and able to stay open to the experience of the participants, to live with degrees of chaos until the concepts emerge, and then be able to conceptualize. This requires hard work combined with creativity. In our study we have put much effort into letting the core problem and processes of the participants emerge (relevance) and into fitting the concepts with data so that they work in presenting what happens in the area we have studied. It has been a process of learning by doing while extending our grasp of GT methodology, which has promoted the development of a beginner into a more experienced grounded theorist.

ACKNOWLEDGEMENTS

We thank the staff on the unit for their cooperation, and we thank the participants for sharing their experiences at a vulnerable time of their lives. This project was funded by Bergen Deaconess University College and Western Norway Regional Health Authority.

REFERENCES

Artinian, B. (1982). Conceptual mapping: The development of the strategy. *Western Journal of Nursing Research, 4,* 379–393.

Backman, K., & Kyngäs, H. A. (1999). Challenge of grounded theory approach to a novice researcher. *Nursing and Health Sciences, 1,* 147–153.

Baker, C., Wuest, J., & Stern, P. N. (1992). Method slurring: The grounded theory/phenomenology example. *Journal of Advanced Nursing, 17,* 1355–1360.

Cutcliffe, J. R. (2000). Methodological issues in grounded theory. *Journal of Advanced Nursing, 31*(6), 1476–1484.

Cutcliffe, J. R. (2005). Adapt or adopt: Developing and transgressing the methodological boundaries of grounded theory. *Journal of Advanced Nursing, 51*(4), 421–428.

Duchscher, J. E. B., & Morgan, D. (2004). Grounded theory: Reflections on emergence vs. forcing debate. *Journal of Advanced Nursing, 48*(6), 605–612.

Fog, J. (2004). *Med samtalen som udgangspunkt: Det kvalitative forskningsinterview* (2nd ed.). København: Akademisk Forlag A/S.

Giske, T. (1993). *Pasienten si oppleving av meining—sjukepleiaren sitt ansvar?* Bergen: Alma Mater.

Giske, T. (1995). Spiritual care in nursing practice. *Christian Nurse International, 11*(4), 4–8.

Giske, T., Gjengedal, E., & Artinian, B. (2009). The silent demand in the diagnostic phase. *Scandinavian Journal of Caring Science, 23*(1), 100–106.

Glaser, B. G. (1978). *Theoretical sensitivity.* Mill Valley, CA: Sociology Press.

Glaser, B. G. (1992). *Basics of grounded theory analysis.* Mill Valley, CA: Sociology Press.

Glaser, B. G. (1998). *Doing grounded theory: Issues and discussions.* Mill Valley, CA: Sociology Press.

Glaser, B. G. (1999). The future of grounded theory: Keynote address from the Fourth Annual Qualitative Health Research Conference. *Qualitative Health Research* 9(6), 836–845.

Glaser, B. G. (2001). *The grounded theory perspective: Conceptualization contrasting with description.* Mill Valley, CA: Sociology Press.

Glaser, B. G. (2005). *The grounded theory perspective III: Theoretical coding.* Mill Valley, CA: Sociology Press.

Glaser, B. G., & Strauss, A. L. (1967). *The discovery of grounded theory: Strategies for qualitative research.* New York: Aldine de Gruyter.

Johnson, M., & Long, T. (2006). Research ethics. In K. Gerrish & A. Lacey (Eds.), *The research process in nursing* (pp. 31–42). Oxford, UK: Blackwell.

Lomborg, K., & Kirkevold, M. (2003). Truth and validity in grounded theory—a reconsidered realist interpretation of the criteria: Fit, work, relevance and modifiability. *Nursing Philosophy, 4,* 189–200.

McCallin, A. M. (2003). Designing a grounded theory study: Some practicalities. *Nursing in Critical Care, 8*(5), 203–208.

Mjølnerød, H. (1997). *Pasientens åndelige/eksistensielle dimensjon slik den uttrykkes hos pasienter i livets sluttfase* [The spiritual and existential dimensions as expressed by patients in the terminal phase of life] (Publikasjonsserie nr. 32). Oslo, Norway: Institutt for Sykepleievitenskap, Universitetet i Oslo.

QSR International. (2002). *Using NVivo 2 in qualitative research.* Doncaster, Australia: QSR International Pty.

Thoresen, I. T. (1993). Hvem trøster hjertene? [Who comforts the hearts?] *Omsorg, 4,* 45–50.

Tønnessen, S. (1999). *Gud og døden snakker vi ikke om: Hvordan imøtekommer sykepleiere pasientens åndelige behov?* ["We don't talk about God or death": How do nurses meet patients' spiritual needs?] (Publikasjonsserie nr. 7). Oslo, Norway: Institutt for Sykepleievitenskap, Universitete i Oslo.

Ueland, V. (1997). *Kommunikativ kompetanse. En beskrivelse av sykepleierens handlingsrettede kompetanse i å samtale om åndelige og eksistensielle spørsmål med kreftpasienter som har kort forventet levetid* [A description of the nursing caretakers' active directed level of skills in dialoguing the spiritual and existential questions with cancer patients with an expected short lifespan] (Publikasjonsserie nr. 28). Oslo, Norway: Institutt for Sykepleievitenskap, Universitet i Oslo.

World Medical Association. (2004). *Declaration of Helsinki: Ethical principles for medical research involving human subjects.* Retrieved November 2, 2005, from http://www.wma.net/e/policy/b3.html

6

Learning Glaserian Grounded Theory Through Mentoring and Scholarly Dialogue

PAMELA H. CONE
TOVE GISKE
BARBARA M. ARTINIAN

Much has been written by Glaser (more than 13 books from 1978 through 2005) and other scholars about grounded theory (GT), including how to learn it and how to do it. All of the scholars in this book have learned through some form of mentoring and/or scholarly dialogue with Glaser and other GT scholars. This exchange of ideas and understanding served to keep the researchers from taking tangential or incorrect directions in the analysis. It helped them all focus on determining the main concern of our participants and discovering how the concern was resolved. This chapter is a discussion of this learning process through group and individual mentoring as well as through dialogue between GT scholars.

MENTORING

In the 1980s, Artinian had the opportunity to learn directly from Strauss and Glaser through a postdoctoral fellowship at the University of California at San Francisco. Strauss was ill at that time, and so she and two other scholars learned the method together by reading *Theoretical Sensitivity* (Glaser, 1978) and engaging in dialogue with each other about it. They spent many hours discussing what they read. A classical Glaserian purist herself, Artinian has published articles and other GT works on various aspects of the method.

Cone and Giske learned primarily from Artinian and Glaser, attending their workshops, receiving their mentoring, and engaging in dialogue with them. They began the mentoring process in the manner of many graduate students: by taking a course in qualitative research. Artinian taught a course at Azusa Pacific University, and other GT scholars taught courses elsewhere that graduate students could attend. For Cone, 15 years of mentoring and scholarly dialogue followed the initial class that she attended. Those years started with a master's thesis, moved through research with a network of scholars, and culminated with a doctoral dissertation from UCSF in 2006 (see chapter 17, "Mutuality: Reconnecting to Overcome Homelessness"). Although Cone chose to use a purist Glaserian approach to GT research, it was not until her postdoctoral study on spiritual care in Norway that she had the privilege of actual dialogue with Glaser.

Giske attended a summer GT course at Azusa Pacific University and enlisted Artinian, the professor of the course, as the methodologist on her dissertation committee. They worked together over several years, and three of Giske's doctoral papers resulting from their work are presented in this book (see chapter 5, "Learning Glaserian Grounded Theory by Doing It"; chapter 7, "Preparative Waiting Patients Hospitalized for Diagnostic Workups"; and chapter 21, "Patterns of Balancing Between Hope and Despair in the Diagnostic Phase on a Gastroenterology Ward"). When professor Artinian visited Bergen, she also mentored the other Scandinavian scholars who are authors in this book and were doctoral candidates at the time. Some attended a workshop conducted by Glaser and were able to dialogue with him about their research and how their understanding of the GT method applied in their doctoral studies.

The American scholars in this book took courses in qualitative research and then moved on to being mentored by Artinian through masters' theses or doctoral dissertations. Their learning processes proceeded through several steps. Reading the works of Glaser was the starting point for each scholar. Discussing GT methodology and when it makes sense to use the method as well as how to phrase a GT question was part of the early process of learning. Discovering when not to use the Glaserian GT method was also an important step in the process. One-on-one mentoring by Artinian through a master's project enabled Cone to grasp the analytical process and capture a basic social process (BSP) in that early project.

Mentoring by an expert GT scholar and dialogue with GT scholars are both important aspects of moving the novice GT scholar toward greater expertise. The move from novice to expert GT scholar requires learning by doing as well as by listening and questioning throughout the analytical process. Later, taking on the role of mentoring new scholars also assisted the editors of this book to become more adept with the Glaserian GT method of research, and to begin to trust their own analytical processes as well as the emerging theories.

SCHOLARLY DIALOGUE

Artinian conducted a series of summer courses on the use of GT method for spiritual care research from 1995 through 2001. These courses, led by Artinian and facilitated by Cone, gave novice and developing GT scholars an opportunity to conduct an ongoing GT study and work on it together for one week each summer. Scholars read *Theoretical Sensitivity* each year and collected data from two participants each. During the research process, many of the scholars formed GT research groups for scholarly dialogue about their studies.

One such group was the research team formed by Van Dover and Bacon Pfeiffer to study parish nursing. Together they identified the BSP of *bringing God near* (2007), which was further developed by Pfeiffer (see chapter 12, "Partnering With God and the Patient"). They have commented that the experience of conducting GT research together, from data collection and analysis through theory development, is interesting and relatively uncommon. This team analyzed data individually, but they also met regularly to do analysis together, comparing notes on how they understood what was emerging through analysis. Their successful teamwork continues to date, and a discussion of their collaborative process will be presented in a future article.

Another group was formed by Vuckovich with several other doctoral students at the University of San Diego. Vuckovich's group met regularly to discuss methodological issues related to their individual research projects. This group was disbanded following completion of their dissertations.

A strong and continuing GT group was formed in Bergen, Norway. Meeting regularly on a monthly basis for more than four years during their doctoral studies, these scholars shared their work with each other, critiquing the work and helping each other stay true to classical GT methodology. A further step in their learning process was the move from descriptive or gerund theories to theories integrated by theoretical codes, and then to theory-based interventional research, an advancement that according to Glaser (2007) rarely happens. A descriptive theory discussed in Part II (see chapter 7, "Preparative Waiting Patients Hospitalized for Diagnostic Workups") can also be found in Part III, "Studies With Emergent Theoretical Codes," and in Part IV, "The Intervention Mode."

Artinian provided workshops in Norway, with participation from Cone, and mentored the Norwegian group during this time period. This Norwegian group continues to meet concerning their ongoing postdoctoral research, developing interventions based on their individual substantive grounded theories. Cone had the pleasure of joining this group during a six-month Fulbright award in Norway.

CONCLUSION

While grounded theory can be learned by reading the works of expert GT researchers or by simply doing the steps as outlined by Glaser (1978), it is clear from the history of the GT method that many tangential methods have been developed by scholars with varying levels of expertise. The authors presenting their research in this book have discovered that Glaserian GT is best and most accurately learned when a Glaserian GT mentor is able to assist the novice GT research scholar. The mentor serves to guide the research process away from the pitfalls of dimensional and situational analysis and from qualitative data analysis. This is not to say that other types of qualitative research methods are not useful; they are simply not the method discovered by Glaser. We have also discovered the value of research groups that meet regularly to analyze data together or to discuss each other's research and writing. The studies in this volume present a purist Glaserian GT approach with the goal of theory discovery and development.

REFERENCES

Glaser, B. G. (1978). *Theoretical sensitivity.* Mill Valley, CA: Sociology Press.

Glaser, B. G. (2007). Doing formal theory. In A. Bryant & K. Charmaz (Eds.), *The SAGE handbook of grounded theory* (pp. 97–111). Los Angeles, CA: Sociology Press

Van Dover, L., & Pfeiffer, J. B. (2007). Spiritual care in Christian parish nursing. *Journal of Advanced Nursing,* 57(2), 213–221.

Studies Using Early Modes of Grounded Theory

PART II

INTRODUCTION: BARBARA M. ARTINIAN

In the early days of Grounded Theory (GT) studies, researchers primarily used either the Descriptive or Gerund Modes to describe the situation of interest. The Descriptive Mode is still used at the beginning of a research study that, with further analysis, can become a fully integrated study. The Gerund Mode, uniquely characterized by using gerund verbs, is used to describe the stages of an identified Basic Social Process. The Emergent Fit Mode is now used to develop a program of research based on previous research in the area.

Although the first introduction of the GT method was published in the book *Discovery of Grounded Theory* (Glaser & Strauss, 1967), widespread use of the GT method began with the publication of the book *Theoretical Sensitivity* by Glaser in 1978. The first study using the GT method that was published in a nursing journal described the basic social process of Limiting Intrusion (Wilson, 1977). This article provided a format for presenting GT research when stages emerged from the data (the Gerund Mode). When patterns emerge with no clear stages connecting them, a description of the patterns or categories that emerged is given (the Descriptive Mode). An example of this is the conceptual map made by Artinian (1983) to illustrate the various career paths a dialysis patient may take (Figure 22.1). Both the descriptive mode and the gerund mode are done within the context of the discovery mode. When the research begins with a theoretical framework, as from a previous study, the emergent fit mode allows the researcher to expand, enhance, or correct the previous theory.

These three modes have been in use since the GT method was introduced and each follows the basic principle of allowing the theory to emerge from the data. All of these modes are still in use today and can produce research that can be published as completed research, or the research can serve as the starting point for more sophisticated analysis of the data. In each of these early modes, analysis of data is based on integrating substantive codes rather than integrating the substantive codes by an emergent theoretical code. Studies using these three modes are appropriate for the researcher new to the GT method and these studies can provide valuable direction for nursing practice.

REFERENCES

Artinian, B. (1983). Role identities of the dialysis patient. *Nephrology Nurse, 5*, 10–14.

Glaser, B. G. (1978). *Theoretical sensitivity.* Mill Valley, CA: Sociology Press.

Glaser, B. G., & Strauss, A. (1967). *The discovery of grounded theory: Strategies for qualitative research.* Chicago, Aldine Publishing.

Wilson, H. (1977). Limiting Intrusion: Social control of outsiders in a healing community. *Nursing Research, 26*(2), 105–111.

I

Descriptive Mode

INTRODUCTION: BARBARA M. ARTINIAN

The descriptive mode presents a description of a setting or life experience. It answers such questions as what types of behavior are going on. The outcome is a report of the major categories or types of behavior. It is a useful way for beginning researchers to gain experience in conducting qualitative interviews and writing memos to begin analysis of the data. This mode precedes the theoretical code mode, which relates variables and patterns to each other to develop an integrated theory.

Two examples of studies in the descriptive mode are presented here. The first is the study conducted by Giske in 2002–2003 describing the behaviors of patients waiting for a diagnosis (see chapter 7, "Preparative Waiting: Patients Hospitalized for Diagnostic Workups"). In-depth analysis sensitized Giske to the theoretical code of balancing, which led her to develop a fully integrated theory (see chapter 21, "Patterns of Balancing Between Hope and Despair in the Diagnostic Phase on a Gastroenterology Ward").

The second example of the descriptive mode is a study of caregiving behaviors of intrapartum nurses (see chapter 8, "Caregiving Behaviors of Intrapartum Nurses"). This study is a beginning analysis of role relationships between nurses and obstetrical patients.

7

Preparative Waiting: Patients Hospitalized for Diagnostic Workups

TOVE GISKE
BARBARA M. ARTINIAN

Hospitalized patients who are undergoing medical examinations aimed at getting a diagnosis endure a challenging time of waiting. They do not know what kind of disease they have, how serious it is, or how it eventually can be treated. Interpretation of both present and future is unsure and open, which leaves them feeling vulnerable and stressed, prey to a deep uncertainty. Selder (1989), writing about uncertainty, states that it forces a person to confront his or her vulnerability and that vulnerability heightens the experience of uncertainty. Mast (1995), McCormick (2002), and Neville (2003) all conclude in their reviews about uncertainty that a high degree of uncertainty is related to high emotional distress, anxiety, and depression. Hospitalized patients waiting for a diagnosis live with uncertainty for a shorter or longer period of time and experience the burden of this reality. Many report that the time of waiting for a diagnosis is the most stressful time of the illness experience (Mishel, 1988, 1997; Neville, 2003; Poole, 1997). Mast (1995) and McCormick (2002) both conclude their articles by summing up the need for further research to help indicate the relationship among interconnected components of uncertainty.

The purpose of this chapter is to present a descriptive grounded theory (GT) of Preparative Waiting that grew out of a study of hospitalized patients waiting for a diagnosis, and to discuss the findings in light of theories of uncertainty.

THE STUDY

Method

A GT methodology, built on Glaser's classic form of GT (Glaser 1978, 2001, 2003; Glaser & Strauss, 1967), was chosen to study how patients hospitalized for diagnostic examination experienced and handled their situation.

Participants

The inclusion criteria were that the participants should be hospitalized for medical examination in the stomach-intestine area, be 35 years of age or older, be mentally and physically able to take part in the interview, and be willing to sign the informed consent form. Eight women and seven men, aged 35–84, participated in the study.

Data Collection and Analysis

Eighteen in-depth interviews, with an average length of 56 minutes, were taped and transcribed verbatim. The interviews were coded line by line and compared with previous coded interviews. After a period of open coding, the interviews were coded selectively, using software NVivo 2.0 (QSR International, 2002). The interviews became more and more specific as our understanding of the participants' situation developed. Throughout the study, memos were written where reflections, ideas, hypotheses, and possible connections were stated. In the end memos were hand-sorted and used in the analysis in which the validation of the patients' main concern, the core category, and the concepts in the theory were developed.

Ethical Considerations

The study was approved by the Regional Ethical Board and welcomed by the medical unit where it was conducted. Patients were informed and asked to take part in the study by a contact nurse at the unit. The interviews took place after the participants had signed the consent form.

FINDINGS

The main concern of the participants was how to prepare themselves for the concluding conference when they would receive a diagnosis, and for life after that. The main concern is both the cause and the mover of the work the patients do (Glaser, 2001).

Engaged in Preparative Waiting

The theory that described how the participants resolved their main concern was named Preparative Waiting (see Figure 7.1).

Preparative Waiting is a core category and all the concepts of the theory are connected and can happen at any time during the process, depending on how a person needs to use them. *Seeking information* and *interpreting clues* move the waiting person forward in trying to make more and more sense of his or her situation. *Struggling with existential threat* and *seeking respite* are more focused on dealing with the threat they experience to self and the importance of keeping themselves on an

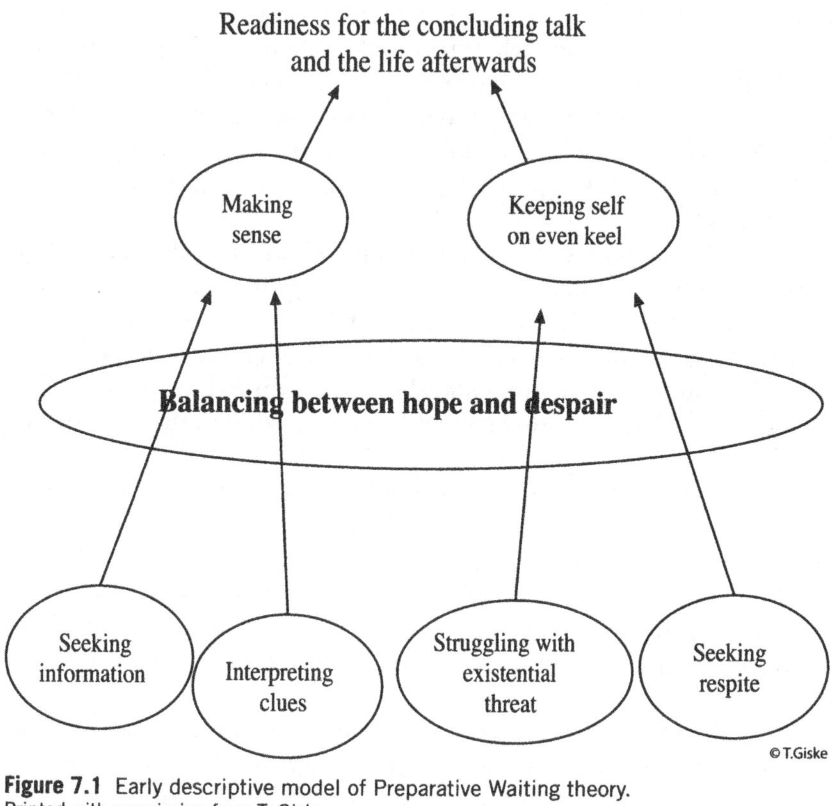

Figure 7.1 Early descriptive model of Preparative Waiting theory. Printed with permission from T. Giske.

even keel. *Balancing between hope and despair* is the filter that everything flows through and describes the way the participants try to keep themselves on an even keel.

Balancing Between Hope and Despair

Balancing is an inner, active work where the patients move between hope and despair. It means balancing emotions to the limits of what is bearable at any time. Balancing is the strategy that filters all the activities of Preparative Waiting and it influences how the patients work on making sense of their situation, how they struggle with existential thoughts, and how they manage to achieve respite. The balancing work makes them "taste" a little of what they fear and what they hope for. If they let despair and their worst fear be too strong, controlling and hiding how painful their situation is and how weak they actually feel becomes very hard. They try to balance and keep themselves strong by actively looking for good reasons for hope. Negative thoughts about the future and their diagnostic outcome are actively forced out of their mind. By doing this they are able to endure the time of waiting and they develop an inner awareness of self so they can prepare themselves for whatever might come. All this is done as in a shadow, in the back of their minds, on and off. The balancing work is preparing them for the concluding interview and for the future.

Living with not knowing and uncertainty about the future, together with pain and the problems of their symptoms, put a lot of pressure on the patients in this study. They told about tension, stress, depression, helplessness, irritation, fear, and uneasiness. The uncertainty was in the back of their minds all the time and they used expressions such as, "It's lying there smoldering" and "I can't relax; it's working in the back of my mind all the time."

These worries intensified as the patients entered the hospital. There they had to face the smells, sounds, and equipment of the hospital, and relate to hospital staff and other patients. The diagnostic examinations they went through in the hospital were interpreted immediately or within hours or days, and knowing that the period of waiting was indefinite, caused the participants to stay in an alert state of mind most of the time.

Being away from family and friends made an obvious difference for them, and some of the participants missed intimate and supportive talk with their spouses. Being hospitalized allowed some patients to relax from the need to worry about their loved ones. Others did not have family or friends nearby. Their loved ones also experienced frustration caused by uncertainty and waiting. For all of the patients, being in the hospital meant being in unfamiliar surroundings and this added to the feeling of being alone.

Their contact with fellow patients varied from mostly avoiding contact to spending time with other patients for talking, learning, or helping out. The participants in our study did more listening and small talk than sharing their own worries with their fellow patients. The amount of contact and the content of conversation were adjusted according to how well the patients could manage listening to problems of others before listening became burdensome and threatened their own balancing work.

Seeking Information

Patients entered the hospital with different expectations, ranging from skeptical to positive, based on previous experiences. Patients admitted on schedule expected a plan of medical examinations and tests upon arrival. Those on emergency admission accepted having their situation evaluated upon arrival, with action taken from there.

In general, content of information exchange was influenced by the degree of trust developed by patients with the individual nurse or doctor. Trust was earned by the patients' informal evaluation of staff qualifications, such as knowledge and experience related to the patient's situation, continuity of contact, and the sincerity of commitment, interest, and care for the patient.

Daily rounds, a major routine in medical units, provided an opportunity for information exchange between staff and patients; however, to use this opportunity, there were many obstacles to overcome. The patients expected doctors to come prepared for the rounds, to have read their case records, to know about results of examinations and tests, and to have a plan for future examinations. Lack of staff continuity and poor doctor preparation undermined quality exchange of information and drained the strength of the patients.

The patients themselves could also be obstacles. Most often, participants trusted the doctors, and they expected the doctors to give them necessary information. Being worried and afraid, however, limited their ability to listen; patients sometimes heard only pieces of information and misunderstood even those pieces, or understood nothing at all. Some were afraid to ask questions, or forgot what they had planned to ask when the doctor arrived at their bedside. This quote sums up how information exchange can go wrong due to misunderstandings:

> I understood (from the doctor) that I most certainly had a malignant tumor. She said they should take a biopsy so the oncological unit could prepare the treatment. (Later I understood that) what she meant to say was that they wanted to take a biopsy to find out whether there was a reason to believe that something was wrong. But it came out all wrong. I could not understand this, but okay, I said, it's you who are the doctor, it's you who knows.

Patients tried to understand their condition by taking in as much information as possible. Information could reduce uncertainty to a minimum and give them better insight into their situation and what to expect for the days ahead. Patients also cared about giving information so the health team could have the whole picture and the right judgment about their situation could be made.

One major patient concern was to gain information on how to prepare for and undergo examinations. Physical preparations such as fasting or vastly increased water intake were unpleasant. The mental preparation included balancing fear and worries related both to going through the examinations and to the actual findings. The longer the patients had been waiting for a diagnosis, the more important it was that test preparations be done correctly to ensure accuracy of results. Lack of accurate information frustrated the patients and diminished their trust in their staff. Delayed or postponed investigations kept patients unrelentingly alert and prevented rest and respite. Patient suffering increased when patients felt that doctors simply saw them as statistics while they awaited an answer that might crush all their hopes and plans. On the other hand, patient hope was strengthened through accurate information and a relationship with committed staff on whom they could lean.

Strategies to Promote Effective Exchange of Information. The participants were vulnerable, were dependent on staff and the system, and tried to prevent conflicts during the investigation process. Some had been through many examinations over time and had learned to fight to make the system work in their favor; others found it most helpful to keep a low profile.

One strategy patients used was to decide how proactive they needed to be to obtain the information they wanted and could trust. This was a balance between trusting staff to know, plan, and remember to pass on needed information to them and realizing that their own questions and proposals were necessary to move their cases forward. Another patient strategy was to make the most out of the opportunity at the investigation unit by asking the doctor for explanations and information. A more passive strategy was just to wait for the doctor they trusted to arrive before asking any questions. Another helpful strategy was to make contact with one particular doctor to improve productivity of contact after discharge. Still another active way of influencing the flow of information was to ask for a meeting with nurses and doctors at the unit where the patient and next of kin could question the accuracy of information they received. To use a trusted next of kin to make contact with the doctor was also a strategy for exchanging information.

Interpreting Clues

Interpreting clues was an ongoing effort in preparative waiting as patients searched for explanations and tried to make sense of their experience. Clues they used could be of inner or outer origin. They tried to figure out the cause of their symptoms and to interpret the symptoms. Since patients had different levels of knowledge and experience with illness and disease, they interpreted their symptoms and resultant seriousness differently. What kind of examination they went through, the priority the examinations were given, and the way the examinations were followed up were all clues that fed into patients' interpretations, and strengthened hope or moved them toward despair. One patient gave this example of how he interpreted what happened to him: "The biopsy taken was decisive and it's obvious that it is considered to be a rather serious affair since it has been given top priority."

Patients' understanding of their conditions ranged from the view that their disease was nothing serious and the health team would not be able to find anything, to the possibility that it might be very serious and would completely change their life. Some moved from one opinion to the other during the examination process as they tried to put all their clues and information together, and some had to deal with the possibility that their problems were psychologically based.

Patients preparing for the concluding interview wanted to save face and be able to make the best use of the medical expertise. Some participants reduced the expectation for themselves and their family in relation to what would be possible to discover about their health problems, and some prepared themselves to simply accept any result. Others felt it was difficult to prepare since they did not know the outcome of the investigation, and they were not emotionally capable of fully thinking through the different possible outcomes. Still others hoped for a diagnosis, but at the same time, prepared for no clear conclusion. One participant had been living with stomach pain and tiredness for years, and had felt the label "psychological" might be applied to her problems: "I'm afraid I will not be able to keep my face straight tomorrow [at the concluding interview], and then it will become: Oh yeah, it was psychological. I have spoken with my husband about this and he said: Well if you cry, what then? Who wouldn't?"

Struggling With Existential Threat

As soon as patients realized that there was a health problem, they began wondering about their future. None of the participants spontaneously discussed their existential considerations. The question chosen to explore their thoughts was formulated as follows "From where do you draw your strength?" Some participants had not given this question much consideration. Some found it a difficult or unfamiliar subject to discuss, while some felt it was easier to express their thoughts after being asked these questions. Often the patients began with sharing the importance of relationships to significant others such as family and friends before moving on to share about their relation to a religious faith. For some, the interview provided an opportunity to formulate what was working inside them, previously unarticulated either to themselves or to others. Sometimes hearing their expressions was like listening to a stream of thoughts pressing outward from deep within.

Facing uncertainty made the participants and their significant others become more aware of what gave value and meaning to life, and which life elements were of real importance. This value clarification could lead to a new perspective, resulting in a positive outcome, such as improved relationships with significant others. One participant reflected, "One gets another perspective on life when one is ill and doesn't know for sure what it is and certainly not the outcome of it. Life turns into another perspective, and some things become trifles." The experience of waiting and not knowing made them also become more aware that their existence might be threatened. Over time, they dealt with thoughts of the possibility of impending death in different ways according to how hopeful or despairing they were. Since they did not know about the future at the time of the interview, they felt their lives were being kept on hold.

About 87% of Norwegians are formal members of a Christian faith community (Statistics Norway, 2008). The personal significance of such membership varied considerably. Many participants experienced waiting for diagnosis as an hour of need; depending on their picture of God, they prayed short prayers filled with pain when they begged for help and turned themselves over to a bigger reality than the medical system could offer. One reflected, "I don't read the Bible and I don't go much to church. But when times are difficult I turn to the little prayer: 'Look after me and don't let it be as bad as I fear.' It's perhaps only in situations like this I use him."

Seeking Respite

The participants told about how they kept themselves going during the time of waiting, by being engaged in daily activities and hobbies, and they expressed the importance of relations to family such as spouse, children, grandchildren, mother, and friends. *Seeking respite* deals with stepping out of the constant tension of uncertainty where they work on balancing their hopes and despairs, trying to make sense of their situation, and dealing with worries for the future, to another mental state where their thoughts are occupied with other things than waiting. In respite they found a mental room where they were disconnected and could get away from the painful tension of uncertainty that "smoldered" in the back of their heads and where they could rest and gain new strength. Rest could help them *recharge the batteries,* as one of the participants expressed, so they could manage to live a little longer with the burden of not knowing. In this way *seeking respite* helped to preserve self.

Patients had different opportunities for seeking respite depending on where they stayed: in the hospital, at the patient's hotel, or at home for the night. Their health condition and medical examinations also influenced the possibility of seeking respite. Conditions promoting respite were influenced by staff and fellow patients. If the patients were given periods of no contact with staff, they could more easily disconnect from the alert waiting mood. Having fellow patients to chat with also helped. Being able to leave the hospital for shorter or longer periods of time offered the possibility to get away from the constant reminder of disease that was triggered by hospital smells, hospital sounds, the sight of hospital staff, and the presence of fellow patients.

At times staff members interfered with patient respite. Some did not respect the patients' need for peace and privacy. Occasionally a staff member provided results about samples and investigations so that patients were forced out of respite and into relating to the process of diagnostic workups. Hospital conditions also hindered respite. Sometimes during periods of high patient population, patients' beds had to sit in the hallway, which made it hard for the patients to withdraw from the daily activity on the ward. Having a private room offered peace and rest, but could also be lonely and allow too much time to think without the distraction from good fellow patients.

Strategies in Seeking Respite. The participants used different strategies in seeking respite. How obedient or undemanding they were to some extent shaped their day. If they sat in the hallway all day waiting for information in a state of *being alert,* or if they took control of their own time, they influenced the nature of their stay. To be able to read and listen to music or to be engaged in a good chat with fellow patients helped the time pass without thinking about the uncertainty with which they lived. One of the participants explained, "I'm doing a lot of thinking here. I brought a book and read it and listened to music to escape into another world while here." To leave the hospital on pass for a period of time could be very helpful and refreshing. Respite could also be found in sleep.

DISCUSSION

Mishel's Theory of Uncertainty

A central theory of uncertainty has been developed by Mishel (1981, 1988, 1990, 1997). She reports that patients undergoing diagnostic procedures experience higher uncertainty than other patient groups (Mishel, 1988, 1997). In her theory, uncertainty is defined as the inability to determine the meaning of illness-related events (Mishel, 1988, p. 225). Her short definition of uncertainty fits with the experience of participants in this study.

In Mishel's theory the "stimuli frame" consists of the component stimuli that provide the patients structure for an understandable cognitive schema. It concerns the patterns of the symptoms, the degree of familiarity of the event, and the congruence between the expected and the experienced event. Mishel (1988) calls the ability for a person to process information *cognitive capacity.* The structure providers such as credible authorities, social support, and education are the resources available for a person to interpret and deal with the stimuli frame.

The participants in this study experienced a great deal of ambiguity with respect to the illness, and it was difficult to find meaning in their symptoms. Their future was painfully unpredictable. Hospitalization and diagnostic workups introduced them to new investigations and preparations together with further waiting for new results. All of these stimuli challenged them to generate new cognitive maps, as presented in the category of *interpreting clues*. The participants' cognitive capacity was influenced by the many symptoms they had such as pain, diarrhea, nausea, and loss of weight. These problems, together with being stressed, suffering fear and depression, feeling helpless, and enduring uneasiness reduced their ability to process information. The educational level of the participants did not come through as an important condition in this study.

Social support is generally thought to assist a person in making sense of the illness experience (Mast, 1995). For most of our participants, social support from family and friends was limited to short visits and phone calls. Our findings indicate that patients received significant support neither from talking with fellow patients nor from involving their social network. On the other hand, credible authorities such as doctors and nurses turned out to be very important in providing information about what to expect during the investigation process and how to interpret the causes and consequences of symptoms. When patients could trust judgments and recommendations made by doctors and nurses, their uncertainty was reduced.

Mishel views uncertainty as an inherent part of life (Mishel, 1990). Uncertainty is a neutral cognitive state until it is appraised for its value and meaning (Mishel, 1997). In our study, uncertainty was appraised as a negative experience because medical investigations could take time, sometimes years. *Balancing between hope and despair* together with *seeking information, interpreting clues,* and *struggling with existential threat* showed internal work in which patients used all their earlier experiences and knowledge to try to interpret their situation. At the same time they looked for reasons to hope for a positive outcome. From our findings we would argue that uncertainty while waiting for a diagnosis is appraised by patients as a danger, but also that uncertainty can simultaneously hold both danger and opportunity. Uncertainty can be a life opportunity when a person realizes that his or her life might be threatened, and out of this threat achieves value clarification and a new perspective on the relationship to significant others. In our research we have seen this new perspective increase mutual family caring and end conflicts that had diminished contact within the family for a long time.

CONCLUSION

Patients going through diagnostic workups are inwardly vulnerable. They seek information and interpret clues in their struggle to define their problems and get help. They want to move on from uncertainty, where they are kept on hold and try to keep calm, to a new phase where they have a diagnosis. A diagnosis will help them to predict more about their future and to relate to their actual situation. In the investigation process they are dependent on staff and system as they try to manage their lives and gain the best understanding of their situation possible. They get existentially awakened, which offers opportunity for value clarification. At the same time they live on hold and this is not the time for sea changes in worldview. To get some relief from the pressure of living with uncertainty, respite is sought. Caretaker efforts at communication, care, and cooperation for these patients must be understood in accordance with the balancing work the patients must do. Sometimes they are strong with hope; other times they are almost crushed in despair. Since patients do their uttermost to keep a steady bearing, caretakers must exert a lot of professional discernment to relate to the patients in the best way.

REFERENCES

Glaser, B. G. (1978). *Theoretical sensitivity.* Mill Valley, CA: Sociology Press.

Glaser, B. G. (2001). *The grounded theory perspective: Conceptualization contrasting with description.* Mill Valley, CA: Sociology Press.

Glaser, B. G. (2003). *The grounded theory perspective II: Description's remodeling of GT methodology.* Mill Valley, CA: Sociology Press.

Glaser, B. G., & Strauss, A. L. (1967). *The discovery of GT.* Chicago: Aldine.

Mast, M. E. (1995). Adult uncertainty in illness: A critical review of research. *Scholarly Inquiry for Nursing Practice, 9*(1), 3–29.

McCormick, K. M. (2002). A concept analysis of uncertainty in illness. *Journal of Nursing Scholarship, 34*(2), 127–131.

Mishel, M. H. (1981). The measurement of uncertainty in illness. *Nursing Research, 30*(5), 258–263.

Mishel, M. H. (1988). Uncertainty in illness. *Image: Journal of Nursing Scholarship, 20*(4), 225–232.

Mishel, M. H. (1990). Reconceptualization of the uncertainty in illness theory. *Image: Journal of Nursing Scholarship, 22,* 256–262.

Mishel, M. H. (1997). Uncertainty in acute illness. In J. Fitzpatrick & J. Norbeck (Eds.), *Annual Review of Nursing Research, 15,* 57–80. New York: Springer Publishing.

Neville, K. L. (2003). Uncertainty in illness. An integrative review. *Orthopaedic Nursing,* 22(3), 206–214.

Poole, K. (1997). The emergence of the "waiting game": a critical examination of the psychosocial issues in diagnosing breast cancer. *Journal of Advanced Nursing, 25,* 273–281.

QSR International. (2002). *Using NVivo 2 in qualitative research.* Donchester, Victoria, Australia: QSR International Pty Ltd.

Selder, F. (1989). Life transition theory: The resolution of uncertainty. *Nursing and Health Care, 10*(8), 437–451.

Statistics Norway (Statistisk sentralbyrå). (2008). *Medlemmer i Den norske kyrkja og medlemmer[1] i trus- og livssynssamfunn utanfor Den norske kyrkja, etter religion/ livssyn. 1. januar* (Tabell 247). Oslo, Norway: Author. Retrieved from http://www.ssb.no/aarbok/tab/tab-247.html

8 Caregiving Behaviors of Intrapartum Nurses

MAUREEN FRIESEN
BARBARA M. ARTINIAN

The childbirth experience is a significant event for women, bringing profound changes into their lives. They often remember these events in detail for many years (Simkin, 1991). Because intrapartum nurses usually have a great deal of contact with couples during childbirth, they are in a position to shape its perceived outcome (Bryanton, Fraser-Davey, & Sullivan, 1994).

Quality nursing care for laboring women combines many skills and caregiving behaviors. The researcher noted that some nurses attempt to manage the childbirth experience without input from the patient, while others seek out and honor patient requests through an agreed-upon plan of care. Even though varieties of caregiving behaviors have been identified, it has been observed that not all nurses use each of them. The differences between the caregiving behaviors used with the laboring patient, and the reasons why nurses choose certain behaviors over others, have not been directly accounted for (Radin, Harmon, & Hanson, 1993).

In this descriptive study, it was found that caregiving behaviors were associated with the development of a nurse-patient relationship. The study showed that certain conditions influenced the caregiving behaviors and the direction of the emerging relationship. It was discovered that these conditions led to the development of a resistive, restrictive, or involved nurse-patient relationship (Friesen, 1999).

THE STUDY

Aim

The aim of this study was to better understand how intrapartum nurses perceived their caregiving behaviors during the labor process.

Method

An exploratory, descriptive design was used in this study, which used the constant comparative analysis of the grounded theory method (Glaser, 1978). Interviews were conducted with the nurses either at the hospital or in their homes.

Participants

The participants of the study included 12 intrapartum nurses between the ages of 31 and 60 with 11 to 25 years of obstetrical experience. They were recruited from a nonprofit, private, tertiary level referral hospital in the Southwest, which had an average of 4,000 deliveries per year.

Data Collection

Eligibility for participation in the study was determined during the initial phone contact. The data collection consisted of a demographic sheet and individual interviews. An open-ended interview guide was used allowing clarification of participant responses and the ability to probe particular statements more in-depth. The following types of questions were asked:

1. What are your goals for the patient during the labor process? Do these vary in particular situations?
2. What is the most satisfying experience you have had in working with a patient in labor?

The questions from the interview guide were expanded when the participants shared new ideas. As new themes and categories emerged, the questions were adjusted to explore those areas more thoroughly. When consistent themes and patterns were identified, the original questions were modified to reflect the ongoing analysis of the study.

Data Analysis

Data analysis began with the transcription of the audiotapes following the interview. After reviewing the transcribed records, memo writing began, and categories began to emerge as the data were compared. The primary categories that emerged from the responses were philosophies of the nurse; supporting activities during labor; and differences in individual nurse-patient interactions.

Ethical Considerations

The study was approved by the institutional review boards of the hospital and Azusa Pacific University. The participants were contacted by the investigator, consent was obtained, and then the interview was completed. Confidentiality was maintained by assigning an individual code number for each participant, and the number was used only to distinguish between participants' interviews, transcriptions, and demographics during data collection and analysis.

FINDINGS

From this study, it was discovered that variation in care was influenced by the type of nurse-patient relationship that developed. Three distinct types of relationships emerged and are illustrated in Figure 8.1:

1. *Resistive relationships,* which were characterized by minimal involvement and were more task-oriented than relational
2. *Restrictive relationships,* which displayed involvement to a limited extent
3. *Involved relationships,* which exhibited a growing bond between nurse and patient

The philosophies and goals of the nurses interviewed were found to encompass common beliefs and values. Each nurse identified the primary goal as maternal-infant safety, and the secondary goal as providing the kind of experience desired by the couple. One nurse expressed it this way: "It is their delivery. As long as it is safe, I don't have a problem with it." Another nurse described one of her goals as providing "a safe

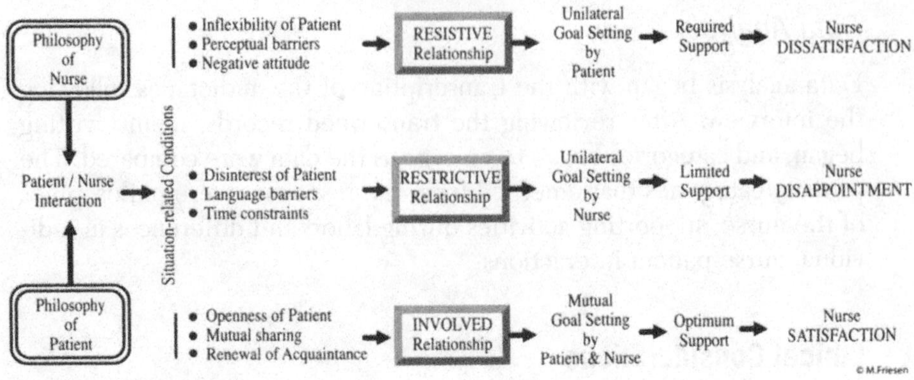

Figure 8.1 Relationships of intrapartum nurses with their patients.
Printed with permission from M. Friesen.

environment for them, so they will feel safe and they will trust me and the care I am giving them."

The patient, through her actions and physical presentation, provided clues about the type of relationship she wanted to develop with the nurse. The responses and interest shown by the patient were found to influence the level of involvement in the nurse-patient relationship. The development of one of the three different types of relationships took place during this interactive process.

Resistive Relationship

Nurses reported that when some patients arrive on the unit, they seem to have "an attitude or a wall already built up." When these conditions were present, the nurses' ability to bond with the patient was particularly low. Resistance was initially demonstrated when a couple made it clear that they had specific nonnegotiable expectations about their childbearing experience. This type of patient was described by one nurse like this:

> [They are] very rigid in their mind how things will be, and sometimes I think it's from the programming that they got from a friend, or from a specific type of labor coaching, a childbirth preparation method that they got, [which promotes] an adversarial relationship from the beginning.

Already established perceptual barriers were attributed by the nurses to external influences, which might include inaccurate information. One nurse shared the views of her patient: "Everybody in the hospital wants me to have a cesarean birth. That's why we tried to do this at the birth center. And now we're here in the hospital. We know what you are up to." The nurse explained, "So that preconceived notion makes it extremely difficult to establish rapport and trust, because they [the couple] are looking for you to deceive them."

In the presence of a negative patient attitude the options for a meaningful relationship were also limited. The response to positive suggestions made by the nurse was described as negative and at times argumentative, as the patient refused to change her position even when it was in her or her baby's best interest. A patient who had this type of attitude was described as "very rigid, and her birth plan was more important than the health of her baby. She was hostile and had difficulty getting along with the staff, including the doctors." When this sort of interaction occurred, the nurses wished for the patient to have a short labor and looked forward to the end of the shift.

The development of a resistive relationship was determined by a series of events, usually outside of the hospital. These external influences shaped the birthing couple's viewpoint, which then created conflicts with caregivers, especially when the couple's or mother's belief systems were different from those of the caregivers. Unilateral goal setting by the patient then took place. One nurse shared an example of a noncompliant patient.

> She was about 43 weeks, maybe 44 weeks. She hadn't seen the doctor in several weeks because she was not going to be induced; she was going to come in when the labor started. . . . She wouldn't let me put a monitor on her when she came in, she wouldn't sign any admission consent form. . . . Then the doctor came to talk with her and he wanted to rupture the membranes to see the fluid. . . . I do recall her saying I would rather have this baby die than to have you intervene in any way [pause] I will have this baby completely natural.

The nursing care then became one of technical support as the patient relied on others for emotional and physical support. So when rapport and trust could not be adequately established, one nurse shared that she felt "a bonding will never take place. . . . It is just not going to happen." When there was no connection between the nurse and the patient, the nurses described that they "are not part of [the birth experience]." In a resistive nurse-patient relationship, the outcome for the nurse was described as "dissatisfaction" with her work.

Restrictive Relationship

During specific circumstances, limitations were found to be imposed by the situation or the patient, making an effective bond difficult to achieve. Limited involvement characterized the restrictive relationship. One nurse shared that she found there are times when "you have patients where you can't even get out of the room because you are talking so much. And other patients when you go in and they don't really want to talk."

Disinterest was seen as a response from the patient who was either unable or unwilling to develop a more involved relationship. A patient who expressed a lack of desire was described by the nurses as being there "to get the job done" and seemed to be "content and not wanting a lot of attention." The nurses described them as "Those patients [who] don't always carry on a long conversation with you when you walk into the room."

When a language barrier was apparent, a restrictive relationship often developed because nurse and patient could not communicate effectively with one another. When a translator was not available, one nurse described the situation in the following way: "It does lack that bond that you have with your patients who do speak English. So, I guess, mainly as long as they know you're there for them, that's all you can do." When there were non-English-speaking patients on the unit, the nurses who were fluent in Spanish offered to care for them. One explained, "I get satisfaction with all cultures, but the ones that don't communicate in English, I feel really blessed to be able to have cared for them. Because that fear of not being able to communicate is just totally. . . . They just lose it."

Time constraints were described as limits placed upon the admission process, as were inadequate staffing, high patient volume, and advanced stages of labor. Sometimes all four factors impacted one another, decreasing the ability for relationship development. The interviewees felt their care, during such times, became more impersonal. This impersonal quality was especially apparent when many deliveries occurred simultaneously, which necessitated multiple nurses sharing the care of the patients. One nurse expressed her dissatisfaction this way.

> I can't stand it when they [the nurses] are switching all over the place and the patient sees five nurses [over the course of her labor]. I mean, some of the patients have the personality that they can do okay with that, it's just

> like no big deal, whoever comes in they get along with everybody. But other patients really need to have some stability throughout the day.

In a restrictive relationship, the nurses were unable to use their entire complement of caregiving behaviors because they were hindered by external constraints. Under these circumstances, the nurse determined which goals seemed realistic to provide for the patient. This relationship was not as personally satisfying for the nurses and interaction was described as limited. The outcome described by the nurses was one of disappointment, since it was "difficult to get to know your patients." One nurse described this disappointment in the following way: "I know for me, a bad day is when I haven't felt connected with any patient. . . . Those days I go home and I feel kind of dissatisfied with my work."

Involved Relationship

Involvement was found to be the relationship that the nurses wanted to achieve with their patients. It was also the one that occurred most often. The basis for this satisfaction was explained as a special connection with the patient and the ability to provide the type of birth experience desired. This experience was described in terms of support, such as using "encouraging and soothing words," "being there," "being in tune with them," "supportive coaching," "gentleness," and "patience." One nurse explained, "I think that it's a matter of clicking. Sometimes you just find a lot in common—you've been with the patient for 12 hours, you have developed this bond, [and] you've become very attached."

One of the conditions noted that seemed to facilitate an involved relationship was openness on the part of the woman. During the interactive process, such a patient encourages the nurse to actively participate in her labor. The nurse described it this way: "So the position that worked for her was kneeling on the floor, leaning against the bed. . . . I breathed with her, and she was just really nice." Through mutual sharing and extended time together, they got to know one another as individuals. One nurse said, "We had this dialogue going on all day. . . . We talked about infant care, we talked about breastfeeding, [and] we talked about what it would be like to deliver. . . . I kept getting feedback from them all day long that this was so helpful."

Another example is when the patient with a subsequent pregnancy requested the same nurse who provided care during a previous delivery. One nurse shared, "The ones that really mean a lot to me are the patients that come back, and I have delivered 2 or 3 of their kids. . . . I've built up a rapport with both the husband and wife. . . . Those are the ones that are very special."

When the interviewees described the development of this relationship, they used words like *attachment, bonding,* or the *establishment of a special relationship.* The connection experienced provided optimum support and facilitated the ability to develop an agreed-upon plan of care. Caregiving behaviors were enhanced within an involved relationship.

As the data continued to be analyzed, it became apparent that spiritual care only occurred within the context of optimum support. Through their interactions, either the nurse sensed the need or the patient expressed spiritual distress. The types of spiritual support provided, as described by the nurses, were prayer, baptism, religious music, and allowing the patient to have religious medals during surgery. When spiritual care was offered, there seemed to be a sense of safety or intimacy in the relationship, where rejection was not an issue. One nurse shared the following:

> I will say a prayer with patients if they want to, or initiate them saying a prayer . . . wanting them to be comfortable if they are a religious family and in the relationship between them and their spouse. Then I want to support that because, to me, having a baby is a religious experience.

Another shared, "She had to have an emergency C-section. She was crying, and she said, I don't have any spiritual music here. I had a gospel tape in the car, and she listened to it in surgery. She said that really made the difference."

The outcome for the nurse became one of satisfaction as the birth experience became more meaningful through this relationship. One nurse put it this way, "There's a lot of joy bringing life into the world. You can't beat this department. You can't beat when a father cries seeing his child born. How can you not think . . . like, oh God, this is the best place to work."

In summary, from the nurses' perspective, relationship development accounts for variations in caregiving behaviors. As the relationship becomes more involved, the ability to provide more suitable caregiving behaviors for the patient becomes possible. Each nurse was capable of participating in all three types of relationship, depending upon the conditions and patients, but ideally the involved relationship was the one sought by the nurses.

DISCUSSION

At the beginning of the study the premise was that caregiving behaviors differed between intrapartum nurses. However, it was discovered that the nursing care offered was done in the context of a nurse-patient relationship. There seemed to be no substantial difference in the caregiving behaviors available, but the conditions for forming a relationship and the type of relationship developed dictated nursing care.

The most dissatisfying of the relationships described by the nurses was the resistive relationship. In this situation, the patient chooses not to have a relationship with the nurse. The nurse either respects the patient's wishes, or attempts to establish some type of relationship. If unsuccessful, the nurse then relinquishes the physical and emotional support to the significant others.

Morse (1991) describes this type of relationship in her study as unilateral. She explains that a connected relationship cannot be decided by only one person, and that involvement denotes a mutual endeavor. "From the patient's perspective, trust and acceptance of his/her situation, that is the hospitalization and the illness experience, are the significant factors. If the patient both trusts the nurse and recognizes the illness and the necessity for hospitalization, then the patient is grateful" (Morse, 1991, p. 462).

In the development of a restrictive relationship, the nurse had limited involvement with the patient. This relationship was found not to be as satisfying as the involved relationship. For various reasons, some of the patients chose to limit their involvement with the nurse. Morse (1991) describes this type of relationship as unilateral, where there is asynchrony between the nurse and the patient. This restricts the relationship, with one person who is unable or unwilling to develop a relationship to the level desired by the other. This uneven desire hinders the process of developing a more involved relationship.

The nurses found it was extremely difficult to establish a relationship when there was a language barrier, and had to verbally communicate through a translator. In psychological studies, research on preferences for particular kinds of providers indicated that the patients tend to prefer those of the same ethnic background (Atkinson & Matsushita, 1991; Lopez, Lopez, & Fong, 1991). The nurses described trying to switch assignments with another nurse who spoke the patient's language in order to provide a more positive birth experience.

Unfortunately, time constraints are beyond the control of both the nurse and the patient. When the patient population is high or when staffing is inadequate, the amount of time to develop a relationship and provide the desired nursing care is decreased. The nurse's role then becomes what the nurses in the study described as a consulting role, rather than a supportive role. Even if the nurses wanted to have further involvement, they were unable to get beyond a minimal level.

Many times the patient had multiple caregivers during her labor, which caused frustration for all involved. Morse (1991) found in her study that relationships are thwarted when the patient has multiple caregivers. She asserted that in a caring relationship, caregivers are not interchangeable, with nursing being the only profession that endorses that notion. She found that lack of time with the patient prevented the establishment of a connected relationship. The nurses confirmed that when there was less time available, they were unable to offer the kind of care that they liked to give to their patients. Under these circumstances nurse job satisfaction was decreased.

A relationship of involvement with the patient was the one most satisfying and most sought after by the nurses. In this relationship, the nurse spent extra time interacting with the patient. This interaction between the two individuals increased the development of trust and rapport between one another. The nurses concurred that in this relationship, they were able to provide the most support for the patient. The findings in this research are similar to the findings of Gagnon and Waghorn (1996), where supportive care was described in the context of physical comfort, and emotional support.

Spiritual care was requested by the patient only after the development of a certain level of trust. It seemed to be provided when the patient expressed the need for spiritual intervention or when the nurse noted spiritual distress. In a qualitative study done by Trojan and Yonge (1993), four different levels of interaction are described, with one level being spiritual. They found that nurses and clients could connect with one another through social, psychological, physical, or spiritual interaction, depending upon their interests and backgrounds.

The nurse-patient relationship as described by Trojan and Yonge (1993) was similar to that identified by Morse (1991). In her study, nurse involvement was characterized as a connected relationship and described as: (a) being committed to helping the patient, (b) bending and breaking rules for the patient, (c) serving as a patient advocate, and (d) believing her care made a difference.

Morse found that the nurse viewed the patient first as a person and second as a patient. This type of relationship is established either through prolonged contact with the patient over a period of time, or is accelerated by the patient's needs. She described this relationship in the context of the patient choosing to trust the nurse and the nurse choosing to enter the relationship to meet the patient's needs (Morse, 1991). Pregnancy was not viewed by the nurses as an illness, but as a short-term situation where the laboring woman needs support. The nurses interviewed expressed their desire to connect with the patient, realizing that the outcome for all involved would be enhanced.

The literature suggests that the nurse-patient relationship can influence the type of nursing care offered to the patient. In contrast, this study revealed that nurses' perceptions of caregiving behaviors provided for the woman in labor are characterized by patient and situation-related conditions, which then determine the development of a specific nurse-patient relationship.

APPLICATION

While the findings from this research study have helped to clarify some differences in intrapartum nursing practice, they have also identified the need to establish an appropriate length of time for orientation. Most of the nurses interviewed for this study felt that during their orientation period, after completing the didactic portion, the patient care focus was on task-oriented duties and the accomplishment of timely documentation rather than on the laboring woman. These nurses stated that their comfort level in caring for patients was not realized until after nine months of working full-time on the unit. Those nurses who described a comfort level before nine months had been assigned to work twice as long with an experienced preceptor. In light of this information, the authors believe that an orientation program should include an appropriate length of time with an experienced preceptor in the clinical setting. The advantage of using an experienced preceptor is that it will allow less experienced nurses to observe interactions, which may encourage them to develop a greater degree of involvement in their nurse-patient relationships.

CONCLUSION

In order for a satisfying nurse-patient relationship to be established, several factors need to be considered. First, the patient needs to be the nurse's focus, not the task. Second, there needs to be time for relationship development. This requires adequate staffing on the unit with policies and procedures developed to provide continuity of care and enhance the amount of time between caregivers and patients. Third, hiring practices need to reflect the demographics of the patient population in order to provide the most appropriate care. When hospitals provide the opportunity for the development of optimal nurse-patient relationships, caregiving behaviors will be enhanced, which should facilitate a more positive birth experience.

REFERENCES

Atkinson, D., & Matsushita, Y. (1991). Japanese-American acculturation, counseling style, counselor ethnicity, and perceived counselor credibility. *Journal of Counseling Psychotherapy, 38*, 473–478.

Bryanton, J., Fraser-Davey, H., & Sullivan, P. (1994). Women's perceptions of nursing support during labor. *Journal of Obstetric, Gynecologic, and Neonatal Nursing, 23*, 638–643.

Friesen, M. (1999). *Intrapartum nurses' perceptions of their care-giving behaviors with laboring patients.* Unpublished master's thesis, Azusa Pacific University, Azusa, CA.

Gagnon, A. J., & Waghorn, K. (1996). Supportive care by maternity nurses: A work sampling study in an intrapartum unit. *Birth, 23*, 1–6.

Glaser, B. G. (1978). *Advances in the methodology of grounded theory: Theoretical sensitivity*. Mill Valley, CA: The Sociology Press.

Lopez, R., Lopez, A., & Fong, K. (1991). Mexican Americans' initial preferences for counselors: The role of ethnic factors. *Journal of Counseling Psychology, 38*, 487–496.

Morse, J. M. (1991). Negotiating commitment and involvement in the nurse-patient relationship. *Journal of Advanced Nursing, 16*, 455–468.

Radin, T. G., Harmon, J. S., & Hanson, D. A. (1993). Nurses' care during labor: Its effect on the cesarean birth rate of healthy, nulliparous women. *Birth, 20*, 14–21.

Simkin, P. (1991). Just another day in a woman's life? Women's long-term perceptions of their first birth experience. Part I. *Birth, 18*, 203–210.

Trojan, L., & Yonge, O. (1993). Developing trust, caring relationships: Home care nurses and elderly clients. *Journal of Advanced Nursing, 18*, 190.

II

Gerund Mode: Basic Social Process

INTRODUCTION: BARBARA M. ARTINIAN

A basic social process (BSP) is a core category that has two or more emergent phases, which resolve the main concern of the group under study. It is used to describe the action of moving though a situation. Glaser writes that grounded theory (GT) is ideally suited to a study that continues over time so that the stages of a BSP can emerge and demonstrate changes that occur over time.

The BSP has been used frequently in carrying out grounded theory studies; it is the most commonly used mode of the GT method (Bryant & Charmaz, 2007, p. 1). Even though the BSP is only one theoretical code among many, Glaser says the BSPs have "emerged as producing rich grounded theory when used as a core variable" (1996, p. ix). Because of the importance of BSPs, Glaser has devoted an entire book to describing their use and giving examples of theories developed using them.

Two gerund mode GT studies are presented in this section. In the first study, Pash explores the experience of dying out of sync as those in middle age go through the process of Letting Go prior to their death (see chapter 9, "Letting Go: The Experience of Dying From Cancer in Young Middle Age"). The second study, conducted by Osuri, found Moving On to be the process that male novice nurses go through in finding their place in the nursing profession during orientation in a critical care unit (see chapter 10, "Moving On: A Study of Male Novice Nurses in the Critical Care Unit").

REFERENCES

Bryant, A., & Charmaz, K. (2007). *The SAGE handbook of grounded theory.* Los Angeles: Sage.

Glaser, B. G. (1996). *Gerund grounded theory: The basic social process dissertation.* Mill Valley, CA: Sociology Press.

9

Letting Go: The Experience of Dying From Cancer in Young Middle Age

LYNDA PASH
BARBARA M. ARTINIAN

The baby boom generation is in its middle age. Adults between the ages of 35 and 55 are considered to be *young* middle-aged (Hardcastle, 1985). The purpose of this study was to learn from young middle-aged hospice patients about the experience of dying "out of synchrony" or "off time" (Rogers & White, 1993, p. 247). Facing death before reaching old age necessitates preparing for loss of the role or roles peculiar to the person's developmental level; death comes before some developmental tasks are completed. Although the majority of hospice patients have been over 65, 20% have been younger (Haupt, 1994). The experiences of this population have not been adequately described in the nursing literature.

Concepts from family developmental theory (Rogers & White, 1993) are important when examining any significant life event. Rogers and White described process norms as those regulating "the timing and sequencing of expectations and behavior" (p. 233). A person who dies before retirement dies out of sequence and also "off time" (p. 239). Dobratz (1993, 1995) asserts that adaptation occurs over time and that time itself may be a factor in adaptation to terminal illness. McCanse (1995) concluded that "death readiness is a developmental state that changes over a relatively short period of time as death approaches" (p. 24). This challenges Dobratz's (1995) finding that the elderly are more ready to die because of their age. Kübler-Ross (1969), in her seminal work with terminal patients, identified stages that can be described as developmental. Her work ends with the stage of *acceptance.* The current study describes a basic social process (BSP) that is found primarily after the acceptance described by Kübler-Ross has occurred.

THE STUDY

Aim

The aim of the study was to learn what unique experiences young middle-aged adults encounter after becoming terminally ill, and what psychosocial and spiritual experiences occur at the end of life in people who face death before old age.

Method

The investigator used classical grounded theory (GT) methodology (Glaser, 1978). This approach focuses on the meanings from the respondents' perspectives. The inaccuracy of caregiver and staff perceptions has been found repeatedly in hospice studies, emphasizing the need for collecting data from the patients themselves (McMillan, 1996; McMillan & Mahon, 1944; Rathbone, Horsley, & Goacher, 1994).

Participants

Sixteen hospice patients aged 38–55 years old who had a diagnosis of cancer were recruited from three hospice organizations in Southern California.

Data Collection and Analysis

Respondents were interviewed by the researcher using a semistructured interview guide. Interviews were taped and transcribed by the researcher. Constant comparative analysis was the method of data analysis, and it began as the first interview was being transcribed and continued through saturation with Respondent 16 (Glaser, 1978). Categories and subcategories were identified and relationships between them analyzed. When practical, respondents were interviewed more than once.

Ethical Considerations

The proposal for this study was approved by the Institutional Review Board of Azusa Pacific University. Written hospice approval was obtained before contact with potential respondents. Prospective respondents signed a consent form after being informed regarding the general nature of the study. Pseudonyms were used to protect patient anonymity.

FINDINGS

Analysis of the interviews uncovered several recurring categories of experiences. Further analysis revealed that eight major categories formed a basic social process by which the study respondents were able to let go of their lives. The process was named Letting Go, as this was seen to best describe the process itself and also the result of completion of the process (Pash, 1999). The study respondents were seen to move from a state of full participation in a very busy life to an apparently complete withdrawal from that life, with an anticipation of what lay beyond. The steps, or stages, in the process are described as they emerged from the interviews. They are depicted in Figure 9.1. Some respondents seemed to experience two or three stages simultaneously, and the stages did not always occur in the described order.

The first stage is *awareness of physical changes and failing health.* Physical changes created changes in the way the respondents were able to live their lives, changes over which they had no control. The next stage, during which the participants realized their *loss of control and independence,* made the stage of *acceptance of death* possible. When the respondents accepted the reality of their deaths, and when others were also made aware of it, there was a noticeable change in relationships. Respondents reported an *increased closeness with others,* and a *desire for openness.* With knowledge of impending death out in the open, and with support from caring friends and family, the respondents made *internal preparations.* This stage included several subcategories: *change in understanding of self and others; positive changes in oneself/learning what is important; learning to receive; changing roles; modifying goals; experiencing pleasure in nature; enjoying the now;* and *appreciating the life lived.*

After these preparatory stages, respondents were found to be *relinquishing responsibilities.* Most of the interviewees actually experienced

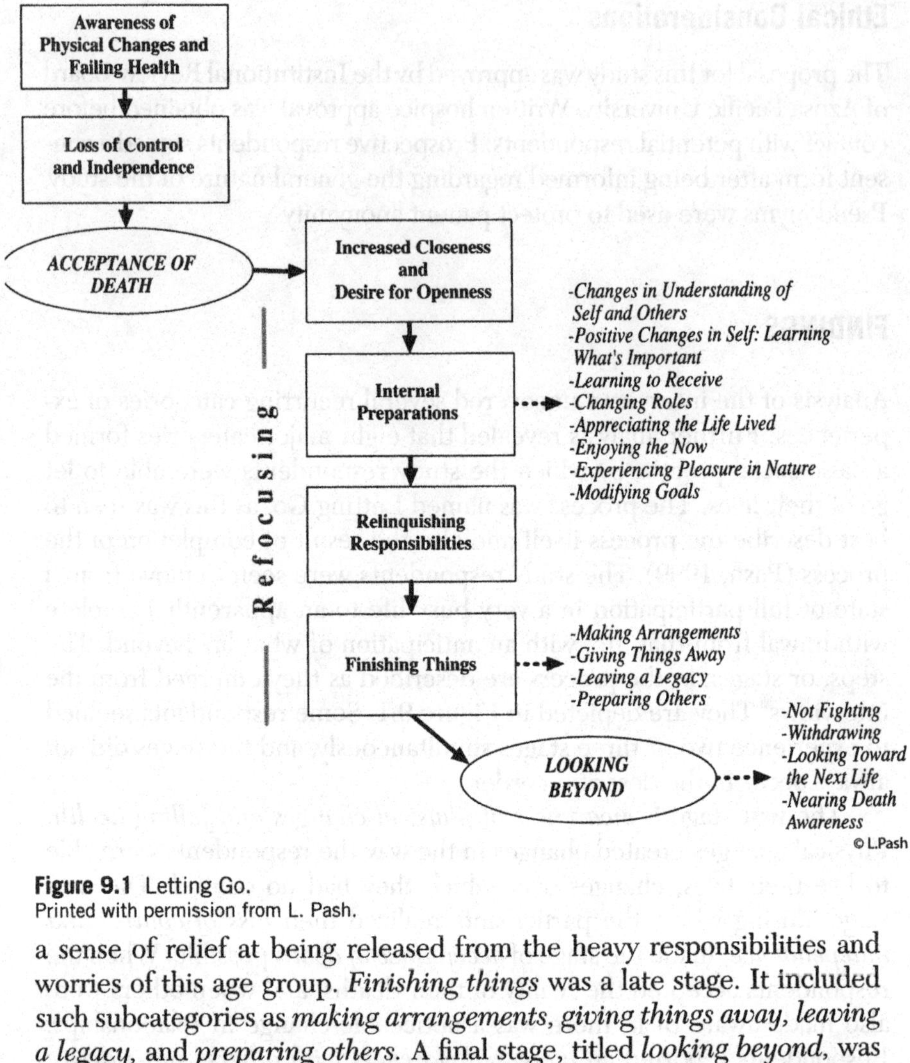

Figure 9.1 Letting Go.
Printed with permission from L. Pash.

a sense of relief at being released from the heavy responsibilities and worries of this age group. *Finishing things* was a late stage. It included such subcategories as *making arrangements, giving things away, leaving a legacy,* and *preparing others.* A final stage, titled *looking beyond,* was a time of withdrawal. At this time, the respondents were not fighting anymore; continuing to live was no longer a priority. They did not think much about what or whom they were leaving behind. They occasionally had a glimpse of where they were going and who was waiting for them.

Awareness of Physical Changes/Failing Health

Most of the respondents recalled having had very active lives before becoming ill, so the loss of physical health and ability to do things was very difficult for them:

- "I've always been a very physically active person. That's been a hard adjustment."
- "And you look at the shower and it looks like Mt. Everest."
- "I used to be a singer and now I can't sing . . . I can't take deep breaths."

Although physical problems caused significant limitations, most respondents came to accept what they realized was a permanent change in their lives. Carla said, "I just finally realized there's certain things I can do and certain things I can't do." This acceptance did not come easily. As Sandy said, "I don't want to accept the idea that I can't go back to doing things." During this early stage, the terminal illness was seen as an unwelcome interruption of one's normal life. There was still a desire to return to a normal active life.

Loss of Control/Loss of Independence

With loss of control over one's body came awareness of loss of one's independence. This was a heavy loss to bear. Debra said:

> What it has done is actually taken away my control. I have always been in control of myself . . . of my own life. Now I don't have that control. Because it dictates to me how I'm going to feel, how far I can walk. You know, just routine things. I really hate that.

Driving seemed to have an especially strong link with feelings of freedom and independence. "You feel so . . . trapped" when unable to drive, explained Laura. "Why can't I run over to McDonald's or out to get my nails done?" "I'm not able to go out and do things on my own," said Chad. "That's one of the things I miss." This man had also lost his ability to be sexually active, but he expressed more regret over not being able to drive.

Acceptance of Death

Although elements of acceptance were found throughout the interviews, it emerged most distinctly following awareness of physical changes and awareness of loss of control and independence. For most respondents, loss of control made acceptance easier. "And then with this, it's all of a sudden out of my hands," Chad explained. "It makes it okay now, to die."

Rosaria said, "I've kind of accepted everything as it is. There's nothing you can do about it." Some people were surprised at their acceptance. "I never thought that I could accept this. But so far, I've been fine," said Sandy.

Religious faith seemed to enhance acceptance in those respondents who professed it. Loss of control of life was not so frightening when the respondents believed a benevolent God was in control. Rosaria said: "You give all control to God. Whatever He wants to do. The people around you . . . there's nothing they can do anymore." Carla said, "God is so magnificent. He is letting me know that he is in control over everything." Forty-four-year-old Pamela told of how frightened she had been of cancer, all her life: "But now I have peace . . . I found if you know the Lord I don't have to be afraid of these monsters that are going to whip me. My life is very happy."

Several respondents expressed the idea of this life as a temporary experience. Laura said, "The physical is such a short thing anyway." Carla told her children, "This is not our home. God said that we are only passing through." After coming to an acceptance of their deaths, the respondents seemed to enter a period of refocusing their thoughts, feelings, and energies. This refocusing affected others as well.

Increased Closeness With Others/Desire for Openness

Knowledge of impending death brought increased feelings and/or expressions of closeness and caring into almost every respondent's life. "My relationships have just blossomed," reported Chad.

Closeness With Family

Marilyn described the phenomenon that was common among the participants and their families: "We're much closer than we ever thought we'd be. You tell them you love them. You cry with them; you share things much more intimately. It's just nice, a very nice way to have relationships." She noted that it was not that her family's feelings had changed, but that they expressed them more. Pamela, whose sister stayed with her for a while, said, "We just had a wonderful time together and said things that we had never said, and hugged and cried together. It was a most beautiful thing." For some respondents, it was not only that the unexpressed was finally expressed. An actual change in feelings also occurred. Charlotte spoke about her sisters taking turns caring for her. "It's been interesting getting to know them." Sandy found that her two adult sons were kinder and more considerate than she ever thought they could be. She worked for 25 years and "I thought I'd lost them." She said that her relationships with her sons became much closer. "I can talk to them much more openly now. It's wonderful."

Closeness With Others

It was not only with family members that respondents reported an increase in closeness and expressions of caring. Chad said that "people are coming out of the woodwork," with an "outpouring of support." In talking about it, Chad cried, "because you can see human kindness in action." The respondents were often touched by the kindness and caring from people that they did not know very well. Carla's landlord lowered the rent so her family could afford their apartment after she quit working. Rosaria's coworkers gave her vacation and sick time so she could keep her insurance. Sandy said she was "just astonished" at the kindness people had shown her.

Desire for Openness

Respondents expressed a need to talk openly about what was happening to them and they wanted others to speak openly as well. Laura said, "Tell them to be open and none of this hush-hush behind doors and treat me like a fragile egg, because you're still *you.*"

Internal Preparations

The interviews revealed positive changes in thinking and refocusing of attitudes that occurred as respondents prepared themselves for death.

Change in Understanding of Self and Others

Debra explained: "Well, we think we know who we are, but now we have more time with ourselves than we ever had before. So now, it's time to think about who you are and what is your spirit." Pamela, age 44, said she came to realize that "my life is not my own; my children are not my own." Sometimes the change was just seeing something that they had not seen before. Debra, commented, "I never knew my baby sister was so strong. I'm seeing a different side of her."

Positive Changes in Self/Learning What Is Important

The respondents described positive changes in themselves that had come as a result of their terminal illnesses. Carla said she quit being a complainer. Richard learned to apologize for his anger. "I *never* would have done that prior to being sick."

Learning to Receive

At first, most of the respondents did not like having to receive help from others. Later, they learned to receive because they had no choice. They also seemed to realize the benefit to others. Laura said, "You've brought joy to people because of what you gave. Now you have to let them have joy by what they can give you."

Role Change

Learning to receive involved a change in role for most of the respondents. It seemed hardest for some of the women. Of her children Rosaria said, "Instead of me taking care of them, they are the ones taking care of me," and "They don't talk to me; they feed me."

Modifying Goals

Terminal illness can disrupt a lifetime of goals and plans. Laura lamented dying before she and her husband could enjoy the comfortable retirement they had expected. She and her husband tried to keep a semblance of their former life. "We've always had a date night. If I can go out we go out; if I can't, we lie here and hold hands and watch TV." Other respondents expressed their ability to adapt to the changes in their lives:

- "You just have to roll with the punches . . . hang in there."
- "I mean, life is life. I sort of take things just as they come."

The respondents seemed to accept the loss of their futures with relative ease. When asked, they would recount matter-of-factly or with mild regret the events they knew they would be missing.

Enjoying the Now

The ability to enjoy the present was seen clearly in the interviews. Charlotte explained, "I just want to enjoy my time. And I am. Like I said, I get excited when I can get out of bed." Chad had a big party "to celebrate the time that we have right now." He summed up the positive features of his life since being diagnosed as terminally ill. "I say this in jest, but not really, that this dying's got living beat all to hell." He was referring to his deepening relationships, his lack of worries about the future, his sense of inner peace, his realization of the goodness of others, and his general feeling of joy in the life he was leading.

Appreciating the Life Lived

Rather than sadness at a life cut short, the respondents tended to express positive feelings about the lives they had lived up to that point. Marilyn, age 52, said, "And I've had a chance to look back and realize I've done an awful lot with my life in such a short time." Pamela said she came to the realization that the fact that she was over 40 years old was "a gift." Keith put his death in historical perspective: "I'm 55. I've outlived Hannibal, Alexander the Great, Caesar, Nero. When you get to thinking about it, in any other time period, I'd be the oldest geezer walking around." Richard, a 50-year-old AIDS patient said, "I've had a good life, an enjoyable life. I wouldn't change anything." Debra said she had "done everything I wanted to do. I feel fulfilled, validated." At 44, Chad said, "Actually, my life is pretty fulfilled."

Finding Pleasure in Nature

Respondents described finding a pleasure in nature that they had not experienced previously. Carla remarked, "Now I love flowers and I want to do some gardening. I never wanted to do none of that kind of stuff before." Debra related her fascination watching a larger seagull assisting a baby gull.

Relinquishing Responsibilities

The responsibilities of this middle-aged group were heavy. Most of the study participants had been working before getting sick, and had various family responsibilities. Many expressed a sense of relief in the relinquishing of their responsibilities and the worry associated with them. During our first interview, when she was still living fairly independently, Sandy worried that her sons would not want to get married because of her own bitter divorce. At the time of our second interview she was much sicker.

Regarding her sons getting married, she said, "There are plenty of girls out there." She had let go of worrying about them. Marilyn, who took care of her demented mother before becoming ill, also had a hard time letting go of this at first. She worried about how her brothers were going to handle everything, but later she said, "You have to tell yourself, well, it's not your concern anymore." Rosaria said she came to realize, "I can't take care of everything."

Physically they could not take care of everything anymore. Pamela had always done the taxes, but she did not let herself worry about it. "My husband's more smart than I give him credit for." Carla found it very easy to give up control. "I was tired of being in control. I was tired of doing all the bills, balancing the checkbook. I don't have to be bothered with all that." She found that she no longer worried about anything. She said, "My only problem is, I have to lay here. I have no other problems." She said it was relaxing to know "it's not my problem." Patients commonly expressed a sense of relief in being able to say "It's not my problem." Chad said it was *very much a relief.* With this illness, "it's all of a sudden out of my hands." He said, "My retirement? Taxes? Old age? I don't have all that kinda futuristic worry." The respondents indicated that the loss of the future also meant loss of the worries and burdens associated with that future. There seemed to be a sense of relief in just living in the now, and letting someone else be in charge.

Finishing Things

While the responsibilities associated with ongoing life were being relinquished, responsibilities associated with finishing up with life's business became more important. Respondents had certain things they felt they needed to finish before they died.

Making Arrangements

Some respondents needed to make arrangements for care of their children or pets. Some of their arrangements were directly connected to the death and what would happen afterward, such as making wills, setting up trusts, and choosing final arrangements. Pamela even bought her burial dress. She said she did it to spare her husband, but "I got a kick out of it, picking out my dress." Chad gave up worrying about a MediCal problem but made a special effort to pay off a personal debt before he died. "Hey, I'm not leaving my brother-in-law a debt. I'm clearing up . . . the wreckage of my past."

Giving Things Away

Some of the respondents gave away some of their possessions. The things of this world were no longer useful (like the car one could not drive), so they let go of them physically and emotionally.

Leaving a Legacy

Some of the respondents expressed a need to pass on what they had learned about life. Debra wanted to tell her grown children things she thought were important. Pamela also spoke of telling her children things she wanted them to know.

Preparing Others

It was important to many respondents to prepare others for the coming death. Preparing children was especially important for mothers. Carla said with satisfaction, "I've prepared the little ones." Pamela said of her talks with her children, "It's gotten them ready."

Looking Beyond

Letting go of worldly attachments, the participants seemed to make a transition toward focusing on what lay ahead of them. They seemed to withdraw from earthly concerns and move toward a more transcendent state of being.

Not Fighting

Death started to seem attractive to some respondents, as the effort of staying alive became burdensome. "I'm at the point where I want to give up right now," said Phyllis. "I'm so tired." "Now I'm getting to the point where I want it to be over with," said Richard, "and I'm just tired and I just don't want to [fight] anymore." Pamela said, "Many times during the night, I tell my husband I wish it was tonight."

Withdrawing

Interest in worldly activities and relationships diminished as the participants turned their attention inward. Richard said, "Bob asks me, why don't you find something you can do, but I really don't have any interest in anything. I just don't have much interest. . . . I just don't want to do anything." Carla wanted her children to understand her need to be alone and quiet. "I like the quietness."

Looking Toward the Next Life/The Afterlife

Thoughts of the respondents turned toward a different plane of existence. There was the anticipation of death and an afterlife. Not all of the respondents professed a belief in an afterlife, but the death that approached was very real to them. Marilyn said, "I'll be in a better place, one of these days." Pamela said, "I'm real excited. I'm really almost looking forward to it." Looking forward to seeing loved ones was comforting for several of the respondents. "I think it makes it easier for me to be accepting of dying now, because I know it's not the end. And the people that you love are waiting for you," said Richard. Carla told her children, "I am going to see my Lord and be with my Jesus." Laura looked forward to seeing the six children that she had miscarried. "Yeah, when I go to heaven I'm going to have six little ones, little people that I didn't know who they were."

Nearing Death Awareness

For the respondents who had let go of their earthly life and were preparing to leave it, the boundaries between a worldly existence and a transcendent existence seemed to loosen. For those who experienced this change in awareness, it was not frightening, nor did it seem unnatural. It was often described as a dream or like a dream. Those that had these episodes seemed to have heightened feelings of anticipation. Richard told the investigator, "Lately I've been having a lot of dreams that Norman and I are together, you know, which is good. I hope it means I'll be seeing him soon. I look forward to it."

In describing her dreams, Phyllis said, "It's going to be very peaceful. And it's okay to let go. And everything that needs to be done is done. I don't know if I've gone to the other side, but I go somewhere." When asked for specifics, she said, "People walking around. One night I had someone sitting at the foot of my bed. Praying. Then I felt an angel in the air over my bed saying it would be okay." Laura told of seeing her father, who had died a few months before:

> All of a sudden there was my dad. Right there at that door. And he was in a brown suit. My mother said that was the suit he got married in. He was just

there with the biggest smile on his face. My dad was kind of a shy person, but here was no shyness. There was just joy and a glow.

DISCUSSION

The basic social process that emerged from these interviews is called Letting Go, because they were letting go of their lives in incremental steps that followed a very logical path. At first the respondents struggled against the changes in their bodies and their lives. When it became evident that the changes were permanent, they accepted the fact that they were dying. Once they accepted their dying, their lives took on new meaning and direction. Relationships deepened; the present took on greater weight. Learning and inner growth took place; responsibilities were released. There was an urge to finish that which needed to be finished; and when the body could no longer go on, the respondents withdrew from any active involvement in this life and actively anticipated death.

The letting go of life was not a passive process. It included the experiencing of what Kübler-Ross (1975) referred to as "the final stage of growth." Byock (1997) states, "Even as they are dying, most people can accomplish meaningful tasks and grow in ways that are important to them and to their families" (p. 32). He calls it "developmental work," and the landmarks are "experienced love of self and others, the completion of relationships, the acceptance of the finality of one's life, and the achievement of a new sense of self" (p. 33). Whereas acceptance was an endpoint—a final stage in a series—for participants in Kübler-Ross's research, it was an early stage for respondents of this study. Most patients had already experienced at least part of the stages preceding the acceptance described by Kübler-Ross by the time they had signed on to the hospice program. Most of the letting go process took place *after* acceptance of death.

Changes in the body were a requirement for the process to proceed. However, one must be careful in using what Benner and Wrubel (1989) describe as an achievement-oriented approach to death. Identifying progressive stages in a process is helpful to understanding, but it also may create expectations that are not realistic for everyone. It is important to use the findings described in this study only as a guide to understanding what may be observed in those who are dying.

Dying Out of Sync

As people grow older, letting go is a normal developmental activity. Letting go is something that happens over years if a person lives to old age.

The participants of this study, at middle age, were forced to squeeze many years of gradually letting go of life into a period of weeks or months. According to Erickson (1963), the goal of old age is *ego integrity.* Ego integrity includes coming to an acceptance of the quality and quantity of one's life and integrating a spiritual sense in which death is not feared. A surprising finding of this study was that the young middle-aged respondents were able to accomplish the tasks of old age that Erickson describes. McCanse (1995) describes death readiness as a developmental process. The current study seems to fit with her assertion that this process can occur over a relatively short period of time as death approaches. Probably the most important implication of these findings is that one does not have to live a long life to die in peace. Relatively young people felt satisfied, even happy, with their shortened lives. The researcher had expected to find more feelings of grief for a life interrupted or cut short. Benner and Wrubel (1989) state that with an extended illness, "Life is not so much interrupted as reshaped. . . . Knowing that one has a terminal illness . . . lends the present a weight that it does not have for other people" (p. 136). Awareness of the weight of the present emerged very strongly from the interviews.

APPLICATION TO PRACTICE

Understanding an end-of-life process is important in the same way that understanding a disease process or the process of giving birth is important. A nurse who understands what is happening when a person is letting go of life will be able to help everyone involved. For instance, if the dying person feels that physical care is a burden for the family, the nurse can help the patient understand that it is a gift to others to allow them to give care. The nurse can help family and others understand the value of expressing feelings openly, and of allowing the patient to speak openly as well. It may be helpful for family members and others to know that they can have a positive impact on the dying experience of their loved one. Even in situations where the dying trajectory is relatively short, an understanding of the letting go process can assist the nurse in guiding and supporting families.

Recently a graduate nursing student with an understanding of this process of letting go took a copy of the conceptual map along with her on a visit to a family in which the mother was dying. There were two adult daughters and two teenage sons. The nurse translated the concepts into

Spanish and explained to the family the steps of the letting go process. For the first time, the family was able to speak openly about some of the events, issues, feelings, and behaviors that had been causing them distress, many of which they had been unable to understand. They described being able to relate the process to what they had seen happening in their own lives. As they spoke among themselves and with the nurse, they related a greater sense of clarity and understanding. The patient died peacefully. Her family reported experiencing a sense of comfort during her last days that they attributed to the nurse's counsel regarding the letting go process.

REFERENCES

Benner, P., & Wrubel, J. (1989). *The primacy of caring: Stress and coping in health care and illness.* Menlo Park, CA: Addison-Wesley.

Byock, I. R. (1997). *Dying well: The prospect of growth at the end of life.* New York: Putnam.

Dobratz, M. C. (1993). Causal influences of psychological adaptation in death and dying. *Western Journal of Nursing Research, 15,* 708–729.

Dobratz, M. C. (1995). Analysis of variables that impact psychological adaptation in home hospice patients. *The Hospice Journal, 10*(1), 75–88.

Erickson, E. H. (1963). *Childhood and society.* New York: Norton.

Glaser, B. G. (1978). *Theoretical sensitivity.* Mill Valley, CA: The Sociology Press.

Hardcastle, B. (1985). Midlife themes of invisible citizens: How ordinary people make sense of their lives. *Journal of Humanistic Psychology, 25*(2), 45–63.

Haupt, B. J. (1994). The National Home and Hospice Care Survey: 1992 Summary, *Vital Health Stat 13* (p. 117). Washington, DC: National Center for Health Statistics.

Kübler-Ross. E. (1969). *On death and dying.* New York: Macmillan.

Kübler-Ross, E. (Ed.). (1975). *Death: The final stage of growth.* New York: Simon & Schuster.

McCanse, R. P. (1995). The McCanse readiness for death instrument (MRDI): A reliable and valid measure for hospice care. *The Hospice Journal, 10*(1), 15–26.

McMillan, S. C. (1996). Pain and pain relief experienced by hospice patients with cancer. *Cancer Nursing, 19*(4), 298–307.

McMillan, S. C., & Mahon, M. (1994). A study of quality of life of hospice patients on admission and week 3. *Cancer Nursing, 17*(1), 52–60.

Pash, L. (1999). The dying experience of young middle-aged hospice patients. Unpublished master's thesis, Azusa Pacific University, Azusa, CA.

Rathbone, G. V., Horsley, S., & Goacher, J. (1994). A self-evaluated assessment suitable for seriously ill hospice patients. *Palliative Medicine, 8,* 29–34.

Rogers, R. H., & White, J. M. (1993). Family development theory. In P. G. Boss, W. J. Doherty, R. LaRossa, W. R. Schumm, & S. K. Steinmetz (Eds.), *Sourcebook of family theories and methods: a contextual approach* (pp. 225–254). New York: Plenum Press.

10 Moving On: A Study of Male Novice Nurses in the Critical Care Unit

PAMELA SIRCAR OSURI
BARBARA M. ARTINIAN

Difficulty in managing successful role transition and professional socialization from the academic setting to the workplace has been a longstanding issue experienced by the novice nurse. Professional socialization is a process that an individual undergoes when entering a new profession. This process has subconscious components, where philosophy, traditions, responsibilities, and obligations of the profession are internalized to achieve professional identity (Tradewell, 1996). The adaptation process to the work setting has been described as traumatic for inexperienced nurses in their first six months of practice (Meisenhelder, 1981).

Inadequate staffing as a result of the nursing shortage and increased workloads nationally has caused health care organizations to seek out novice nurses to fill vacancies in specialty units. The critical care setting is one of many specialty units that sought out novice nurses to specially train and integrate into the intensive care unit (ICU), in response to a projected shortage of 400,000 nurses in 2000 (Coleman, 1990). The novice critical care nurse faces many challenges in meeting expectations of the health care organization, the administrators, and the patients (DiGiacomo & Adamson, 2001). The ICU is a high-demand setting, where the novice critical care nurse performs nursing interventions in the midst of frightening alarms, assists with routine emergency bedside procedures, and works with sophisticated ventilation equipment and complicated invasive monitoring. Given that the level of stress is high in this setting, the novice critical care nurse experiences job strain that can cause both immediate and long-term physical, emotional, and psychological problems (DiGiacomo & Adamson, 2001). When coping skills are not effective in dealing with this type of stress, burnout can occur, which can ultimately affect the quality of patient care.

Little is known about the process of professional socialization of the new nurse graduate, and even less is known about the socialization process of the novice critical care nurse. By analyzing the process of professional socialization, it was anticipated that an improved awareness of the challenges faced by the novice critical care nurse would be gained and recognized. With this knowledge, the discipline of nursing can address the challenges with a clearer outlook on and better approaches to the issues affecting the novice critical care nurse during professional socialization. These approaches will potentially combat detrimental outcomes seen during the socialization process, such as burnout and frustration, and instead will lead to an increased degree of job satisfaction for the novice nurse.

THE STUDY

Aim

The purpose of this study was to investigate professional socialization among novice critical care nurses within their first six months of practice.

Method

The methodology used was Glaserian grounded theory (Glaser, 1978, 1998, 2001).

Participants

The subjects were novice nurses who had graduated recently from nursing school and had newly, within the last 12 months, been employed in an adult critical care setting. Criteria of inclusion of novice nurses included: (a) no prior experience in nursing, (b) an associate and/or bachelor's in nursing, (c) current employment in an adult critical care setting, and (d) no more than one year of experience in the critical care setting. Nurses that fit the stated criteria were interviewed.

Data Collection and Analysis

Data were collected using a semistructured, open-ended interview guide to investigate the socialization process of novice critical care nurses. However, the interview process was not limited to these outlined questions. Instead each study participant was encouraged to discuss situations that were significant to his or her socialization process.

Interviews were tape-recorded with the consent of the study participants. Following the interviews, the investigator transcribed the interviews to written form. The study participants were provided with an informed consent prior to the interview process. Study participants were interviewed from four different for-profit hospitals in a Southwestern state. A total of 16 study participants were interviewed, and 25 interviews in total were conducted with these 16 study participants. Nine of the 16 were female novice nurses, while the remaining 7 were male novice nurses. The ages of the study participants ranged from 23 to 45 years, with the average female novice nurse's age being 30.8 and the average male novice nurse's age being 31.7. Three study participants were bachelor's prepared nurses, while 13 had graduated with an associate's degree in nursing. Seven study participants were Caucasian, 6 were of Asian descent, 2 were Hispanic, and 1 was African American.

Ethical Considerations

The proposal for this study was approved by the Institutional Review Board of Azusa Pacific University. Data were kept confidential and destroyed at the end of the study.

FINDINGS

The critical care setting is full of challenges for the novice nurse. The novice nurse is taught to manage the care of high-acuity patients, while getting familiar with basic nursing interventions, collaborating with the members of a multidisciplinary team, and educating the individuals in the patient's support system. Each individual task that the novice nurse must undertake in this setting is demanding and requires much time and effort. The combination of these tasks can prepare the novice nurse to practice with excellence, or these tasks can overwhelm the novice nurse.

If the socialization to the critical care setting is fruitful for the novice nurse, the training received in this setting will allow the novice nurse to function and practice with confidence and competence:

> I really didn't know what to expect, I had been in the ICU about six times in school, and so I knew that I would really like it. I figured with time I would feel comfortable and that is true, I have become more comfortable.

However, feelings of comfort or being overwhelmed did not influence the study participant's decision to become established in the critical care setting. A strong predictor of establishment into the critical care setting was related to gender. It was found that male novice nurses had set different goals in professional growth and advancement for the future. Male novice nurses verbalized their interest and plans to move on into other areas of nursing.

A category that emerged from the study data revealed the basic social process of *moving on.* All novice nurses experienced socialization in a similar manner; however, male novice nurses verbalized a desire to move on to other specialties in nursing. The multiple responsibilities simultaneously expected of the novice nurse were wearisome for the novice male critical care nurses, leading them to express a need to move on. One male novice nurse replied:

> I really like it (in the ICU), but probably in the long run I am thinking about doing something else, like going to the emergency room to be an ER nurse. . . . I want diversity, I have always wanted to be a critical care nurse and an ER nurse.

Even though much of what novice male nurses revealed in their interviews was similar to that of female novice nurses, the verbalization of *moving on* set them apart.

The Basic Social Process: Moving On

The basic social process of moving on has three stages (Figure 10.1): *setting direction, being socialized in critical care,* and *reevaluating career choice* (Osuri, 2004). This basic social process, Moving On, began as the

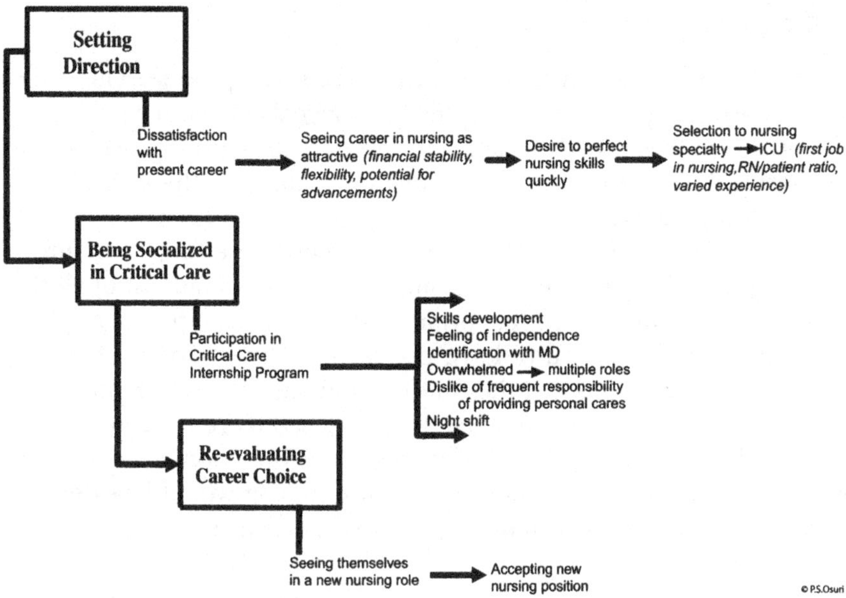

Figure 10.1 Moving On.
Printed with permission of P. S. Osuri.

male study participant explored his career options. The first stage, *setting direction,* involved evaluating the reasons for pursuing a career in nursing, which began prior to nursing school, and the reasons for selecting the intensive care unit as a first clinical position. The stage of *being socialized* in critical care is comprised of nursing experiences that the male novice nurse underwent in the critical care setting during orientation and after the orientation process, when the male novice nurse had began independent practice. It was in this stage that the male novice nurse gained an extensive view of what went on in the critical care setting. The novice male nurses had a better perception of the skills, knowledge, and responsibilities needed to function satisfactorily as a critical care nurse and began verbalizing their dissatisfaction with the multiple roles that they had to perform. The third stage, *reevaluating career choice,* demonstrates the action taken by the male nurse, who is dissatisfied with the nurse's role in the critical care setting. Ultimately, impelled by his dissatisfaction, the male novice nurse moved on to other specialties of nursing that better matched his career interests.

Setting Direction

Setting direction is the first stage of the basic social process. This stage involves assessing and evaluating the career goals of the novice nurse. The novice nurses revealed their purpose in entering the profession of nursing, and also disclosed the reasons for coming to the critical care setting after graduation.

For each novice male nurse, the consideration of setting a new direction came long before entering nursing school. In fact, almost of all the men who were interviewed had prior occupational experiences as paramedic personnel, hospital orderly, psych tech, and pharmacy tech, to name a few. This means that they entered nursing at a more mature age than their female counterparts, and that they had more life experiences to guide them in their appraisal of setting a new direction. As verbalized by one male novice nurse, moving on into nursing would broaden his occupational horizons into more expansive experiences:

> It kinda related to what I used to do as paramedic, and I wanted to expand the sicker type of patients. Because I was used to seeing sick patients, but I wanted to see how it was like to treat them and work with them on a longer basis than just what you would get in the ER. It would be more beneficial for me for when I want to move on in my career.

Even though broadening one's horizons was important for occupational growth for these men, job security, financial reliability, flexibility, and diversity in occupational responsibilities were essential components to setting direction in a new career. One study participant summed it up in one statement by saying:

> One of the major things is job security. With nursing you have a lot of freedom; there are many different fields of nursing that you can go into; you can be an ICU nurse, an operating room nurse, a dialysis nurse, there are so many different areas you can go into, and the pay is all right.

Being Socialized in Critical Care

In the second stage of the basic social process, male novice nurses were exposed to actual critical care nursing experiences. In this stage, the male nurses learned the skills, knowledge, and responsibilities needed to function as a critical care nurse. It was found in this stage that males in contrast to the female participants gave their attention to other areas of patient care:

> It was different than what I expected it to be. I was expected to pay more attention to trends with the patient, and recognizing trends, analyzing lab work, reading up the history. I was more or less trying to keep up with what I was doing rather than figuring out what was wrong with the patient, and now that I'm more comfortable with what I'm doing I can kinda piece all the different parts together, so things become more of a treatment than just playing nurse mate.

Unlike the female novice nurses, the males talked about a dislike for performing basic nursing skills. They were more interested in seeing the whole picture and putting the pieces of the puzzle together. As one male novice nurse said:

> I choose ICU just because you have, the patient ratio is two to one and you have pretty much a lot more time to focus on your patient, whereas if you work on a medical surgical floor where you have a six to one ratio, you pretty much don't get the whole picture of the patient, you pretty much are task oriented and you really don't have that time to focus on what is going on with your patient—physiologically.

In evaluating the satisfaction of the male novice nurses, they revealed that their socialization to the critical care setting taught them a great deal and put them in the midst of many challenges. In spite of the enthusiasm for their experiences in this setting they also disclosed that these critical care nursing skills would be beneficial for a well-rounded nurse who wanted to experience several facets of nursing.

Reevaluating Career Choice

Like the female novice nurses interviewed, the novice male nurses stated that their socialization process was positive and the experiences assisted them in gaining confidence in the setting. However, a distinction could be made between genders when the novice female nurses expressed their satisfaction with the socialization process in the critical care setting, and conveyed an interest in establishing longevity in their current position, as made known by this study participant, who stated, "I think I'll be here for quite a long time, until my back gives out."

The male novice nurses did not express their interest in building a career in the critical care setting. Instead every single male interviewed stated in one way or another that he planned to move on to other specialty areas of nursing. The males stated that the skills learned in the critical care would be beneficial in moving into other areas of nursing care, as verbalized by this male novice nurse, who said, "I can see myself moving on to another area of nursing, using the experiences from the ICU to do something else."

Novice male nurses discussed a need for diversity in their nursing experience. However they characterized their socialization to the critical care setting as quite valuable to their professional growth; as one male novice nurse said, "I like it in ICU. I don't have a full sense of where I want to go. I've thought about a lot of different options . . . if you have a lot of experience in the OR, ICU, or ER you can work anywhere."

A surgical intensive care novice male nurse believed that his critical care orientation would equip him to transition into many other areas of nursing: "I feel I will be ready to change my specialty in two years from now. I want to try ER, OR, and even cardiac care. I feel the orientation I received in the SICU will make the transition smooth as I move into other areas."

The need for diversity in patient care was a prevailing finding in the male novice nurses' responses. More than one male novice nurse stated that he had more than one job to maintain diversity in his nursing experience, as quoted here: "I no longer just work in the ICU. I now have a job in the ER and find the challenge of having diverse experiences really makes a difference for me."

All the males interviewed had had 3–12 months of experiences. Even though they were new to nursing and to the specialty of critical care, they all verbalized the need to move on into other areas during their first interview as a study participant. They all used terms such as *move on, change, challenge, variety, diversity,* and *transition* to describe their interest in making a shift to another nursing area.

It was found that male novice nurses enjoyed the technical challenges of the critical care setting. However they hastily left the setting when faced with the implicit requisite of providing holistic nursing care to critical care patients. When reviewing the basis for moving on into different areas, the reasons and responses initially seemed diverse. However, as these male participants were re-interviewed in regard to their experiences, they stated an interest in specialty areas that demanded reduced patient contact, and required less physical labor. When these male study participants were asked about areas they sought to move on into, they mentioned obtaining jobs in the emergency department, dialysis centers, the operating room, cardiac care units, cardiac catheterization lab where angiograms are done, the neonatal intensive care unit, and employment in transport nursing.

Another factor that leads males to move on into other specialty areas is related to the physical expectations other nurses place on them in the critical care setting. Patients in the critical care setting, due to their labile state, chronic disease process, and state of sedation, can be considered dead weight and difficult to position. Male participants in this study stated that they were constantly asked to assist with position changes and take on heavier patient loads based on their ability to manage such loads.

Summary

Of the seven male study participants interviewed, all of them considered their orientation to be excellent and comprehensive. Although the male novice nurses' experiences were positive, they all verbalized the need to move on to other areas of nursing. They also said that the experiences gained in this setting would assist them in transitioning smoothly into other specialty areas of nursing. Many males conveyed their interest in diverse job responsibilities, which could only be found in gaining experiences from more than one nursing area.

DISCUSSION

As nursing students move into the role of novice nurses, they undergo a transformation in their perception of how the profession of nursing is seen. These novice nurses enter into actual experiences that influence patient's lives, where once their decisions and actions only influenced hypothetical practice. This transformation is defined as socialization. Socialization, as described by Nesler, Hanner, and Melburg (2001) is the process of obtaining professional attitudes, values, and beliefs that are internalized by the novice nurse, leading to the outcome of occupational identity.

In general, nursing has long been perceived as a female profession, where attributes of tenderness, caring, and nurturance have been identified (Egeland & Brown, 1989). Even with perceptions of this kind, the number of males in nursing has grown slowly each year. It is believed that 7% of nurses currently are males, up from 3% in 1980 (Domrose, 2003). Currently, males are choosing to enter the profession of nursing in slow but increasing numbers; however, males enter nursing for very different reasons than females. Unlike female nurses, who value the caring aspect of nursing, many male nurses attach importance to nursing positions that provide prestige, authority, practical motivation, and occupational mobility (Boughn, 2001; Davis-Martin, 1984). Male nurses have been found to enter nursing at a later age than females, and have been identified as having a higher educational level (Grossman, Arnold, Sullivan, Cameron, & Munro, 1989). Salary has a large influence on male nurses when choosing their area of specialty, and has been shown to be a factor in career growth for males (Boughn, 2001).

There is a higher quantity of male nurses in some specialties than in others, a result of occupational limitations and compatibility of occupational responsibilities to attributes. Generally, men entering nursing chose specialty areas that were compatible with their character traits, and that allowed for autonomy and technical prowess (Evans, 1997).

The contributions of male nurses to the profession of nursing are different from the female nurse. For that reason it is important to further investigate male nurses' role in nursing. More so, it is essential to get a better grasp of the general socialization process of the male nurses, and learn in more detail the socialization of males to specific areas of nursing, such as the intensive care setting. As learned in this study, the socialization process for males in the critical care is different from the socialization of females to this area. Males bring to the intensive care different attributes, and seek out different nursing experiences than do female nurses. Even though differences were found in the interviews conducted in this study, it cannot yet be assumed that these findings apply to all novice male nurses in this setting; instead more investigation is needed to have a comprehensive view of this basic social process.

CONCLUSION

Novice male nurses enter into the critical care setting to increase their skills by managing critically ill patients, but are negatively affected by the basic nursing skills that must be performed in conjunction with nursing skills specific to critical care. Novice male nurses perceive this as a barrier in their socialization, which leads them to experience burnout and frustration. On account of the feelings of dissatisfaction male nurses seek to move on. It is through a change in role that these men find their fit in nursing.

REFERENCES

Boughn, S. (2001). Why women and men choose nursing. *Nursing and Health Care Perspectives, 22*(1), 14–19.

Coleman, B. (1990). Advanced nursing apprenticeship program: A strategy for retention of experienced critical care nurse. *Heart & Lung, 19*(3), 236–242.

Davis-Martin, S. (1984). Research in males in nursing. *Journal of Nursing Education, 23*(4), 162–164.

DiGiacomo, M., & Adamson, B. (2001). Coping with stress in the workplace: Implication for new health professionals. *Journal of Allied Health, 30*(2), 106–111.

Domrose, C. (2003, August 25). Men at work. *Nurseweek (California Edition), 16*(18), 15–18.

Egeland, J. W., & Brown, J. S. (1989). Men in nursing: Their fields of employment, preferred fields of practice, and role strain. *Health Services Research, 24*(5), 693–707.

Evans, J. (1997). Men in nursing: Issues of gender segregation and hidden advantages. *Journal of Advanced Nursing, 26*, 226–231.

Glaser, B. G. (1978). *Theoretical sensitivity: Advances in the methodology of grounded theory*. Mill Valley, CA: Sociology Press.

Glaser, B. G. (1998). *Doing grounded theory: Issues and discussions.* Mill Valley, CA: Sociology Press.

Glaser, B. G. (2001). *The grounded theory perspective: Conceptualization contrasted with description*. Mill Valley, CA: Sociology Press.

Grossman, D., Arnold, L., Sullivan, J., Cameron, M., & Munro, B. (1989). High school students' perceptions of nursing as a career: A pilot study. *Journal of Nursing Education, 28*(1), 18–21.

Meisenhelder, J. B. (1981). The new graduate socialization. *The Journal of Continuing Education in Nursing, 12*(3), 16–22.

Nesler, M. S., Hanner, M., & Melburg, V. (2001). Professional socialization of baccalaureate nursing students: Can students in distance nursing programs become socialized? *Journal of Nursing Education, 40*(7), 293–302.

Osuri, P. S. (2004). *Moving On: A study of the socialization process of male novice nurses in the critical care unit.* Unpublished master's thesis. Azusa, CA: Azusa Pacific University.

Tradewell, G. (1996). Rites of passage: Adaptation of nursing graduates to a hospital setting. *Journal of Nursing Staff Development, 12*, 183–189, 224.

III Emergent Fit Mode

INTRODUCTION: BARBARA M. ARTINIAN

The emergent fit mode starts with an existing theory or with variables thought to relate to the phenomenon under study. Its purpose is theory clarification or extension. The emergent fit mode "allows the researcher to build on the work of another researcher or to expand personal work by exploring in depth some aspect of previous research findings" (Artinian, 1988, p. 139). There are many dangers in using the emergent fit mode. If the variables were derived from a review of the literature, they may be wrong. In the past, students were required to conduct a literature review prior to receiving institutional board approval to do a study. From her literature review, Woodward (1982) hypothesized that patients with a colostomy would have lowered self-esteem and social isolation resulting in depression and suicide attempts. However, by using the Glaserian grounded theory method, she discovered the process of Revaluing of Self, which allowed the patients to integrate the colostomy into self and accept self as normal with a physical problem.

If the emergent fit mode is used with a basic social process that has been identified using grounded theory methods, "it cannot be assumed that the core variable of the original study will be the same for the new unit being studied and that it will explain the variation in behavior in the new unit" (Glaser, 1978, p. 108). Nevertheless, Glaser argues for its usefulness when a basic social process needs further development. Using an existing theory "enables the researcher to focus more quickly on a selected portion of the experience of the subjects since the parameters of the larger phenomenon have been identified" (Artinian, 1988, p. 142).

If the researcher follows the principles of grounded theory, any earlier thoughts and misconceptions can be corrected as aspects of the original theory are refuted or modified, or variables are added that were not originally included. In this way a program of research can be developed that adds to a body of knowledge rather than producing unrelated grounded theory studies. Wuest (2000) has used emergent fit to develop a theory of women's caring by building on her previous studies.

In the first example of emergent fit presented here, Thompson identifies four variables in the literature thought to be necessary to nurture hope. Using grounded theory methods she was able to develop the basic social process of Nurturing Hope (see chapter 11). The second chapter in this section describes Pfeiffer's study, which expands and modifies one stage, *opening to God,* which is the third stage in the theory of Bringing God Near (Van Dover & Pfeiffer, 2007). Pfeiffer has used the emergent fit mode to develop the theory of *partnering with God and the patient* (see chapter 12).

REFERENCES

Artinian, B. (1988). Qualitative modes of inquiry. *Western Journal of Nursing Research, 10*(2), 138–149.

Glaser, B. G. (1978). *Theoretical sensitivity.* Mill Valley, CA: Sociology Press.

Van Dover, L., & Pfeiffer, J. B. (2007). Spiritual care in Christian parish nursing. *Journal of Advanced Nursing* 57(2), 213–221.

Woodward, B. (1982). *A descriptive study on the phenomenon of revaluing of self in colostomates.* Unpublished master's thesis, California State University, Los Angeles.

Wuest, J. (2000). Negotiating with helping systems: An example of grounded theory evolving through emergent fit. *Qualitative Health Research, 10*(1), 51–70.

11 Nurturing Hope in Patients With Cancer

MARY THOMPSON
BARBARA M. ARTINIAN

> I am grateful for each day that I can live. Each morning I wonder if I'll be able to face the nausea and pain, but then I start thinking about the nurses, about the friends who will come and how we will share together—then I want to get started with my bath and do what I can do for myself.

Seeking to understand how to foster hope in patients was the motivation for this research. Hope makes a difference in nursing for many reasons. First, illness, accompanied as it is by pain, emotional turmoil, helplessness, and temptation to give up, can destroy hope. Lack of hope thwarts the healing process. Hope not only enables a person to live with illness, but is necessary for life itself. Hope is a powerful motivator. Pervasive feelings of hopelessness can lead to losing the will to live, a passive form of suicide.

Nurses also need hope. Daily encounters with illness and death, as well as pressures on the job and in relationships, can reduce a nurse's level of hope. That sense of diminished hope contributes to stress and diminishment of job satisfaction.

Review of recent nursing literature indicates ongoing interest in instilling hope in nursing practice—among suicidal patients (Cutcliffe & Barker, 2002), nursing home residents (Touhy, 2001), chemical dependency clients (Walker, 2004), medical-surgical patients (Smith & Kautz,

2007), in psychiatric/mental health nursing (Cutcliffe & Koen, 2007), rehabilitation patients (Kautz, 2008), and end of life care (Miller, 2007). We anticipate that the body of knowledge about hope will continue to develop.

THE STUDY

Aim

The aim of this study was to investigate hope from the perspective of patients with cancer who were either experiencing hope or feeling its absence.

Method

A field study method was chosen. Data collection included three in-depth interviews with each of the 10 patients, and observations of behavior. Grounded theory methods were used to analyze the data (Glaser, 1978).

The study illustrates the emergent fit mode. The research began by reviewing classical literature to describe and define hope: Hope is the expectation of attaining a goal (Stotland, 1969), the knowledge and feeling that there is a way out of difficulty (Lynch, 1965). Other literature also revealed repeated themes to describe concepts in hope. These concepts became variables in the study, and interview guides were developed to gather more information about the experience of hope. Participants in the study provided rich examples. Analysis of the data resulted in the development of a basic social process: *nurturing hope.*

Participants

Participants were 10 people who had a diagnosis of cancer, for whom hope was a vital issue in their experience. They lived at home. They included an equal number of men and women, and their age range was 40–70.

Data Collection and Analysis

Interviews of participants took place in their homes during three visits over 2–3 weeks. Transcribed tapes of the interviews and field notes were used to analyze the descriptive data. The final process was evaluating the interrelationship of all the variables in the study. The aim of this process was to understand the experience of hope.

Ethical Considerations

The study was approved by the California State University School of Nursing faculty research committee. An oncologist, who was given information about the research, gave permission for the investigator to contact several of his patients. The investigator met with people interested in participating to explain the study. She gave them a form that described the research process: three visits with interviews that would be tape-recorded, confidentiality, and freedom to discontinue the visits. Participants signed and dated the form.

FINDINGS

Results of the study were focused in four areas: The overall analysis of data led to a beginning conceptualization of hope. Evaluation of *expressions and responses of hope,* which were variables of *expectation* and *action,* provided a framework for assessment of hope. Examination of the *context of hope,* variables of *love from others and God, mutuality, freedom,* and *newness,* provided understanding of the concept of hope. The experience and beliefs of patients identified some specific physical, psychosocial, and spiritual priorities for nursing intervention to facilitate hope (Thompson, 1980).

Conceptualization of Hope

The following conceptual map describes the basic social process of Nurturing Hope. The BSP resolves the patient's concern of having hope while being treated for cancer. It is based on analysis of patient interviews and literature on hope. Development of hope begins with awareness of love from others and/or God that moves into mutuality, freedom, and newness. These variables, facilitators of hope, are assimilated by the person and are then expressed through expectation and action, which are expressions of hope. The relationships among the variables are depicted in a conceptual map (see Figure 11.1). Discussion regarding each of the variables will follow, including describing components of the variables.

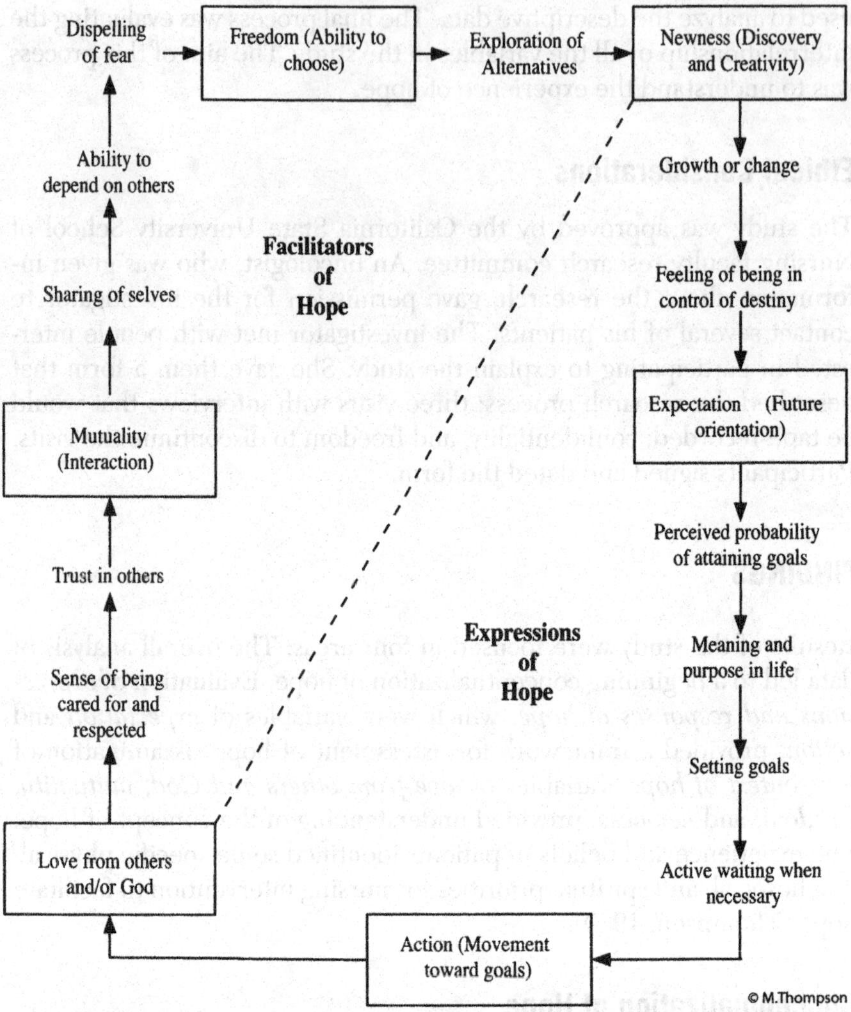

Figure 11.1 Phenomenon of hope showing facilitators of hope and expressions of hope. From "Nurturing Hope: A Vital Ingredient in Nursing," by M. Thompson, 1994. *Journal of Christian Nursing, 94*(3), 10–17. Printed with permission.

Description of Variables That Are Facilitators of Hope

These variables came from literature, research participants, and memos written by the researcher.

Love

Participants described ways nurses communicated the active concern of love. Thoughtful acts of kindness demonstrated *care.* A patient with breast cancer shared: "In my last experience in the hospital I was taken care of by a student nurse who came in and talked with us like we were human. She made special efforts to make our beds smooth and do it fast, just all the little things that make you comfortable."

Patients perceive nurses as *taking responsibility* when nurses fulfill the patient's idea of a nurse's role—and when their problems become the nurse's problems. One female patient described an example:

> After surgery, one nurse tried everything she could to get my stomach settled. She also gave me extra pillows to make me comfortable. It was kindness, not just dumping something and saying, "There you are; it will be all right." Instead, her attitude was, "I'll do whatever you need; I'll help you get through this."

Nurses communicated *respect* by acknowledging the uniqueness of another: calling a person by name, recognizing talents and rights. One respondent suggested: "People show respect in the way they treat me: they acknowledge that I am on earth. What bothers me is to have someone ignore me completely. They should know me, and they don't."

Nurses also expressed love through taking the initiative to *know and understand the patient's perspective.* One woman gave examples of how nurses showed her they understand: "They listen, ask questions, and spend time. They don't rush out of the room. A few times nurses came by and asked if I wanted to talk about anything. It was nice that they were thoughtful enough to ask."

When asked about sources of love, patients mentioned family, friends, nurses, and the physician. Some patients also mentioned God as alleviating fear of death and countering depression, which helped them to feel safe and enabled them to look toward the future with self-respect. A male patient with a recent diagnosis of bladder cancer talked about God's love: "God is understanding and forgiving. I would not have much to look forward to in the hereafter if I did not know that he loves me. I am not afraid to die." A female patient also spoke of the significance of God's love to her: "God's love helps me to respect myself. It gives me responsibility to have patience with those around me. God is concerned about my health and everyday walk in life. He supplies my needs, knows everything, and is everywhere present. That makes me feel safe."

In summary, love provides a positive perspective, one aspect of hope. It reinforces and supports, and gives confidence. Love provides a reason to have plans and think about the future. Love mobilizes what is inside a person and frees us to move. It has a generating quality. Hope begins with love.

Mutuality

Mutuality involves a three-step process. First, it is helpful for a person to experience *perception of a reciprocal relationship*. Attitudes of caring, communicated through warmth and initiative, indicate that a helping person is truly interested in another. Relating experiences of similar interests or circumstances can communicate a common humanity between patient and nurse. Identification with the background of another decreases isolation and promotes a sense of ease and trust. One woman explained: “It is easier to share with people who have had similar experiences in life. They understand that patients are, after all, human. We are not perfect.” Another person began to experience mutuality through reading books about people who had gone through similar circumstances. Still another identified with the suffering of Jesus, taking comfort in the thought that he understood her suffering.

Sharing personal interests and common life experiences with someone often awakens the desire to reciprocate, encouraging a patient to *express needs and concerns*, the second step of mutuality. Physical and mental factors influence this part of the process. A person’s physical weakness may hinder reaching out to others, even though the perception of caring and a reciprocal relationship exists. The inability to reach out to others may be one factor that depresses hope. Mental factors may also hamper mutuality. Inward forces, including fear, lack of trust, lack of communication skills, or choosing privacy rather than interaction with others, influence a person’s state of mind. One man suggested: “My sharing with others depends on my mental attitude and physical state at the time. Sometimes our minds can close up and shut us off from help. It is only when we open up, and read or ask for help, that things will change.”

Expressing needs leads to the final step in the process of mutuality: *sharing personal resources with another*. Reaching out to others may result in sensing personal strengths and developing a sense of worth and meaning in life. It also opens up the person to relationships with others where resources may be found. Patients found mutuality with family, friends, physicians, nurses, and God. One man explained: “I tried to encourage people who were in the same room. Sometimes the nurses would bring other patients who were going through similar things to talk with me. They wanted to help the person but couldn’t, and they knew another patient could, so they asked me. That was good for me." A woman added: "When I was in the hospital I discovered that I could cheer up my friends. They came to cheer me up, but I helped them instead. This encouraged me too."

In summary, interdependence comes from prior experiences of love and trust. Through reciprocal relationships, a person experiences the rewards of reaching out to others and realizes some control over the environment. The process of reciprocal relationships also provides stimulation, opening more alternatives in a situation. Mutuality enables a person to move toward freedom.

Freedom

Perception of choice comes from a sense of independence and power to make decisions, which involves the ability to think and problem solve. Some patients shared how people can have a state of mind in which they believe they can make decisions. One man stated emphatically: "Illness does not control me; I can decide what I want to do." Although illness curtailed his activities, he showed initiative and creativity in maintaining relationships over the telephone. He consistently made choices about life and fulfilled his role as a father. Other patients began to lose hope when they felt that illness, other people, or circumstances were invading their freedom to make decisions about the basic aspects of life.

The second component of freedom comes from *perception of control,* believing that the decisions we make will give us some control over the events in life. One man appreciated that his physician explained the alternatives for treating his cancer, allowing him to decide which course to take. In contrast to choice and control, other situations produce feelings of powerlessness and helplessness. Powerlessness occurs when a person experiences decreased independence in making decisions. It arises when there is not enough information to make a decision or when a person is not given permission to make a decision. The hospital environment can foster a sense of powerlessness when regimentation and routine overshadow a patient's needs and personal lifestyle.

One man told of his frustration when the nursing staff would push his bedside stand away and forget to put it back. He was in traction and could not reach it. He would also feel helpless when he got no response after pushing his call light.

A climate for freedom includes allowing the patient to make choices about personal care, as well as decreasing the unknown through clear explanations. Having a call light answered promptly can help a patient feel some control over the environment.

In summary, the perception of freedom emerges from reciprocal relationships, which stimulate and support the person to look beyond limited alternatives. These relationships enable a person to see an environment that is not confining. Instead, the person believes that he or she can make choices and exercise control over events in life. This belief enables the person to use stimuli in the environment to develop creative solutions, a process that leads to newness.

Newness

Discovery and past experiences with creativity provide a foundation for newness. One man had been involved in creative projects since childhood; his parents encouraged a sense of curiosity in discovering new things. As an adult, this provided a framework for viewing the world that included an impetus for discovery and creativity. He had a consistently hopeful perspective. Another man found discovery in the Bible and stated: "When I read the Bible, it opens up new things." A woman described a craft catalogue that gave her ideas and stimulated plans. Another woman found stimulation in interpersonal relationships that helped her discover new things.

The next step in finding newness is gaining *insight:* viewing self, the world, other people, or God with a new perspective. One woman described her delight in discovering that she could use the foot pedals on the organ with her leg prosthesis. One man felt trapped and helpless after surgery because of all the equipment and procedures. He gained insight when the physician explained that the machine was not trapping him but helping him get better so he could go home. Insight also comes through reading books written by people who have gone through similar experiences.

Insight stirs the mind toward *creative plans* that can result in changed behavior and restored hope, further described in the next section of this chapter, which details *expressions of hope.* In summary, the discovery and creativity dimensions of newness enable people to focus beyond the confines of circumstances. They direct people toward meaningful social and mental involvement that begins a forward momentum, resulting in viewing the future with expectation. *Love, mutuality,* and *freedom* culminate in *newness.* Together they comprise the facilitators of hope that lead to expressions of hope.

Description of Variables That Are Expressions of Hope

Expectation

Expectation also has been called imagination or wishing (Lynch, 1965). Participants illustrated components of expectation. When asked to describe hope, one man stated, "Hope is a state of anticipation, a condition of mind in which you *expect results.*" A former school teacher on chemotherapy for breast cancer added, "Hope is anticipating that *prospects for the future are going to be positive.*" She acted on this expectation by *making plans* to substitute teach the following semester.

People living with cancer also face the reality of death, and seek day-to-day hope as well as ultimate hope. One woman stated: "Nobody wants to die. But hope in God, knowing that you can have everlasting life—that cannot be taken away." Her belief introduced the perspective that not even death terminates the future. Consequently, because the future is ongoing, expectation also continues. An ultimate future is part of the spiritual dimension of hope. Some people believe that life ends at death, and that death is the end of all future hopes. Writers of Christian literature on hope, and some participants in the study, believe there is ultimate hope in which death is the beginning of a new phase of eternal life.

In summary, expectation, a cognitive expression of hope, leads to action, a behavior dimension of hope. Hopeful people live with active participation in relationships, work, and hobbies. In contrast, hopeless people tend to be detached and inactive.

Action

Using the variables of expectation and action as expressions of hope, the researcher formulated an operational definition of hope: Hope is a mental state indicated by future expectation and goal-specific action. Expectation is evidenced by verbalizations reflecting the presence of (a) goals and plans in areas involving coping with illness, activities of daily living, relationships with significant others, relationships and activities beyond significant others, and goals for life; (b) positive probability of attaining goals; and (c) positive perception of the future. Action is evidenced by behavioral or cognitive movement toward goal attainment. This operational definition of hope was used to develop a framework for assessing hope in patients.

DISCUSSION

The primary purpose of this research study was to describe the phenomenon of hope. Even though definitions of variables from the literature of hope formed the beginning framework for this study, by using the constant comparative approach described by Glaser (1978), analysis of the patient responses allowed the beginning definitions to be corrected or enhanced. From analysis of the data the relationships among the variables emerged. The basic social process of Nurturing Hope was discovered, which has two stages—facilitating hope and expressing hope. Findings of this study have been used in the content in current nursing practice. A framework for assessing hope emerged, as well as priorities for nursing interventions to instill hope in nursing care. Information about the findings of this study has been communicated in seminars and a publication (Thompson, 1994).

Hope continues to be a relevant issue in our world as people face uncertainty about the future. Multiple factors block the presence of hope, and many people experience anxiety and diminished hope in their lives. Nurses are present with others in crisis situations where people (including nurses) are searching for hope. Insights from a growing body of current as well as historical literature, and examples from patients and families, can help to instill hope into our lives and nursing practice.

REFERENCES

Cutcliffe, J. R., & Barker, P. (2002). Considering the care of the suicidal client and the case for engagement and inspiring hope. *Journal of Psychiatric and Mental Health Nursing*, 9(5), 611–621.

Cutcliffe, J. R., & Koen, C. V. (2007). Hope and interpersonal psychiatric/mental health nursing: A systematic review of literature—Part Two. *Journal of Psychiatric & Mental Health Nursing, 14*(2), 141–147.

Glaser, B. G. (1978). *Theoretical sensitivity*. Mill Valley, CA; Sociology Press.

Kautz, D. (2008). Inspiring hope in our rehabilitation patients, their families, and ourselves. *Rehabilitation Nursing*, 33(4), 177.

Lynch, W. (1965). *Images of hope*. Baltimore, MD: Helicon.

Miller, F. (2007). Hope: A construct central to nursing. *Nursing Forum, 42*(1), 9–12.

Smith, A. D., & Kautz, D. D. (2007). A day with Blake: Hope on a medical-surgical unit. *MEDSURG Nursing, 16*(6), 378–382.

Stotland, E. (1969). *The psychology of hope*. San Francisco: Jossey-Bass.

Thompson, M. (1980). *An investigation of love, mutuality, freedom and newness with the perception of hope in patients with the diagnosis of cancer*. Unpublished master's thesis, California State University, Los Angeles.

Thompson, M. (1994). Nurturing hope: A vital ingredient in nursing. *Journal of Christian Nursing, 94*(3), 10–17.
Touhy, T. (2001). Nurturing hope and spirituality in the nursing home. *Holistic Nursing Practice, 15(4),* 45–56.
Walker, J. (2004). Journey into hope: A therapeutic relationship. *Journal of Christian Nursing, 21*(2), 19–22.

12 Partnering With God and the Patient

JANE PFEIFFER
LESLIE VAN DOVER

Parish nurses (PNs), by definition (International Parish Nurse Resource Center [IPNRC], 2000), are nurses who combine professional nursing and expertise with theological concepts to facilitate healing, particularly emphasizing pursuit of wholeness and addressing spiritual concerns that may accompany illness. Van Dover and Pfeiffer (2007), using grounded theory methods (Glaser, 1978), developed a substantive theory of the process PNs use to provide spiritual care to parishioners in Christian churches. In order to extend and refine the theory, a decision was made to explore each of the phases in greater detail. During a research course at Loma Linda University, Pfeiffer used the emergent fit mode to explore the third phase of the theory Bringing God Near.

A brief overview of the context of the theory of bringing God near states:

> Bringing God Near states as nurses assess spiritual needs and concerns of patients and families in the context of their health situation and address these through spiritual intervention . . . PNs accept the Christian reality that God is always near. They also understand that people do not always reach out to God or respond to the divine presence, especially in times of illness or crisis (Lewis, 1976). At these times, PNs help patients and families to approach or enter into the presence of God. (Van Dover & Pfeiffer, 2007, p. 216)

The theory of Bringing God Near has five sequential phases: trusting God, forming relationships with the patient or family, opening to God, activating or nurturing faith, and recognizing spiritual renewal and growth. Through the process, the nurse's attention is on both God and patient (see Figure 12.1).

Trusting God anchors the PN's practice in a strong personal faith that has developed over time and has grown into a mature walk with God. This faith is not unshakable, but it has weathered many storms of life and stood the tests. The nurses talk about the need to keep the relationship "alive and vital and growing" and do this through "praying and talking to Him." This dimension is discussed in greater detail in Van Dover and Pfeiffer (2005). *Forming relationships with the patient and/or family* is the second phase. Beginning or renewing relationships occurs with attention to being "present" and engaging the patient in "collaborative assessment" of the challenging situation. The third phase, *opening to God,* involves acknowledging God's presence in the patient's life here and now, and looking to God on behalf of the patient. Next, the *activating or nurturing faith* phase focuses on doing something tangible with the patient such as praying, touching, or using scripture or religious music. Through these activities, "new or revitalized meanings were created that encouraged and supported their faith and enabled them to embrace even the most difficult struggles in life" (Van Dover & Pfeiffer, 2007, p. 218). In the final phase of this process, the PNs are *recognizing*

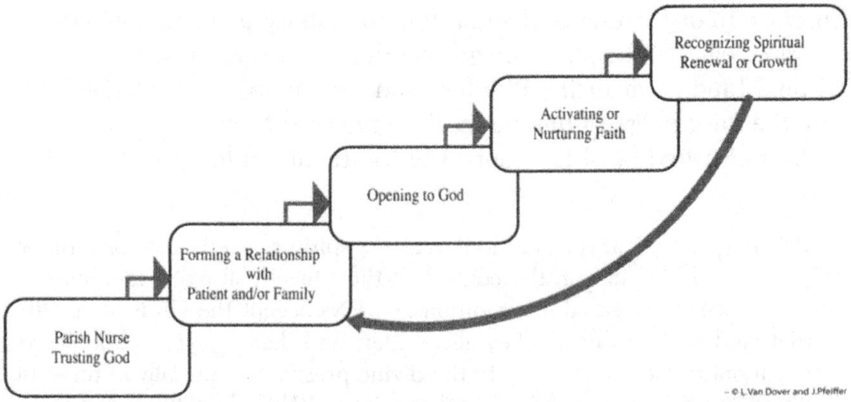

Figure 12.1 Bringing God near: A theory of spiritual caregiving in parish nursing. Printed with permission from the *Journal of Advanced Nursing. L. Van Dover and J. Pfeiffer.*

spiritual renewal and growth in their patients. These outcomes include observable changes in patient "attitudes, emotions, and faith." God and the PN attending to them in their troubles reorient patient perspectives (Van Dover & Pfeiffer, 2007).

Nurses of any faith and in any context have opportunities to welcome God's presence and partnership to provide spiritual care. The PN's personal faith journey and relational focus with the patient and God are foundational to the caregiving process of bringing God near. Understood as "a reservoir of faith" available to the nurse and, by extension, to the patient, *trust in God now* opens the door for "effective spiritual care that honors the individuality or uniqueness of *this* patient, in *this* situation" (Van Dover & Pfeiffer, 2007). While this trust is ongoing throughout the process, and PNs in Van Dover and Pfieffer's study could speak of it fluently in the first two phases, they consistently reported difficulty explaining what really happened when God's presence or guidance was discernible in the *opening to God* phase, though it was very real to them.

Trying to describe in words the third phase of this theory, this intersection of (a) nurses joining the patient on their journey and (b) the presence of God becoming real to nurse and/or patient led to the development of the research question by Pfeiffer: How will Christian PNs describe more fully the experience of God's presence and direction in the nurse-patient relationship in the process of bringing God near?

THE STUDY

Aim

The purpose of this study was to explore the third phase, *opening to God*, of the substantive theory of bringing God near. It was done to clarify and further develop the concept of God's leading and guidance as experienced by Christian PNs while giving spiritual care.

Method

Artinian (1988) and Wuest (2000) assert that the emergent fit mode facilitates a more focused exploration of previously gained unit-specific knowledge. Thus, to expand the understanding from *what* PNs described as an opening to God to *how* they experienced God's leading and guidance in the process of giving spiritual care, the emergent fit mode of grounded theory was used.

Open coding of emergent data, verification, and consolidation of those codes into themes and substantive codes were, by constant comparison, checked for fit with preexistent categories. Glaser (2005, p. 9) and Wuest (2000) both caution "staying open" (p. 51), to both guard against a forced fit of emergent data, or to disqualify the extant category(s) as having undue influence over the researcher. The following terms referring to God's interaction with the PN are assumed to be interchangeable in this study: leading, guidance, presence, and direction.

Sample

After institutional review board approval was obtained from Loma Linda University, four PNs were interviewed individually, and six PNs were part of a focus group interview conducted by the researcher. All but one were volunteers, averaging 6–12 hours a week, with a range of 2–15 years of experience in the role. Several of the focus group PNs were also eucharistic ministers in their local parish. There were four denominational affiliations represented in these PN participants, and four of the interviewees began their PN practice upon retirement from other nursing positions.

Data Collection and Analysis

Interviews with six subjects were approximately 45–90 minutes in length. The interviews were semistructured, open-ended, tape recorded, and transcribed verbatim. Parish nurses were asked to think of a time they gave spiritual care to a patient, and were then asked to describe that encounter. Sample questions included, "How did the relationship and the situation develop? What was going on?" "Describe how you sensed or experienced God being present as you were working with the patient. Tell me more about how you experienced God's presence or guidance or direction as you were there."

Initial coding and memoing showed both similarity and innuendos of difference compared to the previous study. Several categories combined to form themes consistent with the previous study and two of notable difference. Additionally, identification of themes consistent with the previous research resulted in emergence of the theoretical code of amplified causal loops, which integrated the categories (see Figure 12.2).

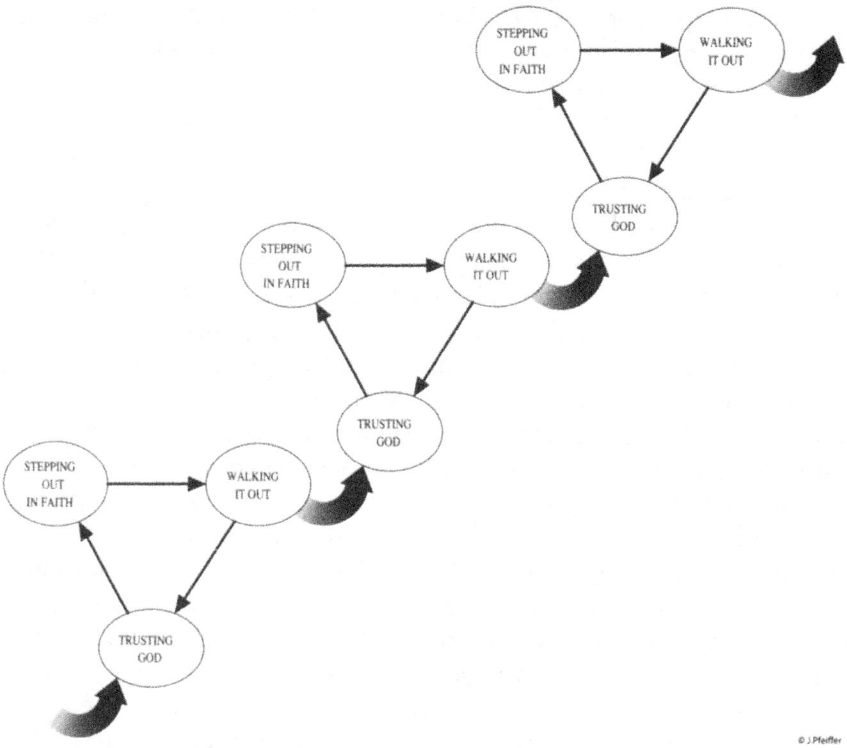

Figure 12.2 Partnering with God and the Patient.
Printed with permission from J. B. Pfeiffer.

This code captured the cyclical nature of responding in faith to the sense of presence in or direction one received from the patient-PN encounter. The theory Partnering with God and the Patient emerged from the data. All data analysis was done by hand.

Initially the similar codes with notably different descriptions concerned me, as if their existence challenged the original *opening to God* phase. However, in construction of theoretical memos it became clear that apparently different descriptions of the process reinforced the previous concept and further revealed the amplified causal loop mentioned previously. Glaser (1978, 2005) in describing the generation of theoretical codes, resultant theoretical sampling, and identification of conceptual indicators explains the ongoing nature of refining and deepening one's grasp of the data, verifying and ensuring fit.

My grasp of the refining nature of theoretical code generation can be illustrated by the example from the responses of two PNs. One PN was very articulate and aware of God's presence *at the time* of interaction with the patient, and this often led her to the next step(s) of caregiving. In contrast, another PN reported awareness of God's involvement most commonly "comes at those moments of silence at the end of prayer [when] you're leaving that spiritual realm in a sense . . . just absolutely knowing that God or a supernatural power is there supporting you to do that." This PN denied any specific unusual sense of being led. Rather her description of what routinely happened in interaction with the patient was characterized by such intent focus on the patient that she would "lose herself" and become totally available to God, only recognizing this had happened towards the end of the spiritual care given, or after the fact.

Glaser (1978) explains the role of theoretical codes as "weaving a fractured [or divergent] story back together again" (p. 72). The first-glance (or apparent) discrepancy of responses was resolved when both above-mentioned PNs spoke of trusting God in the moment, stepping out in faith and walking forward in that confidence, which reinforced trusting God for more leading and guidance. Here, use of the constant comparative method both facilitates the discovery of concepts in emergent and extant (previously collected) data, and prevents forcing new data to fit previously labeled categories. The emergence of a theoretical code, partnering with God and the patient, revealed widely divergent descriptions of the moment or time when guidance is experienced within the deeper conceptual idea of the PN's partnership with God. This led to outcomes in which the PN, and sometimes the patient, shared their awareness of God's presence or guidance. The *how* of this partnership almost always involved the integration of physical and spiritual dimensions of the person, an intensity of focus on the patient, use of scripture and/or prayer, and taking cues from the patient for exploring concerns. Wuest (2000) aptly details the constant comparative method's role in protecting the emerging data from being restricted from its full findings. The method also protects against one's own bias and against any theoretical bias picked up through research of the literature.

Ethical Considerations

Participants were assured of confidentiality, and national guidelines were followed for all data collected, stored, and used for transcription, analysis, and publication. The Loma Linda University Institutional Review Board approved the study. PNs voiced the desire to have study results presented to them once findings were analyzed and the investigator agreed to do so. The same stringent ethical and confidentiality guidelines will be followed in consolidating emergent and extant data sets.

Triangulation was accomplished with individual and focus group interviews, faculty input, and comparison to literature findings. Rigor and credibility were addressed by expert consultation, and by comparing to previous research findings. Validation was sought from the PNs who were interviewed individually by having them read the write-up after theoretical coding was done.

FINDINGS

Two of the emergent themes fit into the *opening to God* category of background to, or nurse preparation for, knowing God's guidance and direction. The first theme was that nurturing or cultivating one's personal relationship with God is foundational to being a fully available PN who could be used by God. The second was that a deeply integrated sense of spirituality manifests as understanding one's "being" as part and parcel with one's "doing." This integration of the physical, social, and spiritual aspects of personhood was consistent with previous research. Yet, there was a nuanced difference, which will be mentioned later.

Other frequently mentioned themes in the PN interviews can be summed in typical quotes: "I *just know, just absolutely know* that God is there." "I had *this sense,* I realized that was what God wanted." "*The words just come!* It's amazing! *There was no doubt* . . . that's where I was being directed to go." The PNs also mentioned a strong *sense of God's presence* (italics to communicate interviewee's emphasis). These themes were heard over and over from multiple PNs and many struggled to further elaborate with verbal descriptions when asked to do so. This sense, this knowing, this definite conviction that God was directing them was present, and yet hard to explain. They did however, comment on learning to release focus on one's self ("What am I going to do or say?") and to relax into the assurance that as they focus on the patient and wait, "The words will come. They always do."

Along with this confidence in God's guidance or presence was the implication of partnership with God in this process. This was expressed as "being the instrument," "being used by God," or "discovering God using me." Several spoke of this as a journey, others of the process, inferring a cycle with the phases of trust: *entrusting yourself and the patient to God → stepping out in faith → walking it out → more will come.*

Nearly every PN voiced some understanding of physical and spiritual needs being intimately related, and understood spirituality as part of the whole versus a separate component of the person. And this seemed to give them freedom to begin, to step out in faith and discover God's leading as they gave whatever care the situation required. All spoke of praying and seeking God's guidance (in multiple and varied forms, or agreed with others who mentioned this).

While previous research found PNs talking about journeying with the patient, the two PNs interviewed individually reinforced the use of that metaphor, of being on a journey. One saw both the patient and the PN being on a journey with God. She suggested the important thing to do was to take one step at a time, best understood as "joining God and the patient on the journey." Note again the implied sense of partnership with God. While this PN spoke of joining God on the journey as primary, it was almost impossible to separate this union with God and his purposes from the patient; there was no excluding the patient at any point in the interaction. One major difference noted in these data was the mention by one seasoned, expert PN of sometimes receiving God's guidance, but being almost unaware *until leaving* the intensely spiritual dimension and reentering the physical dimension that they had most assuredly been in the presence of God, that God had obviously been directing that encounter. In the words of the PN:

> The only time where I can really say that I can feel a particular presence or a strong sense of guidance, so to speak, is when I'm praying; and at the end of the prayer, and just kind of that moment, or in those several moments of silence as you're ending a prayer and you're leaving that spiritual realm in a way, and kind of returning to the present physical world, there's a sense of just absolutely knowing that God or a supernatural power is there supporting you. . . . I think . . . when you get good at it, it becomes almost to the point where you lose yourself and you become just this feeling of compassion—and of caring—it becomes so strong that it's no longer yourself that's there, it's God working through you. It's that supernatural time that's hard to explain.

At the outset of the experiences she is trying to describe, she was operating unaware, functioning in that deeply integrated mode of "being and doing" previously mentioned. This corresponds with the principle, mentioned above, of taking the step immediately in front of her, trusting that as she cared for this patient or that, they and/or their concerns would be brought before God. More of God's leading and guidance would follow. This trust in current and future spiritual help is an important nuance to understanding God's guidance and direction in the caregiving process.

A theoretical concept seen in these data is that of partnering with God and the patient. PNs experience God's guidance and leading as an overflow of their personal faith relationship with God. Consequently, the first phase of the previous study, *trusting*, is descriptive of where this partnership begins. It is also consistent with the PN's deeply integrated understanding of person (nurse and patient) as holistic, indivisible beings. Partnering explains the process already under way as the PN comes to the third phase of *opening to God*, and here amplifying casual looping is seen as the PN continues the process of partnering, now with God and the patient. The diagram shows how the leading and guidance of God is experienced as the PN-patient relationship now expands to include a more explicit awareness of what the PN-patient-God relationship is. Although this three-way relationship was already happening, what was backgrounded now comes to the foreground. Here the PNs take a step → walk it out → [and trust] more will follow →. This process reinforces the PN's initial trusting in God and the process continues until the patient's concerns are adequately addressed.

A second concept present was that of *joining God and the patient on the journey* to facilitate the work of God being done (begun, continued, or accomplished). This resonates with the theoretical code of amplifying causal loops that describes the ongoing process of partnering with God and the patient, reinforces it, and is operative throughout all the phases of the theory of bringing God near.

DISCUSSION

The importance of the nurse's own journey and joining the patient on his or her journey is consistent with the interactive nature of relationships within nursing, and with God. This also opens the possibility that whether the patient is a God seeker, a God follower, aware of his or her place on this journey, or none of these, their spirituality can be accessed, affirmed, and strengthened just by the presence of the nurse and by the care given.

Christian nurse scholars have portrayed two different, not necessarily exclusive, views of how the nurse interacts with the divine in giving spiritual care (Shelly & Miller, 1999; Taylor, 2002). O'Brien (2001) describes one of these as derivative of Catholic mystics, such as St. Vincent De Paul, and St. Francis of Assisi. Speaking of St. Vincent, she writes, "His spirituality was centered on seeing Christ in the person of the needy" (p. 30). This suggests the nurse comes closest to the divine when she touches the life of God *in the face and body of the patient.* From this perspective come the great traditions of compassionate care, with preferential treatment given to the poor and marginalized. Jesus in the Gospel of Matthew illustrates this principle: "I tell you the truth, whatever you did for one of the least of these brothers of mine, you did for me" (*Holy Bible: New International Version [NIV]*, 1983, Mt 25:40).

A second view of interacting with the divine incorporates the theological concept of a transcendent life, focusing on the indwelling Christ, and interaction with the divine Other, that is, God (Shelly & Miller, 1999). Stoll (1990) describes spirituality as having both a vertical dimension based on the person's relationship with the transcendent God, and also a horizontal dimension to people, which is a reflection and expression of one's relationship with God. The implication is that a spiritual encounter that acknowledges only the horizontal dimension will be impoverished, lacking input from the wholly *Other*, transcendent God, and more akin to a humanistic view of spiritual care.

Cone, in her chapter on the experience of giving spiritual care, explains the differentiation of psychosocial and spiritual care as follows:

> [A]ctual spiritual care would be any care that enables patients to exercise their beliefs, values, practices, and affective responses and would be differentiated from psychosocial care by the enabling of the vertical facet of the person rather than the horizontal. It is the "supernatural aspect of spiritual care" that distinguishes it from other care. (1997, p. 272)

Inferred is the centrality of the vertical dimension of the nurse's own spirituality as a means of interacting with God and subsequently expressing her relationship with God in care given to the patient.

Both of these views recognize spirituality to be one inseparable and indispensable dimension of wholeness or spiritual well-being. Taylor (2002) stresses authenticity, self-awareness, instinct, and intuition as essential human components to "presencing." Spiritual formation specialist and academic philosopher Dallas Willard challenges the Christian to add to this wonderfully human capacity the experience of being addressed by the living voice of God. This he further describes as "the distinctive quality, spirit, and content that we have learned through experience to associate with the personal presence of God" (Willard, 1999, p. 184). Willard locates this training, this development of spiritual capacity, in one's day-by-day, practiced interaction or communion with the personal, living God. This brings us full circle to the importance of the nurse's own spirituality being nurtured and renewed in ongoing ways, in order to be fully available to God and the patient in all caregiving. This becomes the basis for knowing and giving voice to what is described in this study: the presence, leading, guidance, or direction of God in spiritual care giving by Christian PNs.

Herein lay opportunities for the nurse and/or patient to step into God's presence, to step beyond the merely physical (no duality intended here) into a more focused spiritual dimension of reality. This sense of stepping beyond the physical corresponds with Willard's notions of learning to recognize and follow God's lead, whether through God's still small voice, circumstances, or inner prompting of the (Holy) spirit. Willard further describes this gentle leading or guidance in this excerpt:

> In the still small voice of God we are given a message that bears the stamp of his personality quite clearly and in a way we will learn to recognize. But in contrast with other cases, the *medium* through which the message comes is diminished almost to the vanishing point, taking the form of thoughts that are our thoughts, though these thoughts are not *from us*. In this way, as we shall see, the human spirit becomes the "candle of the Lord" [Proverbs 20:27]. (Willard, 1999, p. 187)

O'Brien's overall construct of the "The Nurse: The Anonymous Minister" describes how nurses perceive meeting spiritual needs as part of their professional role in nursing. She also explains that in caring lie opportunities to be led or guided by promptings of the Holy Spirit. O'Brien quotes the Brothers of Taizé Community (1992) to explain that we are not expected to actually see or experience the Spirit who dwells in us: "What is asked . . . is that we believe in the Holy Spirit, that we trust in Him, that we abandon ourselves to Him. Far from being another demand made on us, this call to faith sets us free" (O'Brien, 1999, p. 103). This approach to living in God's guidance is similar to the PN partnership with God, previously illustrated. This process of partnering with God and the patient is seen throughout bringing God near, and phase three, *opening to God,* seems to be where the PN and/or patient become most aware of it: step out → walk it out → and in the resultant freedom, previously mentioned, more sense of God's presence or direction is likely to follow → leading the nurse and patient to open to God in ever increasing ways.

CONCLUSION

While this sample size is very small and the findings are not directly generalizable to any other population, the findings could contribute to other spiritual caregiving studies. The combination of two prominent themes mentioned in the interviews, journeying with the patient and partnership with God, offers helpful focus in spiritual caregiving practice. Additionally, understanding God's guidance and leading as an overflow of relationship reinforces the importance of nurses nurturing their own relationship with God in order to partner well with the God to whom they entrust themselves and their patients. This is a study in process, and further research will likely clarify the current findings.

The theoretical code of amplifying causal loops gives shape to nurses perceiving the guidance of God as an interactive process with God (and/or others) in which they are helped to step into his presence. As Dallas Willard (1999) describes, sometimes this happens as we step fully into our humanness, or sometimes as we step beyond the mere human dimension and PN and/or patient begin to experience one's true essence, the often unrecognized spiritual dimension of humanness. Based on this understanding, the dynamic of the amplified causal loop could become step in or out → walk further in or walk it out → and discover more of God for PN and/or patient, with a sense of ongoing access to the God who is present.

It seems the invitation to experience God and humanness more fully is present in parish nursing and nursing in general. PNs bring God near as they trust, form relationship, and gratefully receive that opening to God, when and however it comes, that leads to activating and nurturing faith with spiritual growth as outcome.

ACKNOWLEDGEMENTS

I would like to acknowledge invaluable help given by two researchers. The first is Dr. Leslie Van Dover, principal investigator in the Bringing God Near theory, who contributed the background portion of this chapter. Without this, the emergent fit study I conducted would not have been possible. Secondly, Dr. Barbara Artinian gave expert counsel during formulation and analysis of the research process in both studies. Many thanks are due to each.

REFERENCES

Artinian, B. M. (1988). Qualitative modes of inquiry. *Western Journal of Nursing Research, 10*(2), 138–149.

Cone, P. (1997). Connecting: The experience of giving spiritual care. In B. M. Artinian & M. Conger, *The intersystem model: Integrating theory and practice* (pp. 270–288). Thousand Oaks, CA: Sage.

Glaser, B. G. (1978). *Theoretical sensitivity.* Mill Valley, CA: Sociology Press.

Glaser, B. G. (2005). *The grounded theory perspective III: Theoretical coding.* Mill Valley, CA: Sociology Press.

Holy Bible: New international version [NIV]. (1983). Colorado Springs, CO: International Bible Society.

International Parish Nurse Resource Center (IPNRC). (2000). *Parish nursing education: Preparation for parish nurse and parish nurse managers/coordinators, basic parish nurse curriculum.* Park Ridge, IL: Advocate Health Care.

Lewis, C. S. (1976). *A grief observed.* New York: Bantam Books.

O'Brien, M. E. (1999). *Spirituality in nursing: Standing on holy ground.* Sudbury, MA: Jones & Bartlett.

O'Brien, M. E. (2001). *The nurse's calling: A Christian spirituality of caring for the sick.* Mahwah, NJ: Paulist Press.

Shelly, J. A., & Miller, A. (1999). *Called to care: A Christian theology of nursing.* Downers Grove, IL: InterVarsity Press.

Stoll, R. (1990). *Concepts in nursing: A Christian perspective.* Madison, WI: Nurse's Christian Fellowship.

Taizé Community. (1992). *Listening with the heart.* Collegeville, MN: The Liturgical Press.

Taylor, E. J. (2002). *Spiritual care: Nursing theory research and practice.* Upper Saddle River, NJ: Prentice Hall.

Van Dover, L., & Pfeiffer, J. B. (2007). Spiritual care in Christian parish nursing. *Journal of Advanced Nursing, 57*(2), 213–221.

Van Dover, L., & Pfeiffer, J. M. (2005). Trusting God: Foundation for spiritual care. *Journal of Christian Nursing, 22*(1), 18–21.

Willard, D. (1999). *Hearing God: Developing a conversational relationship with God.* Downers Grove, IL: InterVarsity Press.

Wuest, J. (2000). Negotiating with helping systems: An example of grounded theory evolving through emergent fit. *Qualitative Health Research, 10*(1), pp. 51–70.

Studies With Emergent Theoretical Codes: Theoretical Code Mode

PART III

INTRODUCTION: BARBARA M. ARTINIAN

The theoretical code mode builds on the descriptive mode or the gerund mode but has the purpose of generating integrated theory. It is the least understood mode. The outcome of this mode is a "conceptualization of the underlying social process at an abstract level" (Artinian, 1988, p. 139). Through theoretical coding and memoing, patterns of behavior are identified and related. The purpose of the research is to identify the main concern of the subjects and how they resolve it. This purpose is accomplished by searching for latent patterns using a concept indicator model and allowing the theoretical code to emerge. Glaser has identified numerous theoretical codes that can show how the substantive codes are interrelated. The theoretical codes are emergent and cannot be forced on the data. It is not necessary to use a theoretical code to develop a grounded theory, but Glaser says grounded theories are best when theoretical codes are used because the theory "will appear more plausible, more relevant, and more enhanced when integrated and modeled by an emergent theoretical code" (Glaser, 2005, p. 14).

In each of the 10 research studies included in this part, a theoretical code has emerged and has been used to relate the variables in the theory. The studies are grouped together according to the theoretical code that emerged. Of the many theoretical codes that have been described, five of them emerged in the selected studies: strategizing, cutting point, amplifying causal loops, role theory, and balancing.

Glaser (2005) says that:

> The goal of a GT researcher is to develop a repertoire of as many theoretical codes as possible. There could be hundreds. The more theoretical codes the researcher learns, the more he has the variability of seeing them emerge and fitting them to the theory. They empower his ability to generate theory and keep the conceptual level. (p. 11)

Each study in this section exemplifies one of these theoretical codes. Through a careful examination of these studies, readers will see how an understanding of the use of theoretical codes to demonstrate the properties of the categories, their relationships to each other, and their manner of achieving the desired outcome have been enhanced by further analysis.

REFERENCES

Artinian, B. (1988). Qualitative modes of inquiry. *Western Journal of Nursing Research, 10*(2), 138–149.

Glaser, B. G. (2005). *The grounded theory perspective III: Theoretical coding.* Mill Valley, CA: Sociology Press.

I Strategizing

INTRODUCTION: BARBARA M. ARTINIAN

The theoretical code of strategizing describes the process used to manage or deal with a situation. Strategizing can be described as the making of plans to accomplish a goal.

In this section, two studies are presented using the theoretical code of strategizing. In a study conducted among rural perinatal patients, West identified the main concern to be having an unattended delivery (see chapter 13, "Strategizing Safety by Perinatal Patients in a Rural Setting"). Unlike most perinatal women, who wait until their third trimester to work on the details of their upcoming delivery, these participants began positioning themselves so to have a safe attended delivery as soon as they discovered that they were pregnant.

The second study was conducted by Satinovic among persons with multiple sclerosis whose main concern was generating a good life. This concern was resolved by Remodeling the Course of Life (see chapter 14). The strategies these participants used were aimed at living as good a life as possible with the MS diagnosis.

The process of strategizing resolved the main concern of each of these groups of patients. Health care providers can gain much insight by learning and understanding the strategies that many patients and their families use in managing their health care concerns.

13

Strategizing Safety by Perinatal Patients in a Rural Setting

KATHARINE S. WEST
BARBARA M. ARTINIAN

The health of mothers and infants is of critical importance to a community. Maternity care must not only be available, but also accessible and acceptable to clients (Bushy, 1994). Availability refers to the existence of a particular service, including the necessary personnel to provide that service. Accessibility refers to whether a person has logistical access to services, including the resources to pay for them. Acceptability refers to whether the service offered is a good fit with the values and beliefs of the client (Bushy). Women living in rural areas have limited access to available prenatal services that are acceptable to them (Conrad, Hollenbach, Fullerton, & Feigelson, 1998; McManus & Newacheck, 1989). A lack of appropriate care can contribute to poor perinatal outcomes (Hoffmaster, 1986). Thus, it is likely that the experiences of rural women differ from urban or suburban women.

Mariposa County has a steady birth rate of approximately 130 babies per year. The majority of Mariposa mothers deliver in one of three

From Strategizing safety: Perinatal experiences of rural women. In H. J. Lee & C. A. Winters (Eds.), *Rural nursing: Concepts, theory, and practice* (2nd ed.). Adapted with the permission of Springer Publishing Company, LLC, New York, NY 10036.

neighboring counties because no physician has provided delivery services within Mariposa County since 1982, when the town's general practitioner retired. A local clinic provided childbirth classes and offered prenatal care every other week by a visiting family practice physician from the next county. High-risk obstetrical care was only available by traveling to one of four neighboring counties. Most women drove a minimum of 1–2 hours one way for prenatal appointments and to reach the hospital of delivery (Mariposa County Health Department, 1999), which one mother called the "1 hour of worry."

At a time when disparities in service delivery between metro and nonmetro areas are increasing, both federal and state governments acknowledge the importance of providing standardized services (California Department of Health Services, 2000a, 2000b, 2000c; Centers for Disease Control, 2000). One way to accomplish this is to provide client-specific information to the local public health nursing service. Mothers may have different definitions and concerns than the government has regarding birth services, and it would be prudent to investigate the mothers' views. It is also desirable to tap into the creative solutions that mothers may have developed for themselves and further develop these ideas for the rural community.

The grounded theory study described in this chapter identifies the basic social process of Strategizing Safety by mothers in rural Mariposa County, California (West, 2006), where availability of and access to acceptable perinatal care is a challenge. Strategizing Safety resolved the main concern of the mothers of an unattended delivery. The findings show how mothers viewed their interactions with the health care team and their experience of having a baby in a rural area, behaviors and emotions that typified a mother's response to managing her pregnancy, and factors that influenced these interactions and experiences. The theoretical code of strategizing integrated the process that resolved the main concern of the subjects, which was to have an attended safe delivery of a healthy baby.

THE STUDY

Aim

The primary purpose of this study was to discover how pregnant women living in a rural area seek and experience perinatal health care. The second purpose was to give a voice to rural women and their ways of knowing and behaving during the perinatal period. The study focused specifically on experiences of women having babies while living in Mariposa County, California, so as to understand and identify internal and external factors that influenced their experiences and pregnancy outcomes (West, 2001).

Method

Grounded theory methodology, with constant comparative data collection and analysis (Glaser, 1978) was used for this study. Participants were interviewed in Mariposa County. The interviews were tape recorded and transcribed verbatim. The transcriptions were analyzed using QSR NVivo™ Version 1.2 (2000) software, which facilitated the recognition and understanding of information as presented in the interviews. The constant comparative method required the interviews to be coded, initially to reflect the substance of what was said and then compared later with subsequent interviews for similarities and differences. Codes were compared, clustered, and labeled until categories for those codes emerged (Glaser, 1978). Voice-recognition software facilitated the writing process.

Sample

The rural setting is unique to the data collection process. The inclusion criteria for the study were women who (a) had current residence in Mariposa County, (b) were pregnant at the time of the interview or had delivered within the county since 1982, and (c) provided written consent to participate in the research study. A convenience sample of 9 women with a total of 18 pregnancies was included; referrals were made by family ministries at churches in the county. Demographic data were obtained at the time of consent. Study participants were selected and interviewed until no new information was forthcoming (data saturation).

Data Collection and Analysis

Collectively, at the time of the interviews, the 9 interviewees had been pregnant 32 times, with 22 pregnancies completed, 9 pregnancies terminated early as miscarriage or abortion, and one pregnancy in progress. Eighteen of the pregnancies qualified for inclusion in this study because they occurred in Mariposa County after in-county deliveries had ceased in 1982. The women each had between one and eight living children aged 8 months to 32 years, including one set of twins, and one term infant who died in the postneonatal period from complications as a result of a congenital birth defect.

Using an interview guide promoted an exploration of the women's experiences to better understand what it is like to be pregnant in a rural county. Questions encouraged the women to share their experiences and to identify what factors influenced their pregnancies without prompting any specific type of answer; attitudes were allowed to emerge from answers regarding social interactions. In a similar manner, concerns of access were not directly addressed but allowed to emerge from the data.

It was found that these women sought to manage their main concern of delivering on a rural highway with its potential complications and problems. An unattended delivery was the mothers' primary concern, and Strategizing Safety was the core category that continually worked to resolve that concern. In one way or another, every mother volunteered concern about the distance and the plans she made to cope with this concern.

Ethical Considerations

The study proposal was submitted to and approved by the Azusa Pacific University Institutional Review Board. To ensure privacy and confidentiality during the interviews, all participants chose pseudonyms for themselves and their families that were used in place of their real names during the transcription process and in quotations used in coding. The identification key for the numeric codes and pseudonyms was kept locked in a separate location from the numbered interview tapes and transcriptions, and all data were destroyed at the conclusion of the study.

FINDINGS

Pregnant women in Mariposa County were confronted with the same decisions as pregnant women everywhere: They strategized (a) selecting a caregiver, (b) choosing behaviors supporting a healthy pregnancy, (c) preparing for labor, and (d) experiencing a successful delivery. Women in Mariposa County had one significant difference: They also had to come to terms with at least 1 hour of rural travel during active labor. The women all voiced concerns about an unattended precipitous delivery.

The Basic Social Process: Strategizing Safety

The basic social process of Strategizing Safety, integrated by the theoretical code of strategizing, has four phases: (a) seeking information, (b) choosing, (c) following through, and (d) fine-tuning (West, 2001; see Figure 13.1).

For the Mariposa women in this study, strategizing safety in pregnancy commenced upon confirmation of the pregnancy and concluded with birth. The first phase, seeking information, involved fact-finding about the various types of obstetrical care that were available, either locally or at a distance. Interpretation of the facts was filtered through personal beliefs and previous experience. The second phase, choosing, included selecting a

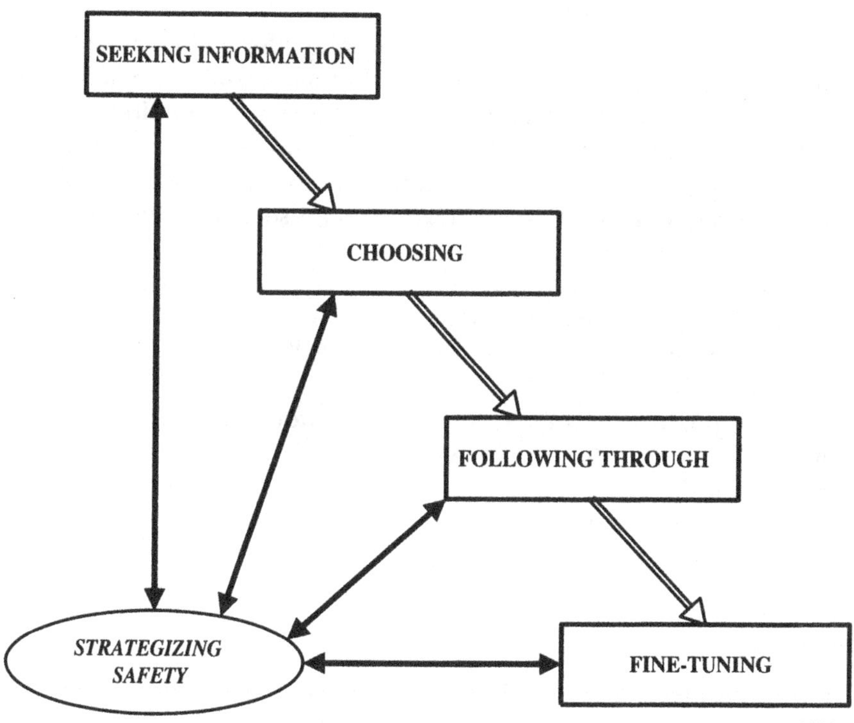

Figure 13.1 Basic social process: Strategizing safety and the four phases of *seeking information, choosing, following through,* and *fine-tuning.*
Reproduced with the permission of Springer Publishing Company, LLC, New York, NY 10036.

caregiver for the pregnancy—either a physician or a midwife or combination of the two. In making her choice for caregiver, a woman committed herself to a location for delivery. The third phase, following through, began with the initiation and continuation of prenatal care. As pregnancy progressed, changes in circumstances or development of complications sometimes required an alteration in strategy. Coping with the pregnancy was managed with the help of the woman's social support network and her own inherent abilities. The fourth phase, fine-tuning, included preparation for labor and the experience of delivery. The labor experience included getting to the right place for delivery at the right time; it was the core of the basic social process. Stressors and circumstances unique to the peripartum sometimes dictated changes in plans. Medical interventions were sometimes guided by the need to resolve "the 1 hour of worry" because of the distance involved from the women's homes to the birthing location.

Seeking Information

The first phase of Strategizing Safety is seeking information. Sometimes a woman found a physician or midwife through friends or relatives or current health care providers. If she was pregnant for the first time or a newcomer in town, she sought additional information about types of health care providers and delivery options before making her choices. Sometimes she sought information based on personal history:

> My grandma had [her] children here, most of them at home. . . . I liked the idea [of a home delivery] because my mom had . . . her children at home, and I thought if she can do it, surely I could do it.

In this first phase, the women were seeking information based on what they knew from people they knew, or where they believed they might find obstetrical services. However, it became evident in the next phase, choosing, that they were already considering the 1 hour of worry as they gathered information.

Choosing

The second phase of Strategizing Safety is choosing, which is accomplished as a direct result of the information obtained in phase 1. Individual choices were influenced by the circumstances of availability of care, and also the meaning and importance of the decision to the mother.

In Mariposa County, women could choose a physician or midwife for obstetric services. Both types of providers were available to attend hospital deliveries, but only in neighboring counties. Only one midwife attended home births in Mariposa County. "I asked [my sister-in-law] if her midwife would come over here, but she doesn't travel that far. But then I asked for a referral. That's how I found out about the midwife here."

Other women made their choices by first deciding on the location for delivery and then finding a caregiver on staff at that location. This was sometimes influenced by the reports from other women:

> I asked people for names and I called around and asked the offices questions. I had made the decision that I didn't want to go to [a particular town] . . . because I heard a lot of bad stories, . . . So, I knew that I wanted to deliver in [another] area.

Prenatal visits were available at the midwifery clinic in a nearby town but the midwife was not available for home deliveries. Most prenatal care was obtained through physicians' offices outside of Mariposa County.

Ultimately, choosing hinged on several factors, but time and distance were always major influences on the final decision. Mariposa women weighed the options in their minds, strategically balancing the pros and cons of travel for prenatal care with considerations for a safe delivery. Travel concern was the constant factor, with the main point being to resolve fear and worries. The 1 hour of worry was the compelling factor that guided their choosing.

Following Through

Following through, the third phase of Strategizing Safety, occurs after information has been obtained and a choice has been made. Following through is evidenced by the woman's behaviors as related to the specific circumstance for which safety must be strategized. Coping and adaptation behaviors that enable one to follow through during this phase are derived from a combination of personal experience, self-care, and social support from friends and family.

During the perinatal experience of the Mariposa women, following through was contingent on the distance the women traveled to reach their caregiver or the distance the caregiver traveled to reach the patient: "Actually [for] my exams, the doctor would come up to a clinic up here. But [for my other pregnancies], I'd just go to her office in town."

Women frequently combined their prenatal visits with other activities. Sometimes, alternative plans were developed in conjunction with the women's support networks and health care providers.

Fine-Tuning

Fine-tuning begins with final preparation for the event that indicated a need for safety in the first place. For pregnant women in Mariposa County, fine-tuning was the phase that was synonymous with labor and delivery. It was the onset of labor when the 1 hour of worry was most acutely experienced and fine-tuning was implemented. Fine-tuning may come about from actions of the person who is strategizing safety or may result from the actions of others, such as the medical staff. Stressors may develop leading to additional fine-tuning. Fine-tuning may also be imposed on the situation by the environment, such as snow-closed roads. Distance and travel needs were foremost in all their thoughts: "The only hard thing is the emergency. [Emergency services in Mariposa are] kind of just a helipad and a band-aid dispenser."

The experience of labor proved whether their particular strategy for safety was adequate. Labor in the right place attended by the right people and a successful birth was the desired outcome. Once labor began for the rural woman, getting there was the observable critical behavior during the 1 hour of worry. Getting there involved more than just transportation; sometimes, getting there required strategizing an alternative route, especially during the winter snow season. One mother who lived between Mariposa and Yosemite reflected that, had the road to town been snowed over, "We could go up to Yosemite, although they don't really have those kind of services; they do have a clinic there . . . and probably the doctor could have helped us there."

The original plan sometimes included an alternative labor support person in the event that the woman could not contact her preferred labor support, such as her mother or a neighbor. If the woman found herself in early labor, and already at or near to the planned location of delivery, the 1 hour of worry sometimes resulted in fine-tuning the labor plan itself. One woman was in early labor at the hospital when she had to restrategize her fine-tuned plans:

> [My doctor] said, "If you had someplace to go here, I would just send you home. But since you live so far away," and he just had to think about us going to a hotel. He just didn't agree with that. That was an issue.

The birth itself sometimes demanded immediate fine-tuning as described by the mother who delivered along the highway on the way to the hospital.

> Actually, I just got on all fours and . . . just kind of squatted down and held on because there was . . . no way to really get comfortable . . . I was pretty upset to think [an emergency medical technician was going to do the delivery] because I wasn't sure what his skills were. So they didn't have to do anything really. Just catch the baby, but they did fine.

Fine-tuning concluded with the birth of the infant. With the arrival of the newborn, strategizing safety was completed with all the corresponding fears of an unattended delivery resolved; the 1 hour of worry had ended.

Summary

The identified social process in this study, Strategizing Safety under the circumstance of rural perinatal care, was completed with the infant's birth. For Mariposa women, the safe arrival of the newborn was the result of nine months of strategizing to optimize the situation surrounding the 1 hour of worry during rural travel. Although it is certainly true that urban women seek safe delivery for their infants, urban women's concern for safety during travel in labor does not usually manifest, if it manifests at all, until the final weeks of pregnancy. In contrast, women in Mariposa County strategized safety from the beginning of pregnancy, throughout pregnancy, occasionally during that significant hour of travel during labor, and sometimes even after arriving at the planned location for delivery. One mother summed up the situation:

> I would love to have my babies where I wouldn't have to travel fifty-five or sixty miles. Maybe because I have healthy pregnancies and deliveries, I don't have that worry so much, but I just think a clinic or someplace to go to have my babies . . . [it] would be wonderful to have a place up here to have my babies.

DISCUSSION

Research about the inner world of the pregnant woman has been published in the nursing and psychological literature since the middle of the

20th century, often based on the work of Rubin (1961, 1967a, 1967b, 1975). According to Rubin's long-accepted seminal research (1975), there is a sequence to the psychological tasks of pregnancy and a different focus during each phase. According to Rubin, the mother's focus is inwardly aligned and the fetus is interpreted as being a part of her physical self. Nesting behaviors and thoughts of delivery help her prepare for birth, including strategizing logistical issues at the time of labor such as transportation. According to Rubin, only in the final weeks of a full-term pregnancy does the mother begin to prepare, or strategize, for the trip to the hospital with thoughts toward alternative plans or contingencies. Rubin (1975) called this set of behaviors *safe passage*.

More recently, Patterson, Freese, and Goldberg (1990) conducted research to explore how women utilized health care during pregnancy. They identified the major concern of women as seeking safe passage, a kind of strategizing, throughout pregnancy and childbirth by means of several processes that were described as largely internal in nature. Patterson et al. also stated that seeking safe passage might consist of a single approach with the ultimate outcome being the enrollment in prenatal care.

Similar processes were identified in this study of rural women with one notable difference. Women in Mariposa County were specifically concerned with the external environment and the attendant implications for safe passage throughout the pregnancy, ending with delivery. Mothers in Mariposa began to strategize for the trip to the hospital, at least mentally, immediately upon confirmation of pregnancy. These thoughts pervaded their entire pregnancy. Specifically, it was the 1 hour of worry—the concern with delivering en route to the hospital—that influenced all their decisions and choices. This was not about seeking safe passage simply to enroll in prenatal care. Strategizing Safety was the process by which these women attempted to bring control to their external environment throughout their pregnancy in anticipation of the birth.

APPLICATION TO PRACTICE

Rural families are hardy people and acknowledge that their choice of residence includes risks and responsibilities. They normalize certain hardships of accessibility and may be more likely to accept conditions perceived as risky by urban dwellers. Knowledge of the Strategizing Safety basic social process in rural areas can be utilized by rural nurses from the perspectives of the pregnant woman and also her providers.

Embracing telehealth technologies could allow local health care providers to provide in-person prenatal visit evaluations as indicated with a real-time consultation with a distant obstetrician as needed. The local hospital could partner with distant obstetrical practices to fund a mobile van staffed by advanced practice nurses to provide regular local access to prenatal care. Telehealth connections via cellular Internet services could provide instant contact with the sponsoring obstetricians.

Understanding that her concerns for safety at the end of pregnancy affect the woman at the beginning of pregnancy, anticipatory guidance usually reserved for the last trimester of pregnancy should be provided during the initial prenatal visit. This initiates a proactive partnership by the health care team, which anticipates the need to resolve her main concern of safety. Anticipatory preparation for an unattended delivery while en route could include assisting the family in the preparation of an obstetrical kit and emergency childbirth training for her partners.

If the delivery date is during inclement months, instruction should be given for discussions with local emergency and access agencies of the potential need for services. One mother was snowed in when her amniotic sac broke and true labor began. Because she did not live near a main road, the county snowplow was not expected to create access to the highway into town. A call to the sheriff department changed the priorities of the community, resulting in priority road access and a sheriff escort to the delivery hospital.

The data revealed that most health care providers for these women were unaware of the distance she traveled. Instructions were provided without regard for the implications, such as being sent home when in early labor. The women, however, proceeded with their own plans and checked into hotels local to the hospital to finish early labor. However, one obstetrician had knowledge of the distance involved and felt compelled to make a medical decision to induce labor before the woman was clinically ready. She recounted a prolonged, painful labor that ended in a cesarean delivery. She stated: "To this day, I just know in my bones, that had I been able to go home and wait until my body was ready, I would have had a much better delivery."

Further research on the Strategizing Safety basic social process should be done to validate this as a rural concern for other health conditions besides obstetrics. Do rural farmers also strategize safety if they have cancer? Do rural families strategize safety if a family member has special needs? Furthermore, do pregnant women living in poverty in suburban areas or the inner city also engage in strategizing safety if the only hospital to provide indigent care requires a 1-hour journey on three crosstown buses? Do they also experience the "1 hour of worry"? How and when do they strategize safety for their babies?

CONCLUSION

Ultimately it is the family's choice to live in rural areas with all the attendant advantages and disadvantages. Because of this choice, rural women understand they are responsible to strategize the safety of their families and babies. Even though their 1 hour of worry influences their health care decisions for the 9 months of pregnancy, the women in this study believed the trade-off was worth it. "It's like having your own path to heaven" to live in a rural area according to one mother:

> But I think I just love being up here so much better . . . it's still worth it. The drive is still worth it. I wouldn't move down there just to get closer to medical care . . . But it would be wonderful if we had someplace close to go for prenatal and postpartum care here at our [own] hospital.

REFERENCES

Bushy, A. (1994). When your client lives in a rural area: Part I. Rural health care delivery issues. *Issues in Mental Health Nursing, 15,* 253–266.

California Department of Health Services. (2000a). *Comprehensive perinatal services program (CPSP).* Retrieved December 24, 2000, from http://www. dhs.ca.gov/prp/mchb/Comprehensive_Perinatal.htm

California Department of Health Services. (2000b). *Federal performance measures.* Retrieved December 24, 2000, from http://www.dhs.ca.gov/prp/mchb/Federal_Performance_Measures.htm

California Department of Health Services. (2000c). *Outcomes measures.* Retrieved December 24, 2000, from http://www.dhs.ca.gov/prp/mchb/Outcomes_Measures.htm

Centers for Disease Control. (2000). 16—Maternal, Infant, and Child Health. *Healthy People 2010.* Retrieved September 7, 2004, from http://www.healthypeople.gov/document/HTML/Volume2/16MICH.htm

Conrad, J., Hollenbach, K. A., Fullerton, J. T., & Feigelson, H. S. (1998). Use of perinatal services by Hispanic women in San Diego County: A comparison of urban and rural settings. *Journal of Nurse Midwifery, 43,* 90–96.

Glaser, B. G. (1978). *Theoretical sensitivity.* Mill Valley, CA: Sociology Press.

Hoffmaster, J. E. (1986). Rural maternity services: Community health nurse providers. *Journal of Community Health Nursing, 3,* 25–33.

Mariposa County Health Department. (1999). *Family Health Outcomes Project (FHOP) report.* Mariposa, CA: Author.

McManus, M. A., & Newacheck, P. W. (1989). Rural maternal, child, and adolescent health. *Health Services Research, 23,* 807–848.

Patterson, E. T., Freese, M. P., & Goldenberg, R. L. (1990). Seeking safe passage: Utilizing health care during pregnancy. *Image—the Journal of Nursing Scholarship, 22,* 27–31.

QSR NVivo™. (2000). Qualitative data analysis software program (Version 1.2) [Computer software]. Melbourne, Australia: QSR International Pty Ltd.

Rubin, R. (1961). Basic maternal behavior. *Nursing Outlook, 9,* 683–686.

Rubin, R. (1967a). Attainment of the maternal role: Part I. Processes. *Nursing Research, 16,* 237–245.

Rubin, R. (1967b). Attainment of the maternal role: Part II. Models and referrants. *Nursing Research, 16,* 342–346.

Rubin, R. (1975). Maternal tasks of pregnancy. *Maternal-Child Nursing Journal, 4,* 143–153.

West, K. (2001). *Strategizing safety: Perinatal experiences of women in a rural California county.* Unpublished master's thesis, Azusa Pacific University, Azusa, CA.

West, K. (2006). Strategizing safety: Perinatal experiences of rural women. In H. J. Lee & C. A. Winters (Eds.), *Rural nursing: Concepts, theory, and practice* (2nd ed., pp. 96–109). New York: Springer Publishing.

14

Remodeling the Course of Life: Moving On in a Changed Life

MILKA SATINOVIC

Knowledge about peoples' own subjective experience of living a life with multiple sclerosis (MS) is of particular importance in nursing care, medical treatment, rehabilitation, and health care planning. There are, however, shortcomings concerning a deeper understanding of quality of life (QOL) as a process in which persons are active participants who meet life's ups and downs and solve problems in their own way.

Questions about what a good life is like and how to live a good life are particularly important when we speak of a chronic illness like MS. Most scientific investigations on QOL have been done through quantitative approach QOL measurements (Benito-Leon, Morales, Rivera-Navarro, & Mitchell, 2003; McCabe & De Judicibus, 2005; Nortvedt & Riise, 2003). QOL measurements show that people living with MS report lower QOL than people with other chronic illnesses. Studies on quality of life using qualitative research (Reynolds & Prior, 2003; Russell, White, & White, 2006; Somerset, Sharp, & Campbell, 2002) give us a nuanced picture of life with MS, shifting between a health and an illness perspective (Paterson, 2001, 2003), and of different strategies used to live a life that is as good as possible (Kralik, Koch, & Eastwood, 2003).

In this study, Remodeling the Course of Life (RCL), I report how participants with MS try to generate a good life while living with this chronic disease. This process has four phases: *keeping up normal life, moving on in a changed life, doing the best in a changed life,* and *preventing illness from controlling life* (Satinovic, 2008). The purpose of this chapter is to describe and discuss the second phase of the remodeling process, moving on in a changed life, which appeared to be a turning point in the process of RCL.

THE STUDY

Aim

The aim of the study was to obtain deeper insight into the experience of living as good a life as possible with an MS diagnosis.

Method

Grounded theory (GT), as described by Glaser and Strauss (1968) and Glaser (1978), was used in this study. In accordance with the methodology, the researcher searched the data for elements that the participants experienced as challenges in life with this serious chronic illness, and how they handled these challenges.

Sample

Participants were a convenience sample of Norwegian people who were (a) diagnosed with MS with any variations in functional status, type of illness, or gender, (b) 18 years and older, and (c) without psychiatric diagnosis.

Data Collection and Analysis

Data collection was done through qualitative interviews and participant observation. Interviewees were recruited from three different health care settings: a rehabilitation unit, people who were in contact with an MS nurse, and people who attended an MS course. Participant observation at five courses for people with an MS diagnosis generated the field notes. Twenty-one interviews, carried out with 17 participants diagnosed with MS, were conducted by the researcher and lasted about 2 hours. They were tape recorded and transcribed verbatim. Analytical procedures, moving from raw data to developed theory, were: open coding, constant comparison, memo writing, saturation, searching for the core category, theoretical coding, and sorting and writing up the theory.

Ethical Considerations

The research protocol was approved by the Regional Medical Research Ethics Committee of Norway. The head nurse at the rehabilitation unit approached patients from that unit who fulfilled the inclusion criteria, to obtain their consent to be interviewed and tape recorded at that unit. The MS nurse at The National Competence Centre for MS asked people who were in touch with her to participate. All those who agreed to participate were contacted by the researcher; interview schedules and written consents were obtained. Attendees at the MS course were invited to participate, and consents were obtained.

FINDINGS

The main concern reported by participants was how to live as good a life as possible with MS. This challenge was resolved through a process consisting of four phases, in which the person tried to remodel the course of life: *keeping up a normal life, moving on in a changed life, doing the best in a changed life,* and *preventing illness from controlling life.* The second phase, *moving on in a changed life,* is the focus of this chapter (see Figure 14.1).

Remodeling the Course of Life is a process through which challenges of sudden change in the course of life are handled, which leads to an experience of a good life with MS. When remodeling is difficult to achieve or absent, suffering and even suicidal thoughts can dominate life. Keeping up normal life as it was before the diagnosis continues as long as the illness is stable and invisible. When the state of health deteriorates, the person will be compelled, more or less, to be open about the illness, and will start to adjust to the fact that it influences life considerably. A transition to a new phase will take place. When the illness suddenly becomes visible, the person can be forced to disclose the illness—so to speak, to get out of the closet. In other situations the transition to a new phase moves slowly as a person gains the understanding that normalizing strategies take most of one's energy and that there is little left to life enjoyment.

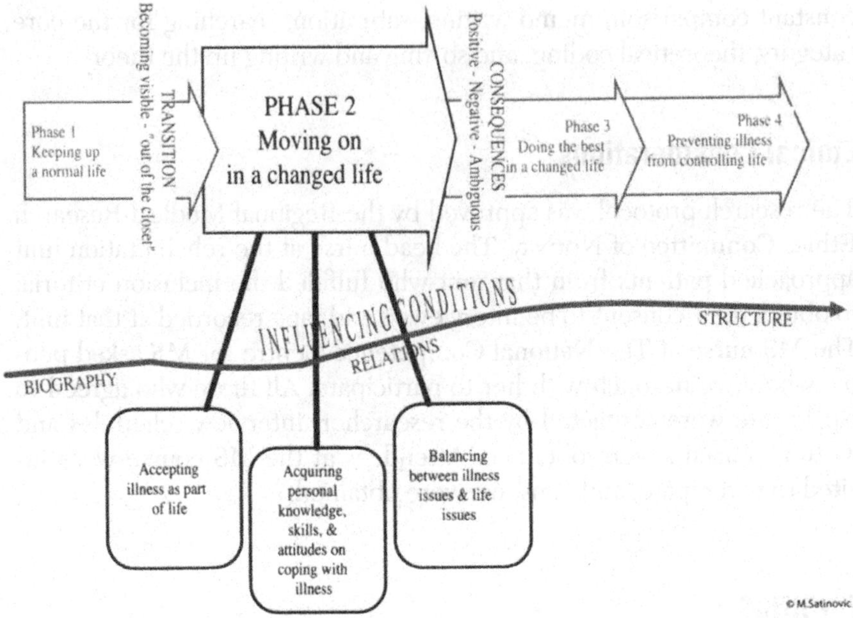

Figure 14.1 Moving On in a Changed Life.
Printed with permission from M. Satinovic.

Moving On in a Changed Life

In this phase, the problem is no longer fear of loss of a normal life but fear of what has to be changed in life, how it can be done, when it has to be done, and what consequences it will have for one's course of life and life enjoyment. The concept of life with MS that was expressed by participants was, "I have MS but I can live a good life if I take MS demands into consideration." The strategies they used to move on in a changed life are: *accepting illness as a part of life; acquiring personal knowledge, skills, and attitudes on coping with MS;* and *balancing between illness issues and life issues.*

Accepting: "You Have to See Life From a Different Perspective"

Accepting the fact that the illness is a part of life seems to be the turning point to the process of Remodeling the Course of Life. If the person cannot accept the illness and necessary changes related to it, he or she will always long for the earlier course of life. This position will hinder handling illness and generating a good life with illness in the long run.

Accepting the illness as a part of life is a process that requires time, energy, experience, and understanding. "I have used three years to accept it to a certain extent, at least that I have MS and that it affects my life considerably" are the words that illustrate the problem which the individual encounters. A chronic illness like MS affects nearly all aspects of life, physically, psychosocially, and existentially. "You lose so much, but you can also get new values by looking at life in a different way, from a different perspective" are statements that express some of the complexity of remodeling the course of life. Accepting the illness is an important step on the road in a remodeling process.

The fact that the individual accepts the illness is not enough. Relationships at home, at work, and in society affect the process. "I think that I can live a good life with MS." But it also has to do with how others experience it. One person illustrates this point in the following words: "My wife accepts it in a way, but in another way she does not accept it." A young man had the same kind of experience with his friends: "They accept the diagnosis, but they don't understand that I can't participate late in the evening because I get tired." Also, coworkers can have a problem realizing what it really means to live with MS even if they accept that the person has the illness. The extent of MS fatigue can be difficult for others to grasp. The expectation that a person should be able to do more than is actually possible can lead to misunderstandings and negative repercussions in the workplace. Clearly, other peoples' views or attitudes toward MS can hinder the personal process of acceptance.

Acquiring Competence: "You Have to Learn to Tackle the Illness"

The second strategy used to move on in a changed course of life is *acquiring personal knowledge, attitudes, and skills* to cope with various MS-related problems within different life domains. It may be important to develop skills to administer medication, to perform self-catheterization, and to use a wheelchair or a car. In addition, one also has to change a negative attitude toward self-catheterization or using a wheelchair. The move implies the shift from seeing the wheelchair as the worst-case scenario to seeing it as a useful means to gain control and be mobile. Competence develops through a variety of means, such as learning by one's own experience, receiving advice from health personnel and others with MS, and through MS courses, rehabilitation, printed materials, and other resources. To be competent means to know one's limits and how long one can stretch the limits of activity. The individual must learn how to prioritize activities and choose how to spend limited energy. The following quotation illustrates the need for development of personal competence: "I was at the seminar about economizing of energy. I didn't get the answer there, but I have found it on my own." One informant described the process in this way, "Nobody can take care of your life during the day; it's only you who can do it. You can ask for advice, but you have to do it yourself."

Thus, acquiring personal competence is a complex and difficult process that takes time and energy and implies much interaction with health care personnel, relatives, other people with MS, and people in general. Acquiring personal competence seems to be crucial in generating a good life with MS.

Balancing: "You have to Balance Between Illness Issues and Life Enjoyment"

As the illness becomes an accepted part of life and the capability to handle problems related to MS improves, the focus changes to a balancing process. The central challenge is to balance between illness issues and life enjoyment. One informant described how she tried to seek balance: "It's important to me to find a balance, so that I don't get sick again and get a new attack. At the same time, I want to do as much as I can at home."

Beginning to use a wheelchair at the right time, not too early or not too late, requires realistic personal assessment. "I have an application for a wheelchair at home, so that I can send it when I want to. But now I feel better, so I will wait." Another participant shared her conscious choice about work. She was forced to choose between her job and disability benefits during a meeting with the insurance office. She stated the reason for her decision: "It's very important to have a job. I could have disability benefits, but I have such an interesting job. So I had to decide: either disability benefits or the job. I chose the job. It is important to have a job you like."

Her story shows how difficult it may be to implement balancing in real life because of the strict rules on disability benefits. Another example is about deciding to give up work, even if on a voluntary basis, and how this led to an experience of relief. The right decision for the individual will vary, depending on the illness type and severity, personal values, and biography on one hand, and the structural conditions, such as welfare, on the other hand. Engaging with too many different persons at different community offices and having too few opportunities of choice between job or disability benefits, or a job-disability combination, can make a process of change difficult to achieve in a satisfying way. Taboos about the diagnosis in the community, at work, or in society in general, may also hinder or delay a person's acceptance of the illness and development of capabilities to tackle illness-related problems and issues.

Consequences of Moving On in a Changed Course of Life

The consequences of *moving on in a changed course of life* are sometimes positive, sometimes negative, and sometimes ambiguous. In the study, positive consequences were described as a better relationship with a spouse, with neighbors, or with coworkers. Other positive consequences included openness, knowledge, and understanding about the illness. Openness can clear the way for relationships with other people for patients who have "invisible" MS, a mild form with symptoms that are invisible to others. During the process of change people can experience growth and development. One patient said, "You have been forced to make up your mind on what to get out of your life." This described how change resulted in personal development even if one was forced to it. Then conscious choices about self-care to address illness were no longer experienced as a threat but as a possibility. One young participant described how he had thought that using a wheelchair or doing self-catheterization would reflect defeat and lower self-esteem. After he started using these devices, he saw them instead as possibilities for choices of when and how to use energy for what was needed or desired.

Losing one's job is a negative consequence of change, because having a job is not only about economic issues. When one loses a job, the loss is more than economy; the loss includes friendships, self-identity, and a social life.

Accepting the change is a turning point in the process of Remodeling the Course of Life with MS. Accepting change in the course of life opens up many doors and introduces the opportunity to test one's own capabilities. The more accepting persons with MS become, the more readily they can embrace the next phase, which is *doing the best in a changed course of life.*

Conditions Influencing the Process of Remodeling

The process of Remodeling the Course of Life is influenced by the life context of the person, such as biography, relations, and structural conditions.

The extent to which these conditions promote or delay the remodeling process will vary among persons and situations.

Biography

The influence of one's biography is related to the person's current stage of life, to personal values, and to experience. The person's life situation will decide which factors have to be remodeled. A person who is diagnosed with MS later in life, with a job and a family, will have different problems and remodeling challenges than those of a youth in the middle of his or her education.

An optimistic, inquiring, and creative approach to the necessary changes appears to promote the process of Remodeling the Course of Life. Examples of this attitude include cracking jokes about how bad it is to sit in a wheelchair, and doing crossword puzzles to delay loss of memory. To be stuck in a depression too long, or continuing to long for what is lost, keeps the focus on the problem, and contributes little to the remodeling process.

Relations

Important relations are those people who are close, like a lover, spouse, family, and friends. Their contribution is crucial when it comes to promoting or delaying the person's efforts in the remodeling process. Reactions such as overacting, making the situation taboo in conversation, showing pity, and stigmatizing may have a negative effect and delay the remodeling process. Parents may cause a delay by treating their adult daughter or son like a child, and making decisions on her or his behalf. On the other hand, people who are close may promote the process by supporting the individual's efforts to cope with the problems of the remodeling process, by helping to tackle grief, or by affirming the individual's ability to make choices concerning activity, lifestyle, or profession.

Structure

Structural conditions that can affect the process of remodeling are treatment options, attitudes and knowledge of MS in the health service and in society at large, the welfare situation, and accessibility of resources. When a disease-modifying treatment such as interferon was offered to a wide range of people with MS, it brought about many structural changes.

These included a new schedule of regular appointments, new training, and other new concerns. In this way structural change in treatment contributed to improved care and increased activity in follow-up.

Summary

The process of remodeling varies concerning use of time, effort, and extent. For some persons, remodeling may be a relatively brief experience; for others, it may take longer. Some people will feel they have to remodel over and over again. The extent of the process of remodeling will also vary; it may be minor with a mild type of MS, or major in the situation of progressive MS. Furthermore, the remodeling process may vary between being a time of personal growth and development and being painful and difficult. The most painful, difficult, and time-consuming phase appears to be phase 2.

Successful remodeling is crucial for living a good life with MS. A person who does not succeed in the process may feel controlled by the illness. For that person, loneliness, depression, and suicidal thoughts may become a part of daily life.

DISCUSSION

Phase 2 in the process of Remodeling the Course of Life is about moving on from a normal life to a life with MS and can be compared with the findings of Kralik et al. (2003) on transition. These researchers found that "the transition is not simply the change, but rather the process that people go through to incorporate the change or disruption into their lives" (p. 324). According to them, the transition process involves (a) the movement between the two points, (b) the transformation either as incorporation, integration, or adaptation, and (c) a process of inner reorientation. They found that the process takes time and comprises personal, relational, and environmental change. These findings are similar to those of the current study. The remodeling process has many similarities to the transition process. It begins with keeping up a normal life as long as possible and moves on when illness worsens and becomes visible, demanding increased energy in order to maintain a normal life.

Eventually, persons with MS are forced to change and move on into the next phase. They do this by accepting the illness as a part of life, by acquiring the knowledge, skills, and attitudes to handle MS, and by balancing between illness issues and life issues. In this way, they develop mastery over a changed life and form a new basis for a good life. The process of remodeling ultimately differs from the process of transition described above in that it comprises more than a shift from one point to another. For a person living with progressive MS, the process of remodeling implies adjusting to a new set of conditions and goals over and over again. In other words, remodeling continues throughout life as health and illness fluctuate (Thorne & Paterson, 1998, 2000). Phases in the process of remodeling overlap each other, and it seems that movement occurs both forward and backward, depending on the context and the situation. For example, persons with MS may be open about illness with their nearest relations, but still conceal the illness from an employer.

The process of remodeling is promoted or prohibited by personal biography, relations, and structural conditions. The knowledge of the process of remodeling is crucial for nurses working with people with MS and other chronic illnesses, because they can facilitate the process by giving support of the right kind and at the right time.

Walker (2004) suggests a model of readiness for change in order to understand life-altering events such as becoming a teenage parent, living with HIV/AIDS, or growing older. Readiness for change consists of three elements: (a) facing uncertainty, (b) accepting changes, and (c) doing what is possible. The process of remodeling shares these elements, but it also adds a new element: preventing the illness from controlling life when it progresses and threatens to dominate life.

The main challenge that people with MS in this study experienced was fear of sudden change in the course of life. This challenge can be compared with the concept of uncertainty (Walker, 2004). Fearing loss of a normal life, job, friends, life evolvement, and one's self-concept corresponds to Walker's concept of "facing uncertainty" (2004, p. 5). According to Walker, people are better prepared for uncertainties after they have evaluated their fear of inevitable life events and processes. The study presented in this chapter confirms his proposition. Individuals' awareness of future uncertainties and the fear of their consequences were strongly present in my data from people with MS. Accepting changes represents a turning point in moving on in a changed course of life for people with MS. My findings correspond with Walker's proposition that people are more likely to take responsible actions when they accept changes in physical appearance, social roles, and abilities.

Readiness for change is attained when people know what to do and do what they can, or as Walker puts it, when they are "doing what's possible." People with MS work on readiness to change by developing personal knowledge, skills, and attitudes to manage MS related issues and establish a balance between illness issues and life issues.

CONCLUSION

Moving on into a changed course of life is phase 2 in the developed substantive theory of Remodeling the Course of Life as a means to a good life with MS (Satinovic, 2008). There is evidence for the usefulness of this concept when comparing it to the concept of "transition" (Kralik et al., 2003) and the concept "readiness for change" (Walker, 2004). In addition, the developed substantive theory can be used in nursing practice to assist persons with MS to facilitate a life that is as good as possible (see chapter 24, "An Intervention Program Using Remodeling the Course of Life Theory Among Persons With Multiple Sclerosis").

REFERENCES

Benito-Leon, J., Morales, J. M., Rivera-Navarro, J., & Mitchell, A. (2003). A review about the impact of multiple sclerosis on health-related quality of life. *Disability & Rehabilitation, 25*, 1291–1303.

Glaser, B. G. (1978). *Theoretical sensitivity: Advances in the methodology of grounded theory.* Mill Valley, CA: Sociology Press.

Glaser, B. G., & Strauss, A. L. (1968). *The discovery of grounded theory: Strategies for qualitative research.* London: Weidenfeld and Nicholson.

Kralik, D., Koch, T., & Eastwood, S. (2003). The salience of the body: Transition in sexual self-identity for women living with multiple sclerosis. *Journal of Advanced Nursing, 42*(1), 11–20.

McCabe, M. P., & De Judicibus, M. (2005). The effects of economic disadvantage on psychological well-being and quality of life among people with multiple sclerosis. *Journal of Health Psychology, 10*(1), 163–173.

Nortvedt, M. W., & Riise, T. (2003). The use of quality of life measures in multiple sclerosis research. *Multiple Sclerosis,* 9(1), 63.

Paterson, B. (2001). Myth of empowerment in chronic illness. *Journal of Advanced Nursing, 34*, 574–581.

Paterson, B. L. (2003). The koala has claws: Applications of the Shifting Perspectives Model in research of chronic illness. *Qualitative Health Research, 13*(7), 987–994.

Reynolds, F., & Prior, S. (2003). "Sticking jewels in your life": Exploring women's strategies for negotiating an acceptable quality of life with multiple sclerosis. *Qualitative Health Research, 13*(9), 1225–1251.

Russell, C. S., White, M. B., & White, C. P. (2006). Why me? Why now? Why multiple sclerosis? Making meaning and perceived quality of life in a midwestern sample of patients with multiple sclerosis. *Families, Systems & Health, 24,* 65–81.

Satinovic, M. (2008). *Omlegging av livskurs, en grunnleggende prosess i et godt liv med multippel sklerose.* Bergen: Universitetet i Bergen.

Somerset, M., Sharp, D., & Campbell, R. (2002). Multiple sclerosis and quality of life: A qualitative investigation. *Journal of Health Services Research and Policy, 7*(3), 151–159.

Thorne, S. E., & Paterson, B. L. (1998). Shifting images of chronic illness. *Image: Journal of Nursing Scholarship, 30*(2), 173–178.

Thorne, S. E., & Paterson, B. L. (2000). Two decades of insider research: What we know and don't know about chronic illness experience. *Annual Review of Nursing Research, 18,* 3–25.

Walker, C. A. (2004). Change readiness: A construct to explain health and life transitions. *Journal of Theory Construction & Testing, 8*(1), 26–33.

II Cutting Point

INTRODUCTION: BARBARA M. ARTINIAN

The theoretical code of cutting point can be described as an event or decision that provides direction for the actions that follow. This critical juncture or benchmark is a turning point in a response to a situation.

This section includes two studies that have decision points marking clear-cut turning points. Vuckovich studied the process of giving medications to psychiatric patients. If the patients refused the medication, the nurse reached a cutting point of deciding if she would further engage with the patient. If the activities of engagement failed, a second cutting point was reached (*impasse*) and coercive actions were needed. The main concern of the nurses was to have a therapeutic alliance with the patient and they resolved their concern by the core category of Justifying Coercion (see chapter 15).

The second study was conducted by Artinian and Hecox among patients with COPD who were trying to manage their chronic disease. Participants in the study experienced two major cutting points. The first benchmark marked the point of downward progression into helplessness when they were forced to leave their former way of life. The second cutting point marked a point of ascent to regaining control by a decision to accept responsibility for their lives. This decision brought them back to a form of life in which they could do the things that were important to them (see chapter 16, "Regaining Control: Managing Changes in Chronic Obstructive Pulmonary Disease").

Understanding various cutting points of decision-making or life events is important for nurses who assist patients in managing chronic illnesses or who deal with patients who are in need of regimen management.

15 Justifying Coercion

PAULA VUCKOVICH
BARBARA M. ARTINIAN

The first author has long been interested in the problems of recidivism and concerned about how nurses manage to develop therapeutic alliances in the context of involuntary care. In her experience, psychiatric nurses are very good at getting their patients, even the involuntary ones, to understand the importance of taking their medication. To better understand this, she began a grounded theory study on the experiences of nurses administering medication to involuntary psychiatric patients. She expected to discover what nurses were doing right. In her study she found no universal process for getting patients to accept medication. Although the nurses in the study were practicing in the framework of Peplau's (1952/1991) nurse-patient relationship, their interventions were as individual as each nurse-patient dyad. There was no one right way. What she did uncover, however, was a basic social process (BSP) (Glaser, 1978, 1992, 1998) that nurses used when, in spite of their best efforts, they were unable to convince patients "desperately in need of medication" to take medication voluntarily. This was the process of Justifying Coercion.

Use of coercive power overtly violates the nurse's understanding of the proper nurse-patient relationship. Nursing is based on the premise that the nurse provides care at the patient's instigation, not that the nurse forces care on an unwilling recipient. The American Nurses Association (ANA) (2001) *Code of Ethics* and standards of psychiatric nursing practice (2000) state that coercion is to be avoided and patients are to participate in decisions about their own care to the extent possible. The participants in the study, like other nurses studied (Smith & Godfrey, 2002), wished to see themselves as "good nurses" and "doing the right thing."

When administering medication involuntarily, psychiatric nurses are confronted with an ethical dilemma. In Western society, autonomy, self-responsibility, and informed consent are valued and supported by law (Aiken, 1994). Beneficence is also valued and is one of the primary values of nurses (Aiken, 1994; Davis, Aroskar, Liaschenko, & Drought, 1997). When beneficence and autonomy are in conflict and coercion is necessary for beneficence, nurses need a way to resolve the conflict and retain their self-esteem. They experience a need to justify their actions both ethically and legally. In California, involuntary medication can only be given in a psychiatric emergency when someone is in imminent danger of physical harm or after a capacity hearing in which the person is judged to lack capacity to consent to psychotropic medication (Los Angeles County, 1998). Except in psychiatric emergencies, nurses only administer medication involuntarily if there has been due legal process and the hearing officer is satisfied that the legal criteria have been met.

Justifying was the label used for providing self and others sufficient lawful and ethical reasons for an act. In accepting and remaining in positions where patients were involuntarily detained, participants had determined that involuntary treatment in itself was ethically acceptable to them. The conflict that arose was whether such treatment was legal and ethical for a particular patient. The code *coercion* indicated "the act of compelling a person by lawful authority or physical force to do what that person was refusing to do." *Coercive acts* are those acts that result in the person's forced acceptance of treatment.

THE STUDY

Method

The study was conducted using the grounded theory methodology described by Glaser (1978, 1992, 1998). Each step of the research was reviewed by an expert grounded theorist and discussed in a peer group of grounded theory researchers to ensure methodological rigor. Two psychiatric nursing experts reviewed the findings for credibility.

Participants

Unstructured audiotaped interviews were conducted with 17 California psychiatric nurses. All nurses involved in the study were from a single state to ensure uniformity of the legal processes governing involuntary hospitalization and involuntary administration of medication. All were employed in psychiatric facilities that admitted involuntary patients.

Data Collection and Analysis

Transcripts of the interviews, the researcher's memos regarding observations, interviews and conversations, transcripts of working sessions of the grounded theory research group, theoretical memos written after consultation with an expert grounded theorist, written comments of the psychiatric nursing experts, and literature reviewed after the theory began to take shape were the data used in analysis. All data were reviewed line-by-line and coded concept-by-concept using NVIVO™ software. Analysis included constant comparison of interviews, codes, and concepts. The research process was captured in numerous memos, which created an auditable record of the ongoing analysis. Although there were data generated regarding techniques the nurses used to reach agreement it became clear that what was emerging was not a social process of reaching medication adherence but something entirely different. Grounded theory methodology is a process that uncovers ways people deal with a situation that is of concern to them, and how it is resolved (Glaser, 1978, 1998). Success in getting a patient to agree that medication was necessary was not problematic; failure was. As the interviews progressed a core category emerged which was labeled Justifying Coercion. Interviews continued over a period of 2 years until saturation was reached with no new data on justifying coercion and all identified concepts explained by justifying coercion.

In grounded theory, a basic social process (BSP) is a core category with at least two clear emergent stages "that differentiate and account for variations in a problematic pattern of behavior" (Glaser, 1978, p. 97). The transition from one stage to another is ordinarily contingent upon one or more things happening. This contingency may be in the form of a cutting point—a theoretical code indicating a point in time when the occurrence or nonoccurrence of a particular critical event will determine whether a new stage is entered (Glaser, 1998, 2005).

Ethical Considerations

The study proposal was approved by the Committee on the Protection of Human Subjects at the University of San Diego. All participants gave informed consent. All data were kept confidential and were destroyed upon completion of the study.

FINDINGS

Justifying Coercion in involuntary administration of medication (Vuckovich, 2003) is the process that the 17 nurses interviewed used to resolve the conflict between ideal treatment and actual patient care. The process has three stages and two cutting points. The stages are *assessment of need, negotiation,* and *justifying and taking coercive action.* The cutting points are *decision to engage* and *impasse* (see Figure 15.1).

Stage 1: Assessment of Need

In the first stage of the process, assessment of need, the nurses considered severity of illness and danger to the patient. The nurses truly valued patient autonomy and patients' rights. One said,

> The problem is how you balance the patient's rights thing and how you balance someone's ability to make a decision for their own self. And that's very, very difficult because basically you are saying he or she can't make the decision for themselves and that's always a tough thing. But you know that if they take medications they'll be a lot better and they'll be grateful, you think.

They prided themselves on quickly acting as advocates to get unnecessary involuntary hospitalizations resolved by getting the hold revoked and the patient either discharged or converted to a voluntary status. They reported that they listen to the patient's accounts of experiences with medication and advocate for the patient with the psychiatrist for management of side effects or a change in prescribed medication. Often the nurses are not convinced that coercion will be necessary. They work on establishing a nurse-patient relationship and convincing the patient that they have the patient's best interests in mind. They believe that if they give a patient time and space and attend to the patient's concerns most of the time the patient will come to see that medication is required.

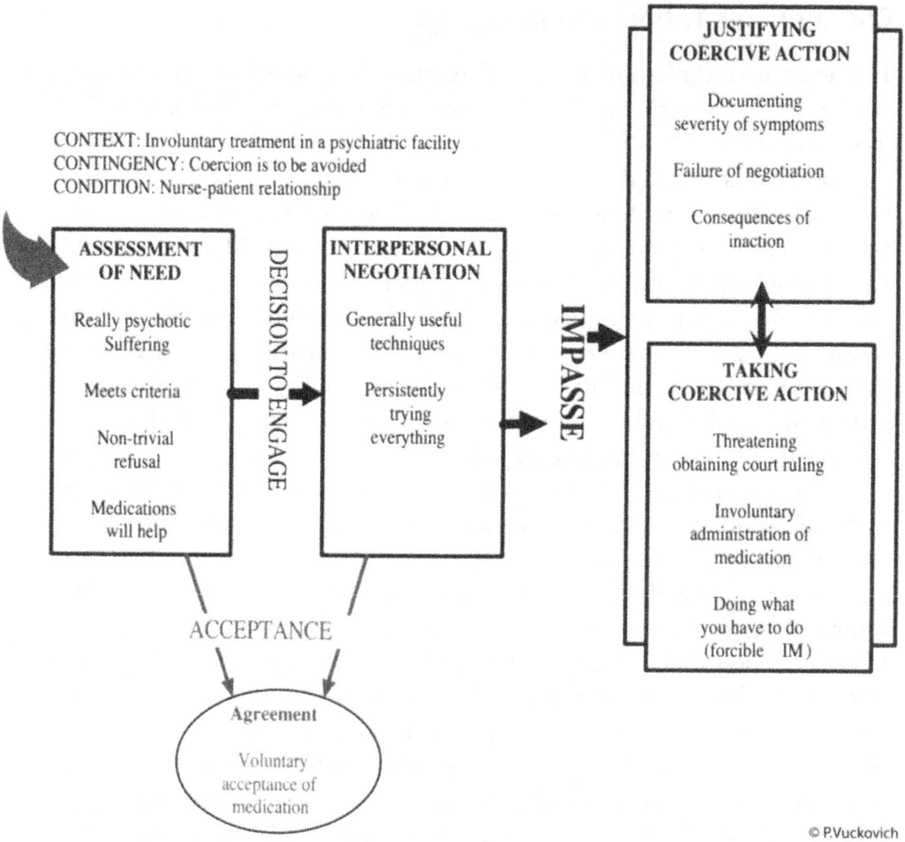

Figure 15.1 Justifying Coercion in involuntary administration of medication. Printed with permission from P. Vuckovich.

At this point many patients take medication as prescribed and are no longer problematic for the nurse.

Only for the "really psychotic," "really delusional," and "really dangerous" do the nurses assess that there may be a need for coercion. They talked of patients experiencing self-degradation and being tormented by hallucinations. They talked of danger to the patient and others. The word most frequently used to describe the seriousness of the situation was "really": really psychotic, really dangerous, really desperate. They emphasized the fact that once the patients were medicated, "They do get better." "It's miraculous, really, to see the change." They were convinced that antipsychotic medications were good and unremitting psychosis was bad for patients. They thought it was dangerous to leave certain patients unmedicated.

Cutting Point 1: Decision to Engage

However, in order to ensure ethical practice the assessment of need must be done for each individual patient and each separate coercive act. Once it was established to a nurse's satisfaction that need existed, the first cutting point was reached and decision was made about whether or not to work with the patient in a special way. The *decision to engage* makes the process of justifying coercion personal and individual as opposed to perfunctory. If the nurse does not decide to engage, he or she will continue to do the necessary teaching and documentation of responses required by law. However consideration of the justification for coercing that individual will be left to another nurse or the psychiatrist. Some nurses acknowledged avoiding very resistant patients or transferring or delegating their care to someone else.

When limitations of time or failure to establish a connection to a particular patient made it impossible to engage, the nurses felt guilty and/or frustrated because they were participating in actions that were not completely justified in their minds. Many of their stories were about interrupting a coercive action in progress and intervening in ways that made coercion unnecessary. A decision to engage means a commitment of time and energy to working with an individual patient to establish a working agreement on the necessity of treatment and thus avoid coercion. Hess (1996) indicates that engagement, which brings the patient's voice into the decisions about treatment, is an ideal rather than an obligation or duty. Engagement means the nurse *actively* embarks on the next stage of the process: *negotiation.*

Stage 2: Negotiation

The stage of *negotiation* involves all the generally helpful nurse-patient interactions that are designed to help a patient understand the situation and get the most out of the hospital experience. The aim is to reach a viable agreement on treatment. If routine interactions do not suffice, these interactions and every other technique that the nurse has in his or her repertoire are repeated over and over until the patient either comes to agree and coercion is unnecessary or the patient and nurse reach the next critical juncture: *impasse.* The agreement the nurse is ultimately seeking is not simply acquiescence to accepting a pill this one time, it is an agreement that the medication is necessary for the patient's well-being and should be continued even after the patient is no longer involuntarily detained. In essence, the negotiation is a negotiation of the patient's understanding of having a mental illness that requires treatment. If this understanding is never reached, involuntary medication is not reasonable unless the patient is going to remain involuntary for a protracted time. Negotiation is limited by the nurse's expertise and experience, time available for individual interaction, the role of the nurse in the setting, the patient's symptoms, and the patient's willingness and ability to engage. Each nurse told proud stories of negotiations that achieved agreement and ended the process without coercion. It was clear that they were persistent and tenacious once they were engaged with the patient in negotiation.

The participants started by treating the resistant patient in the same manner that they treated any patient. Each nurse had preferred ways of initiating a relationship and doing medication education that they believed were generally successful. They modified their approaches depending on the response. If a nurse-patient relationship seemed to be developing in a therapeutic direction, or if the nurse was motivated by the suffering he or she observed, the nurse would intensify the effort and persistently try the same or additional techniques, hoping to reach agreement. The usually helpful technique included verbal interventions such as talking to, explaining, educating about their disease and condition, medication education, pointing out, limit setting, talking with, listening, persuading, offering options, and inducements. Nurses also reported nonverbal interventions such as giving time and space, spending time, coming back repeatedly, and staying with a patient for extended periods.

When no nurse on a unit made a decision to engage, negotiation was limited to the presenting of required medication information and offers of medication. Extensive negotiation is only undertaken when the nurse sees hope of a positive outcome and the patient's suffering or dangerousness impels the nurse to act. The nurse's belief in the efficacy of medication and the conviction that without medication a particular patient's life will be disastrous provides the motivation for negotiation, but only hope for eventual adherence maintains a noncoercive negotiation process over a long period of time.

Cutting Point 2: Impasse

When things came to a point that further negotiation appeared futile, impasse was reached. Impasse is the point at which it becomes clear that no matter what the nurse does there will be no voluntary agreement. Without reaching an impasse a nurse cannot legitimately go on to the final stage of *justifying and taking coercive action*. Thus this is a cutting point at which, without a certain condition, the process stops. If the patient agrees to take medication without coercion or the nurse did not perceive an ongoing or imminent danger and backed off, there was no impasse. A nurse said, "I think we have to respect a patient's decisions. If they are not really, really a potential danger to themselves, others or gravely disabled . . . I think we need to respect that and support that and try to make it happen." The nurses participated willingly in the next stage of the process when they were convinced that if the patient continued psychotic and was not medicated it would be significantly harmful to the patient and/or others.

Stage 3: Justifying and Taking Coercive Action

Justifying coercive action and *taking coercive action* are distinct subsections of the final stage but are so intrinsically linked both in time and behavior that they constitute a single stage. Framing nurse's notes to show incomprehension and psychotic resistance rather than reasonable doubts about necessity and efficacy is the beginning of coercive action. At times this beginning coercion is clear to both nurse and patient as the nurse tells the patient, "I'm going to chart that." Publicly justifying the need for coercive action in a written document or in testimony before a hearing officer is therefore in itself a coercive action.

Throughout the first two stages of the process, the nurses document every attempt to reach agreement and the results of each attempt. They also continuously document the patient's behavior and their assessment of the patient's psychiatric condition. Initially, part of their interaction is what they term "pointing out reality" during which they reiterate the circumstances of the patient's involuntary hospitalization and advise the patient of the legal situation. They advise the patient that accepting medication would better his or her situation, telling patients of the positive consequences of compliance and warning of the negative consequences of medication refusal.

Pointing out reality gradually begins to be more coercive, at times approaching threats as the nurses reiterate what they see as the truth. For example: "If you continue refusing medication the hearing officer is going to agree with the doctor and say you have to stay in the hospital." The nurses don't consider these statements threats. They call it persuasion. They have already justified in their own mind the need for the patient to comply. They would prefer that the patient understand the necessity of taking medication but they will settle for acceptance of the pills being offered. They wish to spare the patient the formal legal process and preserve the patient's dignity by allowing the patient to be the one who decides to comply. But most of all they wish to avoid forcible administration of medication.

The decision by the nurse to forcibly administer a medication is both an internal justification and an external act. "The words "Do it!" or "Now!" which often signal the team the decision has been made and it is time to take physical hold of a patient often follow so quickly on the decision that the justification and action are inseparable. Once the action has been taken, documentation of the justification continues in the medical record so that although internal justification precedes action, public and formal justification often follows action.

Even when a nurse has justified in her own mind and to the satisfaction of the legal system that a patient requires involuntary medication administration, the nurse will still negotiate for oral acceptance of medication. The nurse responsible for medication administration goes through the process in a truncated fashion every time medication is to be given. The participants felt that for patients to be held down and have garments removed to allow forcible administration of medication was the ultimate in humiliation. They did everything in their power to avoid this final level of coercion. If refusal persisted and forcible injection was required, the nurses attempted to do it as privately and gently as possible without punitive overtones. Many chose to stay with the patient after the event, assuring him or her that the intent was to help and the staff was not going to abandon him or her.

DISCUSSION AND IMPLICATIONS

Justifying Coercion is a process used by individuals and organizations when coercion, which is generally regarded as wrong by their culture, is the only feasible way to accomplish something that is seen as necessary. This study focused on involuntary administration of medication, but other forms of coercion used in the care of involuntary psychiatric patients were part of the data. The process of justifying all forms of coercion was the same. To justify coercion, the required condition is that the action to be taken must be considered beneficent and failing to take action grossly maleficent. There must be an expectation that the end result of the action will be good and not acting will cause significant harm. One nurse said,

> It's not that I want to force medications on people. It's just that the difference is so dramatic when you take medications. It ends the suffering. I mean the suffering, that's the bottom line, the suffering. It's inhumane not to give treatments to people when there's a high likelihood that one of these medications is going to at least help them get out of this acute state.

Nurses use coercion only as a last resort. When they find no need for coercion, or discover circumstances that increase the patient's resistance, they advocate for changes in the treatment plan or medication regimen that will promote patient autonomy and participation in the treatment plan. They see coercion as violating a patient's dignity and as disrespectful, violating the principles laid out in the *Code of Ethics* (ANA, 2001). The legal system uses a rights-based determination of justification for involuntary treatment and the nurses do their best to make sure that rights are not violated and that the criteria are met. However, nurses' discussions of using coercion reflected Olsen's (2003) relational approach to the ethics of forced treatment rather than a rights-based approach. They judged the necessity of involuntary treatment in the context of the nurse-patient relationship and worked to change a patient's status to voluntary if they believed it was warranted.

It is the decision to engage that creates an opportunity for the patient to have a voice in the decision making. The nurses were undisturbed by keeping a patient in treatment involuntarily if they saw the need, but profoundly disturbed when they had to use force in a way that disrupted their relationships with the patients. They were proud of their successes at avoiding coercion and felt a sense of failure when such avoidance was impossible. They did everything they could to mitigate coercive actions. Their intent, like the nurses in Olofsson and Norberg's studies (Olofsson, Gilge, Jacobsson, & Norberg, 1998; Olofsson & Norberg, 2001), was to mitigate the coerciveness by caring interactions before, during, and after a coercive act. The participants seemed to be more concerned about patient's rights and more likely to advocate against coercion than the nurses in Scandinavian studies (Hummelvoll & Severinsson, 2002; Olofsson et al., 1998; Olofsson & Norberg, 2001) but the attitudes toward protecting the patient's dignity and preserving the relationship appear to be much the same. In the United States the acceptance of the need for coercion is supported by the due process afforded by state laws. A nurse described this acceptance:

> I don't have much question or doubt or concern about the Riese (California's name for the hearing for capacity to consent to medication). If the doctor

would go all the way, to have to go through the court—to go through so many steps to fight to get the patient to take medication, that pretty much says how much they think the patient needs medication. So I support that. I think it's being done appropriately and it's necessary.

CONCLUSION

Justifying Coercion is a process that psychiatric nurses use to reconcile themselves to the use of involuntary procedures when the symptoms of psychotic illness make it impossible to rely on a therapeutic alliance. Even Hummelvoll (1996), who advocates for the nurse-client alliance model, says that sometimes it is necessary to use "genuine paternalism" and "caring deprivation of liberty" (Hummelvoll & Severinsson, 2002) to treat those psychiatric patients that truly lack the capacity to consent. Coercion is undesirable but sometimes necessary. Psychiatric nurses in this study prided themselves on using their relationship and negotiating skills to avoid coercion but suffered ethical distress and felt the need to justify their actions when avoidance was impossible.

There needs to be more guidance in psychiatric nursing for making the decision of when coercion is justified. Coercion should not be presented only as an ethical dilemma. If it is uniformly perceived as an unethical practice or as a failure of care as opposed to a reasonable choice when circumstances dictate its use, many caring and compassionate nurses will avoid practicing in involuntary psychiatric units. Involuntary units need to provide sufficient staff and enough support for nurses to engage with patients in protracted individual interaction so that genuine negotiation is possible. Perfunctory negotiation does both the patient and the nurse a disservice. Nurses who rarely or never have the opportunity to practice according to the standards of the profession either become disillusioned and leave, or develop into "bad" nurses who use coercion without adequate justification.

Further research into negotiation techniques and the circumstances that enable engagement with patients is necessary to answer the original question: How do psychiatric nurses avoid coercion? It is apparent from this study that the participants did avoid coercion on many occasions. They did not take coercion for granted as inevitable, but rather genuinely did their best to establish rapport, develop a trusting therapeutic relationship, and negotiate a mutual agreement on treatment.

Justifying Coercion is a BSP not limited to psychiatric nursing. Discussions with parents, pediatricians, and nonpsychiatric nurses working with both children and elderly adults regarding the research and whether the process applied to them was answered uniformly, "Oh yes." Throughout the period of research, and during the postdata analysis literature search that is part of the grounded theory methodology for integrating grounded theory into the existing body of knowledge (Glaser, 1978, 1992, 1998), the media were full of debates on the war on Iraq. The language and arguments used to justify war were very similar to those the nurses used to justify forcible medication administration, and the ethical literature regarding justifying war (Elshtain, 2003; Evans & Sahnoun, 2002; see Figure 15.2). The ethical literature revealed the same general process.

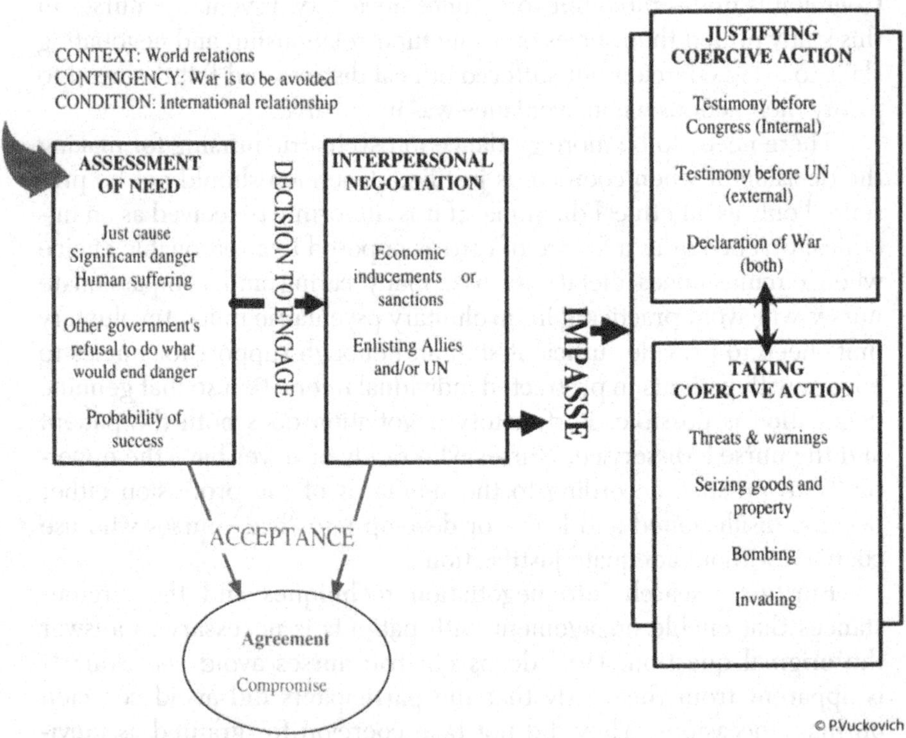

Figure 15.2 Justifying Coercion in war.
Printed with permission from P. Vuckovich.

REFERENCES

Aiken, T. D. (1994). *Legal, ethical and political issues in nursing.* Philadelphia: F. A. Davis.

American Nurses Association (ANA). (2000). *A statement on psychiatric-mental health clinical nursing practice and standards of psychiatric-mental health nursing practice.* Washington, DC: American Nurses Publishing.

American Nurses Association (ANA). (2001). *Code of ethics for nurses with interpretive statements.* Washington, DC: American Nurses Publishing.

Davis, A. J., Aroskar, M. A., Liaschenko, J., & Drought, S. (1997). *Ethical dilemmas and nursing practice* (4th ed.). Stamford, CT: Appleton & Lange.

Elshtain, J. B. (2003, 19 February). Will it be a "just war" or just a war? [Commentary]. *Los Angeles Times,* B15.

Evans, G., & Sahnoun, M. (2002). The responsibility to protect [Electronic version]. *Foreign Affairs, 81*(6), 99–111.

Glaser, B. G. (1978). *Theoretical sensitivity.* Mill Valley, CA: Sociology Press.

Glaser, B. G. (1992). *Basics of grounded theory analysis.* Mill Valley, CA: Sociology Press.

Glaser, B. G. (1998). *Doing grounded theory: Issues and discussions.* Mill Valley, CA: Sociology Press.

Glaser, B. G. (2005). *The grounded theory perspective III: Theoretical coding.* Mill Valley, CA: Sociology Press.

Hess, J. D. (1996). Ethics of compliance. *Advances in Nursing Science, 19*(1), 18–27.

Hummelvoll, J. K. (1996). The nurse-client alliance model. *Perspectives in Psychiatric Care, 32*(4), 12–20.

Hummelvoll, J. K., & Severinsson, E. (2002). Nursing staffs' perceptions of persons suffering from mania in acute psychiatric care. *Journal of Advanced Nursing, 38,* 416–424.

Los Angeles County Department of Mental Health. (1998). *LPS designation handbook.* Los Angeles: Author.

Olofsson, B., Gilge, F., Jacobsson, L., & Norberg, A. (1998). Nurses' narratives about using coercion in psychiatric care. *Journal of Advanced Nursing, 28,* 45–53.

Olofsson, B., & Norberg, A. (2001). Experiences of coercion in psychiatric care as narrated by patients, nurses, and physicians [Electronic version]. *Journal of Advanced Nursing, 33,* 89–97.

Olsen, D. P. (2003). Influence and coercion: Relational and rights-based ethical approaches to forced psychiatric treatment. *Journal of Psychiatric & Mental Health Nursing, 10,* 705–712.

Peplau, H. E. (1991) *Interpersonal relations in nursing.* New York: Springer Publishing. (Original work published in 1952).

Smith, K. V., & Godfrey, N. S. (2002). Being a good nurse and doing the right thing: A qualitative study. *Nursing Ethics, 9,* 301–312.

Vuckovich, P. K. (2003). *Justifying coercion: Nurses' experiences medicating involuntary psychiatric patients.* Doctoral dissertation, University of San Diego. *Dissertation Abstracts International, 64,* 1690B.

16 Regaining Control: Managing Changes in Chronic Obstructive Pulmonary Disease

BARBARA M. ARTINIAN
JUDITH MILLIGAN-HECOX

Today, chronic obstructive pulmonary disease (COPD) is one of our nation's rapidly growing health problems. It is a disease with severe social and economic impact. Management of this illness has been a tremendous challenge to health care providers. Goals of therapy have traditionally focused on reduction of airflow obstruction, prevention of complications, and improvement in the patient's quality of life. In addition, rehabilitation programs assist the patients to reach their highest level of health through education, accurate diagnosis, therapy, and emotional support.

In this paper, we report the theory of Regaining Control that describes how patients improve behavioral and psychosocial adaptation to the disease. Grounded theory (GT) researchers search for theoretical codes that can conceptualize and integrate a substantive theory (Glaser, 1978, 2005). In this study, the theoretical code *cutting point* was found to organize the data. Subjects in this study experienced two major cutting points—the benchmark event that forced them to leave their former way of life and the benchmark of accepting of responsibility for their lives, which led to the decision to *get with the program*. This brought them back to life, although in an altered form. The theoretical code of cutting point marked the point of downward progression into helplessness and exploring options and the point of ascent to regaining control by accepting the responsibility for change.

COPD encompasses a number of conditions, but the most common are bronchitis and emphysema (Schultz, 1994). Classic emphysema develops over many years and the effort to breathe increases so that breathing becomes a difficult chore. Dyspnea is the major factor that influences quality of life (Riley, 1996).

Pulmonary rehabilitation programs provide COPD patients the opportunity to receive therapy and treatment aimed at reduction of symptoms and increased participation in activities of daily living. For this study, patients from an inpatient hospital program were interviewed during their participation in the program or after their discharge. In this program the team implemented the therapy, treatments, training, and counseling necessary for the patients to initiate a change in lifestyle and most importantly to incorporate the changes on a long-term basis. The usual duration of the program was two to four weeks.

THE STUDY

Aim

The aim of this study was to learn how patients with COPD managed their disease.

Method

Classical GT was chosen as the method for this study (Glaser, 1978, 1998, 2001, 2005). In GT, data collection and analysis are performed concurrently. Parallel studies were conducted by the two authors, both using the discovery mode. Insights from the separate studies were shared in the form of memos.

Participants

The focus of the study was the program in a rehabilitation hospital in a southwestern state in the United States. The participants in the study were 10 subjects who had participated in the rehabilitation program at an earlier time and were currently in other programs and 24 patients currently participating in the rehabilitation or who had been discharged from that program within the previous year. The subjects were between the ages of 35 and 95, had the diagnosis of COPD, and spoke English.

The study included family members or significant others if they were available. In addition, the first author made observations several times a week over a 1-year period in the rehabilitation class held at the hospital.

Data Collection and Analysis

The first author transcribed the 10 tape-recorded interviews of former patients, and the second author transcribed the 24 tape-recorded interviews with recent patients. All observations in the rehabilitation classes and home settings were recorded in field notes. The interviews were analyzed initially by open coding with words such as *pacing* and *depending* occurring frequently. Selective coding began when the participant's main concern was found to be how they could again participate in society. Memos from both the interviews and the observations were written to aid in theoretical coding. For example, *losing control* was a memo that led to understanding how a subject could regain control. Data were tracked by computer and larger categories were constructed; patterns were searched for. By comparing similar incidents, basic properties of a category were defined and relationships among the categories were clarified.

Analysis by the two authors resulted in two separate theories. Artinian (1995) developed the theory of Regaining Control after prolonged ventilation. It had four phases: *glimmer of hope, getting with the program, accepting mentoring*, and *taking charge*. This paper was presented at the California Society of Pulmonary Rehabilitation at a conference in San Francisco. Milligan-Hecox developed the theory of Coming to Terms, which had the stages of *ignoring to normalize, changing and clarifying values*, and *living the challenge* (1996). This theory is presented in Figure 16.1.

For the purpose of this chapter, elements of the theory of Coming to Terms were merged into the theory of Regaining Control to modify and enhance the Regaining Control theory. Both theories describe how patients improve behavioral and psychosocial adaptation to COPD.

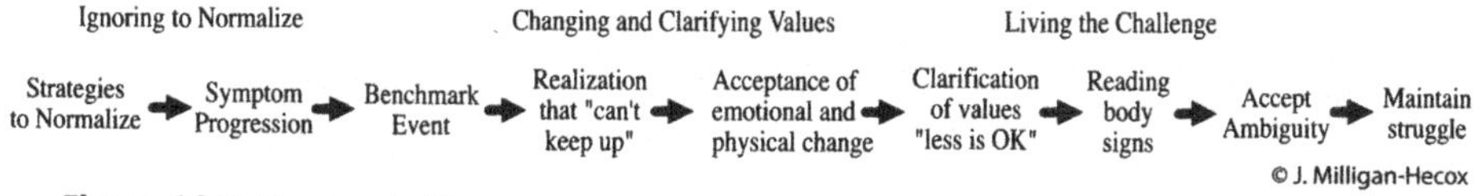

Figure 16.1 Coming to Terms.
Printed with permission from J. Milligan-Hecox.

Ethical Considerations

The institutional reviews boards at Azusa Pacific University and the participating hospitals approved both studies. After receiving approval for the study, subjects were recruited by the clinical nurse specialists at the three hospitals. The investigators contacted all those patients who agreed to participate and interviews were scheduled. A written consent form was signed at the time of the interview.

FINDINGS

The Theory of Regaining Control

From the analysis of the data about the patient's experience in going through the rehabilitation program, the basic social process of Regaining Control was identified. It has five stages: *ignoring symptoms to normalize, experiencing helplessness, feeling a glimmer of hope, getting with the program,* and *taking charge of life.* Each stage progresses into the next stage as patients come to terms with their disease through acceptance and acknowledgement of the life changes of COPD (see Figure 16.2).

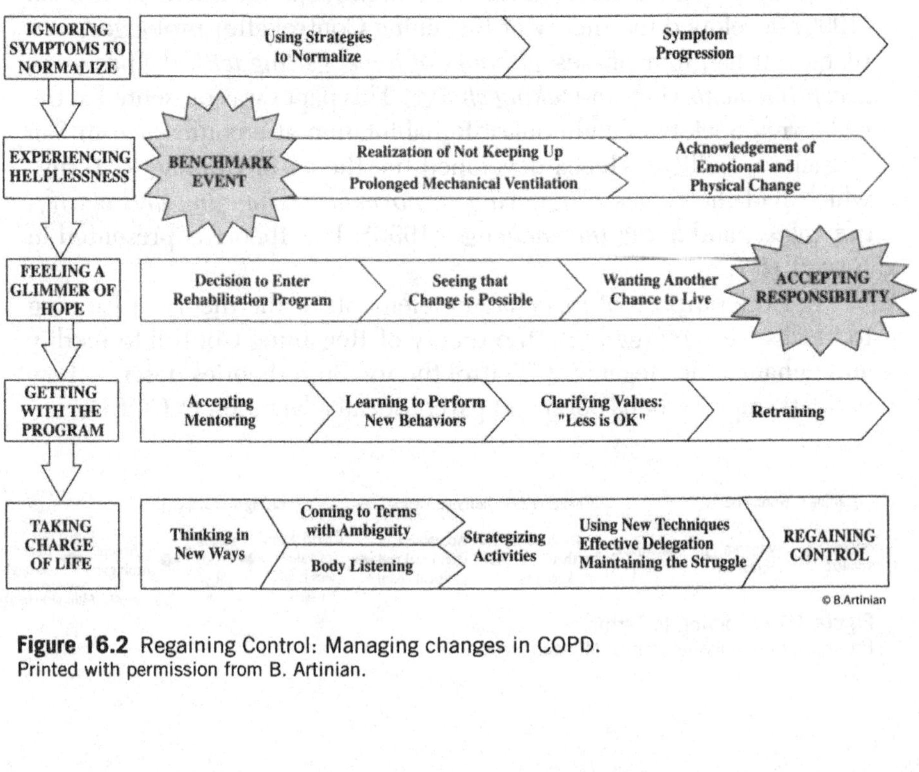

Figure 16.2 Regaining Control: Managing changes in COPD.
Printed with permission from B. Artinian.

The first stage is described as *ignoring symptoms to normalize*. This is a strategy to make life appear normal that subjects used until they realized that the life they once lived was no longer possible. The physical and emotional changes posed by their disease made them feel helpless (stage 2). Entry into a rehabilitation program presented them with a way out of the helplessness they were experiencing. After starting the program, the improvement they saw in their physical condition offered them a glimmer of hope and that was what made them realize that they must accept responsibility for their own improvement (stage 3). At this point they committed themselves to the program and were willing to give up their own autonomy and accept the mentoring of the staff in both behavioral retraining and adopting new attitudes (stage 4). As they completed the program they were ready to again take charge of their lives and incorporate the new ways of thinking and strategizing into their daily lives (stage 5). In this way they were able to retain control of their lives within the constraints of COPD.

Stage 1. Ignoring Symptoms to Normalize

The first stage, *ignoring to normalize*, was described in the data as an intense experience in which the subjects developed strategies around their work or social environment, which made them feel normal in spite of their discomfort. Symptoms slowly and surely progressed as they struggled to maintain normalcy. Finally, a benchmark event occurred that brought them to terms with the realization that they could no longer ignore this illness.

Strategies to allow these patients to feel and to be seen by others as normal were described as intense and even frightening experiences as they clung to what they perceived as normal. One female patient who was experiencing end-stage disease at the time of the interview said she had only retired from her job four years before. She felt she looked quite normal then. This patient stated:

> I could fake it. People weren't aware I really felt 100% disabled. I really couldn't function well at all. But by limiting what I did and what I exposed myself to, I misled a lot of people. When I finally retired, no one really knew how ill I was but me.

Other patients described strategies to normalize more in terms of maintaining feelings to remain normal and rationalizing and minimizing the symptoms being experienced. Symptoms continued to progress in COPD, leaving patients frightened and uncertain. Yet as long as they could continue to ignore and strategize, they clung to what they perceived as normal.

An elderly male patient who struggled for years to maintain normality described hiding his oxygen tank in the car when he had to be out in the community doing errands. He described his strategies in the face of symptom progression in the following way:

> I fudge quite a bit. I leave my oxygen tank in the car. I kept driving until about two weeks ago. I would drive myself to the bank, pay my rent, and leave my oxygen in the car. I wouldn't stay very long when I was out. I could do without the oxygen long enough to do my errands.

By using these strategies patients found ways to manage their progressive symptoms to preserve what they believed to be as near a normal life as they could maintain. This was so meaningful to them that the possibility of harmful consequences of these strategies was not perceived as dangerous. It was a repeated habitual behavior if they were going to have their very own normalcy in life.

Eventually a situation happened, a benchmark event, that brought them to terms with the realization that they could no longer out-strategize this illness on their own. It triggered a comprehension and a realization that the normalcy they once fought to preserve and maintain would no longer be possible.

The patient previously described who limited what she did and thus misled a lot of people until she decided to retire described the behavior or benchmark event that finally brought her to terms with the major life change of leaving her job. She related the experience in the following way: "Well, I guess you can only fake it for so long. You can sit there at the desk and look like you're okay. But if you have to get up and walk around, which is what I could no longer do, then you can't fake it anymore."

For one woman her ability to maintain her job and help support her family was vital to her sense of normalcy. For her the benchmark event was described in the context of work:

> I began to lose jobs. As I look back it all falls together. I couldn't keep a job. I'd get a good job and then I would lose it. I kept questioning what I was doing wrong. But this all goes together. It hit me. I couldn't keep a job, I was too slow. I couldn't remember. I wasn't getting enough oxygen to my brain and that was why I was too slow.

Stage 2. Experiencing Helplessness

As symptoms progressed and they were no longer able to keep up or they were unable to wean from a mechanical ventilator after surgery, an accident, or a serious illness, patients experienced the benchmark of *experiencing helplessness*. They could no longer strategize on their own to maintain the normalcy they saw as giving meaning to their life and they were forced to acknowledge the emotional and physical changes that had occurred. This was a profound experience in which they realized that new ways to cope with illness must be found. One patient said, "It was almost like mentally or somehow my body knew." When a patient who was ventilator dependent was asked, "What is hard about being on the ventilator?" he replied, "Nothing, it is getting off that is hard."

Stage 3. Feeling a Glimmer of Hope

The decision to enter the pulmonary rehabilitation program was a step in moving from the downward descent of helplessness. While in the program patients observed other patients making progress and they saw that change was possible. They also observed that they were feeling stronger and able to do more as they began the therapy. This gave them the courage to desire a second chance at life, but they realized that they would have to accept the responsibility for behavioral change.

Stage 4. Getting With the Program

It required firm determination on the part of the patients to give up the autonomy they possessed as adults and accept the mentoring of the staff. This decision to accept responsibility for changing their behaviors and attitudes led them to enter the rehabilitation program and was the benchmark that moved them in the direction of reclaiming control of their lives. In the program they had to accept mentoring to learn new behaviors and change their values about life. Not all the patients who tried out the program were able to do this and they continued in their state of dependency and did not remain in the program. One patient who entered into the spirit of the program said, "I don't have time to be frightened anymore. I've got to learn. I've got to practice what I learn if I'm going to live. Otherwise you'd freak out, panic, and everything would close up. Then you could hyperventilate, and snap, and you would be dead."

It is not an easy program. During the class, if a patient would lean down to pick up something without doing the pursed lip breathing technique, the therapist would stop the class, ask the person what had been done wrong, and then require the person to perform the action correctly. One patient commented on the program in this way:

> [It] is all regimented and on time, you know, exercise, they come in and take your test at a certain time. Everything is regimented, everything is orderly. Good food down there, real nice people, good atmosphere. The exercising does you good, and I do the same exercises now as when I came out.

In addition to the behavioral changes, patients are also helped to clarify their values and agree that "less is OK." This is part of the retraining of the program.

Stage 5. Taking Charge of Life

There are huge emotional and physical changes patients must come to terms with if they are to survive. Their view of self and the values they once centered their lives on must change. They must come to terms with the experience that to do less now becomes acceptable. There is a resignation on their part that allows this to happen. One patient expressed how things that were important are now not as important as before: "Oh, I can't run or anything anymore, but I can walk, cook, or whatever. So, it's minimal, the difference."

Many of these patients had previously been able to live their lives without depending on family and significant others. Coming to terms with the need to depend on others can be a painful process. Patients were afraid to either jeopardize close relationships or drive a loved one even farther away. It is a period of personal change that is described by one patient in the following way: "Well, someone has to do it for you now. That's hard, that's embarrassing." Family members were encouraged to participate in the program so that they could learn to think in new ways. It was difficult for them to learn how to live with the patient. One patient described how her husband treated her differently now. "A lot of times now I go to do something for myself and my husband is right there to do it before I can because he doesn't want me to do it. He's going to have to learn to let me do what I can do. He's very protective of me."

A major difficulty the patients described was the ambiguity the disease presents. They felt that they could not plan ahead because they would have to wait to see if this was going to be a good day or a bad day. One patient said that she was afraid to make plans with friends because she did not know if she could go through with them. Even being able to walk could not be taken for granted: "There are days I can walk and there are days when I can only walk half as much. I can be like somebody ran over me with a truck." The patients handled this by coming to terms with the ambiguity and focusing on the moment: "It's just letting things jell together, just one day at a time; just doing as much as I can do. Because I can't even say tomorrow, I'm just thinking about today."

The struggle and ambiguity of this illness made these patients very aware of what their bodies were telling them. They became acutely keen to any change and structured their lives around these signs. Patients told how they did what their bodies told them:

> Yeah, you pace yourself. You have to pace yourself. Well, you get it, you feel it. You know when it is time for a rest period. You know when. Mostly, I think, listen to your body and don't ignore it and if it says you're tired, so you're tired. Tired is okay.

Even though life was filled with ambiguity and struggle, patients realized that if they were to survive, they needed to develop strategies to manage their lives. One man said, "It's not a life that I would grant to anybody, that I would wish for somebody else to have, because it's not a good life, but it's the only one I've got and I've got to hang on to it or I won't be around."

One strategy they used was to incorporate into their lives all the new techniques they had learned in the rehabilitation program:

> Anytime you are doing anything—walking, walking up steps, picking up something, any kind of exertion, purse-breathe, purse-breathe." "I walked fast and now slowly. Don't move from lying to sitting so fast, do it slowly, pace yourself. I think this is the one thing that is important.

Another strategy was to simplify clothing to what could be put on easily and to rearrange the house so that everything was convenient even if it didn't look as good. Yet another was to delegate those activities they could no longer do. In explaining how she did her shopping, one woman said:

> They have electric carts now. So, I run around in this cart and do my shopping. If I need help, they have one of their employees go along with the cart. They load it in the car and when I get home, I use my wheelchair to put my groceries away. If I can't manage at home, I have to wait for my son to help me.

These and many other strategies were used to manage their constant struggle to live. Patients knew that the only way to survive was not to give up. Patients described their struggle in these ways:

- I am a fighter and I think working as long as I did, I made myself stay well somehow, or well enough. You have to work at it. That's what you have to do, if you don't work at it, you won't get there.
- You have to help yourself. God teaches us that. Help yourself. I do everything I am supposed to be doing.
- Survival is good. I want to get stronger. There are still things I would like to do. I have a problem with crowds and closed places, but I want to get back to my church.
- Struggle, keep going, don't let the mucus settle or it will turn into pneumonia. You've got to keep it up. You've got to keep going. You have to exercise. It's a lifetime battle. Unfortunately you can never stop. You've got to keep thinking ahead. Everything you do, you have to think what you do. You have to think positive. If you don't think positive, no one else will do it for me. Plan ahead. It's hard and it's easy to be dead.

Even though life was not the life they had once lived, the patients who were able to incorporate the retraining and new patterns of thought into their lives experienced regaining enough control so that they could do the things that were important to them.

DISCUSSION

Although most of the research literature about pulmonary rehabilitation deals with the physical management of the signs and symptoms of COPD, several authors discussed the psychosocial aspects of the disease. Just as in our sample population, many patients tried out the rehabilitation program but were not willing to get with the program. Perry (1993) noted that this form of rehabilitation requires a "selected and highly motivated individual" (p. 861). Tiep (1987) spoke of the "spiral of the disability" of COPD (p. 18). Tiep described patients who had options to further retreat into their illness or to organize and enter active treatment. However, Tiep did not describe what happens to the patient who enters a rehabilitation program and the changes that occur that lead to a successful outcome. Kaplan, Eakin, and Ries (1993) suggested that it is the personality of a particular patient that leads to adherence or nonadherence, but they noted there is no empirical evidence relating to this.

In our study, it was the interaction of patients with each other and staff support that provided the impetus for behavioral and psychological change. The support provided was not that of a sympathetic caregiver, which Kaplan et al. (1993) say may reinforce comfortable but noncompliant behavior. Rather, the support provided in the program was that of a taskmaster. We found that patients were willing to accept the regimentation of the program because they saw that the end goal of regaining control of their lives was more important than the momentary humiliation of being singled out in a group and instructed how to do an activity. It was their desperation to live that made them cooperate with program objectives rather than the belief that they could do it (self-efficacy theory) as suggested by Kaplan et al. (1993). This study represents a beginning attempt to understand the behavioral and psychosocial changes that take place in an effective pulmonary program.

CONCLUSION

Glaser states that a theory once developed is abstract of time, place, and people (2001, p. 129). Therefore, this theory of Regaining Control can be used to direct interventions for any patients with chronic illness that can be improved with rehabilitation. To illustrate this, the first author describes the intervention being providing for a young woman with the chronic condition of obesity. In the stage of ignoring symptoms to normalize, during a period of depression, this young woman gained 70 pounds. She would not allow anyone to discuss the weight gain with her although she briefly attended Weight Watchers. She experienced her benchmark event when she made a visit to a nurse practitioner for a medical problem, discovered she weighed 202 pounds, and felt that her body was falling apart. She acknowledged the changes that had occurred and was willing to accept the advice from the nurse practitioner to find a personal trainer, begin an exercise program, and return to Weight Watchers. Before she could actually start working with the trainer she started walking more and changed her eating habits. This led to a weight loss of 10 pounds and made her see that change was possible (*feeling a glimmer of hope*).

Her next benchmark was accepting responsibility for herself and getting with the program. She has been told that the first weeks of training would be the hardest and that she should expect her muscles to be sore. She would also have to accept mentoring to learn new behaviors and ways of eating. If she perseveres in completing the retraining, she will enter the next stage of *taking charge of her life*.

In her case, it is hoped that there will be no long-term problems and she should be able to think in new ways and listen to her body. She will also need to strategize her activities to continue to use the new techniques and maintain the struggle. If she is successful in following the new program, she will be able to regain control of her life. The use of the theory of Regaining Control describes the stages of the rehabilitation process and gives guidelines about how to proceed through each stage.

REFERENCES

Artinian, B. (1995, April). *The process of regaining control: Outcome of a pulmonary rehabilitation program with advanced COPD.* San Francisco, CA: California Society of Pulmonary Rehabilitation.

Glaser, B. G. (1978). *Theoretical sensitivity: Advances in the methodology of grounded theory*. Mill Valley, CA: Sociology Press.

Glaser, B. G. (1998). *Doing grounded theory: Issues and discussions.* Mill Valley, CA: Sociology Press.

Glaser, B. G. (2001). *The grounded theory perspective: Conceptualization contrasted with description*. Mill Valley, CA: Sociology Press.

Glaser, B. G. (2005). *The grounded theory perspective III: Theoretical coding*. Mill Valley, CA: Sociology Press.

Kaplin, R. M., Eakin, E. G., & Ries, A. L. (1993). Psychological issues in the rehabilitation of patients with chronic pulmonary disease. In R. Casaburi & T. Petty (Eds.), *Principles and practice of pulmonary rehabilitation* (pp. 351–365). Philadelphia: W. B. Saunders.

Milligan-Hecox, J. (1996). *A qualitative study of managing changes in chronic obstructive pulmonary disease.* Unpublished master's thesis, Azusa Pacific University, Azusa, CA.

Perry, T. (1993). Pulmonary rehabilitation in perspective: Historical roots, present status, and future projections. *Thorax, 48*, 855–862.

Riley, P. (1996). Effects of a pulmonary rehabilitation program on dyspnea, self-care, and physiological functioning of patients with COPD. *Rehabilitation Nursing Research*, 5(2), 43–52.

Schultz, D. (1994). *American Lung Association Lung Disease Data 1994.* New York: American Lung Association.

Tiep, B. L. (1987, July). Rehabilitative hope for patients with chronic lung disease. *Continuing Care,* 18–23.

III

Amplifying Causal Loops

INTRODUCTION: BARBARA M. ARTINIAN

The theoretical code family of causation explains processes that have causal consequences. While there are many types of causal relationships, the emergent theories addressed in this section involve amplifying causation as the process that moves a situation toward its outcome. Amplifying causal loops can be described as the iterative interaction in which "consequences become continually causes and causes continually consequences" (Glaser, 2005, p. 9). The progressions can be in the form of worsening or improving escalations.

The first study presented in this section was done by Cone among formerly homeless mothers (see chapter 17, "Mutuality: Reconnecting to Overcome Homelessness"). Further analysis of the theory of reconnecting identified mutuality as the causal factor that resulted in the consequence of an amplifying investment on the part of the mother in her own trajectory out of homelessness.

In the second study, Artinian explores the special relationships that nurses form with some cancer patients (see chapter 18, "Risking Involvement With Cancer Patients"). The main concern of the nurses was to provide nurturing care to cancer patients within a personal comfort zone. This was resolved by either of two amplifying loops that emerged from the data: *practicing involvement* and *resisting involvement*. The more a nurse practiced one way of interacting with dying patients, the more he or she continued to practice the type of behavior that provided comfort.

Understanding these causal loops, both negative and positive, can inform nursing practice and assist nurse leaders to provide the support that nurses need in order to continually provide support to patients. An understanding of causation and the amplifying nature of some causal-consequence relationships can be of benefit in a broad application to nursing practice.

REFERENCE

Glaser, B. G. (2005). *The grounded theory perspective III: Theoretical coding.* Mill Valley, CA: Sociology Press.

17 Mutuality: Reconnecting to Overcome Homelessness

PAMELA H. CONE
BARBARA M. ARTINIAN

Homelessness negatively affects the spirit, mind, and body of those who experience it (Averitt, 2003). It includes everyone who does not have a regular nighttime place to live (NCH, 2004). In U.S. cities, there is a slight majority of homeless men, but the fastest-growing segment of the homeless population is single mothers, a vulnerable, at-risk group (Weingart Center, 2001). Greater Los Angeles had 91,000 homeless every night at the time of this study (Netburn, 2005). Homeless families have complex needs, including limited access to health care and fragmented social support (Urban Institute, 2000). Because of this, single homeless mothers and their children who have no social network face the challenge of recurrent homelessness (Toohey, Shinn, & Weitzman, 2004). Current strategies for care of the homeless focus primarily on providing food and shelter, strategies that keep these families alive but give only temporary help (Whitehead, 2002). A review of the literature found no qualitative research about the experience of getting out of homelessness from the perspective of homeless mothers. This led to a Glaserian grounded theory (GT) retrospective study among formerly homeless women who had had children at the time of their homeless experience.

The basic social process (BSP) of Reconnecting to Overcome Homelessness (Cone, 2006) emerged as the process that resolved the main concern of the participants: getting off the streets into stable housing. Glaser

MOVING OUT			OVERCOMING		
1 Becoming Ready	**2 Connecting with SOMEONE**	**CUTTING POINT**	**1 Revaluing SELF**	**2 Mutually Finding SOLUTIONS**	**3 Reintegrating into SOCIETY**
• Hitting bottom • Feeling ready to change	• Accepting contact • Reaching out for help • Getting connected		• Choosing to listen • Claiming identity • Reaffirming self-worth • Taking action	• Establishing long-term support • Mutual problem-solving • Getting practical help	• Finding a home • Becoming financially stable • Settling in • Giving back to society
CONTEXT: Homeless motherhood					
CONDITIONS: Living in some sort of temporary situation then Reconnecting					
OUTCOME: Getting and staying off the streets after obtaining stable housing					© P.H.Cone

Figure 17.1 The stages of Reconnecting.
Printed with permission from P. H. Cone.

(2001) states that grounded theories are modifiable and can be analyzed in more depth to allow the theoretical codes to emerge. Initially understood as having four stages, Reconnecting was further analyzed and a cutting point emerged as a decision point within the process that signaled the start of the move out of homelessness. This changed the focus to two stages of Reconnecting, *moving out* and *overcoming*, that are separated by the moment of decision (see Figure 17.1) to make a one-on-one connection.

Further analysis revealed that the *mutuality* of this connection is what enabled mothers to overcome homelessness. This mutual connection emerged as an amplifying causal loop. Glaser (1998) explains that reanalysis can move a substantive grounded theory to more abstract theory, to refine and modify theory, and to test hypotheses in further research. When a BSP has emerged through the discovery mode, the move from concrete, situated concepts toward those that are more integrated and abstract from time, place, and people can be time consuming and difficult, so it is often left undone (Glaser, 2005). This chapter discusses efforts to further develop the substantive theory of Reconnecting.

THE STUDY

Aim

The purpose of the original study was to discover the process whereby formerly homeless mothers got off the streets into stable housing (Cone,

2006). The aim of further data analysis was to clarify initial understandings of the Reconnecting process and to develop the emergent substantive theory into a more integrated theory through the identification of the theoretical codes that moved the process to its outcome.

Method

Classical Glaserian GT methodology was used for the original study as well as for more in-depth analyses (Glaser, 2005). Data collection for the original study occurred in the Los Angeles area from 2003 to 2006 with interviews of formerly homeless mothers. These interviews were conducted in the participants' homes or in a public place selected by the participants. Constant comparative analysis began with open coding of the first interview and continued until themes emerged. Theoretical sampling was done in another large metropolitan area in the Southwest of the United States. Data collection ceased upon category saturation. The qualitative software developed by QSR International, NVivo, was used to manage data. Conceptual maps assisted with data analysis.

Sample

Inclusion criteria for participants were:

1. Women at least 18 years of age
2. Had children at the time of their homeless experience
3. Identified themselves as formerly homeless mothers
4. Spoke English

The Stuart B. McKinley Act (NCH, 1999) defined a homeless person as anyone who does not have a regular nighttime residence. Nunez (2001) further defined homelessness as being homeless for more than 6 weeks. He based this on literature that revealed a change in thinking occurs when one has been homeless for 6 weeks or more. Participants in this study had been living on the streets from less than a year to more than 20 years. All had been out of homelessness for more than 6 weeks at the time of the interview. The sample included 18 participants and 12 firsthand accounts from the literature ($N = 30$). The ethnically diverse sample reflected the general demographics of the homeless in 2005 of the Los Angeles Homeless Services Authority report (Netburn, 2005).

Data Collection and Analysis

Originally, data were collected through a series of semistructured interviews using an interview guide that asked participants for their stories of homelessness. Field notes and memos about the in-vivo codes, the process, and identified categories were also considered data. Constant comparative analysis of the rich data revealed the multiplicity and complexity of needs that mothers faced during their homeless experience, as well as the process whereby they got out of homelessness. Glaserian GT methods were used both in the original analysis and in further analysis (Glaser, 2005) as data were compared and reanalyzed. Since categories were saturated in the initial study, there was no further data gathering at the time of reanalysis. However, all data, including conceptual maps, were reexamined in greater depth.

Data were reanalyzed with special attention given to memos that indicated early understanding of the theoretical concept that explained the movement through the process of Reconnecting. Further analysis revealed both the cutting point of the decision to connect with someone and an amplifying causal loop of mutual connection. As the care provider invested time and energy in the homeless mother's life, there was increasing mother involvement in her journey out of homelessness. New memos were written to track researcher thinking and to capture insight into the theoretical codes. Theoretical concepts replaced many of the in-vivo codes as the theory became more abstract. Conceptual mapping helped to develop and display the concepts, their relationships, and the process. An early map drew attention to the importance of reconnecting (see Chapter 4, Figure 4.1).

Ethical Considerations

In the United States, major universities such as the University of California at San Francisco (UCSF) use national guidelines for ethical research but have their own research oversight committees for the approval process. After approval was received from the UCSF Committee for Human Research, interviews were scheduled and informed consent was obtained from participants. All of the participants agreed to have their interviews audiotaped and transcribed and to choose their own pseudonyms. Demographic data and transcriptions of the tape-recorded interviews were deidentified, and tapes were destroyed upon completion of the study.

FINDINGS

Reconnecting: A Process of Overcoming Homelessness

The participants' main concern, of getting out of homelessness into a stable life with their families, emerged through initial analysis. Reconnecting with society was the process that resolved their main concern. The importance of connections to a caring person and a social network was understood as necessary for restabilization to occur and repeat homelessness to be avoided. Through conceptual mapping, it became evident that there was more to the emergent concepts than simply a process.

From Process to Theory

Theory development began with clarifying the process and theoretical codes and then moving it to a more abstract dimension. As analysis continued, several assumptions became clear. Based on the analytical process, reflective memos, logical reasoning, and philosophical literature, five assumptions regarding reconnecting are posited.

1. Human-to-human connections are essential to motherhood and to life in society.
2. Human connections can be and often are severed in today's society; the fabric of American society is as fragile as the family itself.
3. Disconnection must occur in order for there to be a need for reconnection; crisis often precipitates disconnection in family life.
4. Reconnecting must be initiated by one side or the other; the side that is strong and caring usually makes the initial contact.
5. Reconnecting is only the initial step in the mending of societal fabric; connections must be sustained through social support in order for human-to-human connections to be maintained and society to be strengthened.

Working effectively with disconnected individuals is possible after a readiness to change enables the individual to make the decision to change and a one-on-one connection with a caring person is established. Overcoming adversity and disconnection begins after the connection is solidified. In an amplifying causal loop, a greater investment on the part of the care provider evident in the early stages of the relationship results in increased investment of the recipient in the process, which grows as it is nurtured by the care provider. The mutuality of the connection is a significant factor in promoting momentum toward the outcome of reintegration into society.

Theory Emerging Through Reanalysis of Data

Glaser (1998) claims that "all is [*sic*] data" (p. 8), including observation, field notes, and memos as important additions to the actual transcribed interviews. During more in-depth analysis, memos were a key factor in clarifying the theoretical codes drawn from selective codes. All memos that mentioned the relationships between open and selective codes were reexamined, and related interview sections were reread. The recurring theoretical concepts were reconnecting, cutting point, mutuality, causation, and amplifying investment. The relationships of all these concepts emerged. The theoretical code of *cutting point* emerged as the decision to connect with a person that made reconnecting to society possible. Finally, the theoretical code, *amplifying causal loop*, was revealed as the concept that propelled the process to the outcome of restabilization and reintegration.

Theoretical Code: Cutting Point

Moving out and *overcoming* emerged as two stages of the process of reconnecting. These stages each have several steps with subprocesses. The cutting point of a decision to connect with someone and to try to get out of homelessness divides the stages. A cutting point is a clear point of decision-making that makes a difference in the trajectory of a process. This point of decision occurred after the participants had begun the moving out process, when initial contact with a helping individual was made. The decision to connect with a caring person, thus reconnecting with a member of society, was the point at which the homeless mother made a decisive move toward overcoming homelessness. Until there was a clear-cut decision to move on rather than to simply survive out in the "jungle of homelessness," these mothers could not overcome homelessness and achieve "homefulness." (See Figure 17.2.)

Moving Out

The first stage in the process of Reconnecting was *moving out*. It involved leaving the survival mode and included the categories of *"becoming*

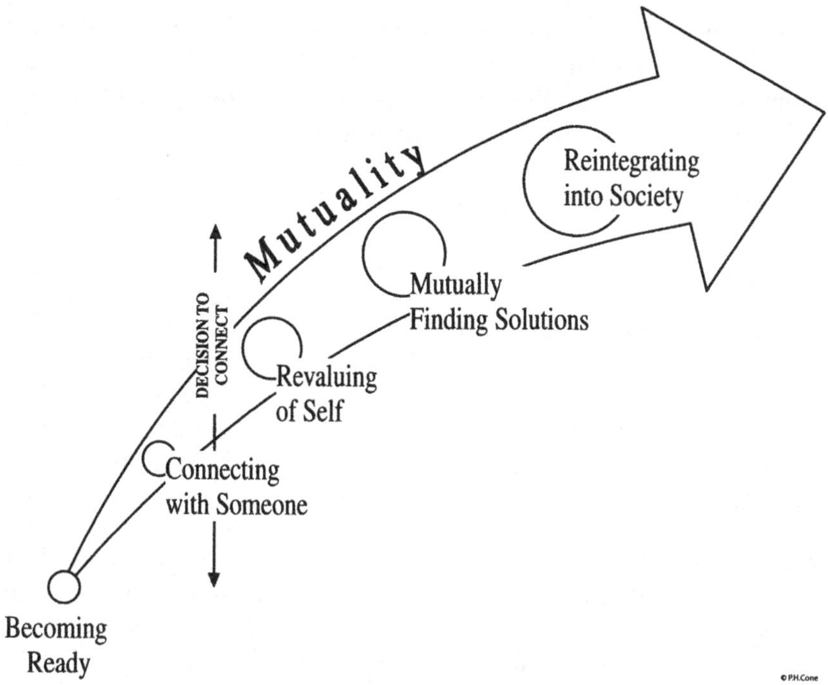

Figure 17.2 Mutuality: Reconnecting to overcome homelessness. Printed with permission from P. H. Cone.

ready" and "*connecting*" with someone. Each category had several steps that moved the reconnecting process toward overcoming.

Becoming Ready. This stage began when a caring individual made initial contact with a homeless mother. At some point, it moved to hitting bottom and feeling ready to change. Caring individuals had to keep on reaching out with kindness, in order for the lack of trust in society to begin to change. Hitting bottom was motivational and helped move the homeless mother toward a willingness to change. Evaluating whether someone was ready to make a change was difficult and not uniform. Over and over again the participants expressed that they had to be the ones to make the choice to move out of homelessness, stating, "You gotta want it for yourself." The readiness to change was necessary before connecting was possible.

Cutting Point: Connecting With Someone. Connections have two sides, and the process of reconnecting involves both. When the mother reciprocated the one-on-one reconnection process initiated by a caring individual, the connection was made. A cutting point occurred when the readiness to change and the one-on-one connection solidified into a decision to move on out of homelessness. Prior to this cutting point, these homeless mothers had been adrift and indecisive about their lives. After this point, they moved steadily out of homelessness. This establishment of a one-on-one connection with a caring individual began the process of overcoming.

Overcoming

After the mothers decided to reconnect with society through a contact with a genuinely caring member of society, they moved into the stage of overcoming. The three steps in the stage of overcoming included: revaluing self, mutually solving problems, and reintegrating into society. Establishing mutual and long-term connections with social supports was important at this stage.

Revaluing Self. This step in the process included choosing to listen, claiming a new identity as a person of worth, reaffirming to themselves and others their self-worth, and taking action on their new identity. Nurturance by the care initiator provided an opportunity for those who had lost dignity, been disrespected, and made to feel worthless to regain a sense of self-worth and to see themselves in a more positive light. This valuing of the mother on the part of the care provider was a key factor in assisting the mother to begin the process of revaluing herself as a worthwhile human being. One said, "I'll never forget her kindness. She made me feel like I was worth her time and help."

Mutually Finding Solutions. Respect for the individual's input throughout the problem-solving process increased dignity, which in turn, influenced the motivation to change. Mutually desired change moved the process toward success. Many mothers in this study wanted to collaborate in the process of finding solutions to their financial instability and their need for a home for their family. Instead of being told what to do, these women wanted to have a voice in the planning and make their own choices for their future. Mutually working on solutions gave them respect and dignity that had been lost.

Theoretical Code: Mutuality

Creative problem solving was far more effective and enjoyable for both mothers and care providers when mutuality was practiced. Mutuality was the key to moving out of homelessness and becoming reconnected (see Figure 17.3).

As the mutual connection with an unconditionally caring person became stronger, and the care provider instilled a sense of belonging, a sense that the homeless mother had a place in society was promoted. When this occurred, most mothers received enough energy to envision a future with a home, and worked to that end.

By this point, these mothers had gradually become more involved in their trajectory out of homelessness, with increased investment of time and energy toward that end. Care providers maintained a strong connection while allowing the mothers to find new connections that could form the basis for a safety net of social support. These women discussed the support networks established with the help of their care providers. One mother said the people she connected with "are still there for me . . . a little bit of a safety net." Consequently, she did not worry about falling back into homelessness. Investing herself in reestablishing and stabilizing a social support network and in discovering the means to sustaining it helped the mother find her place in society. For example, friendships that developed with church volunteers led to new support networks through the church family, a family previously lost to these women through disconnection.

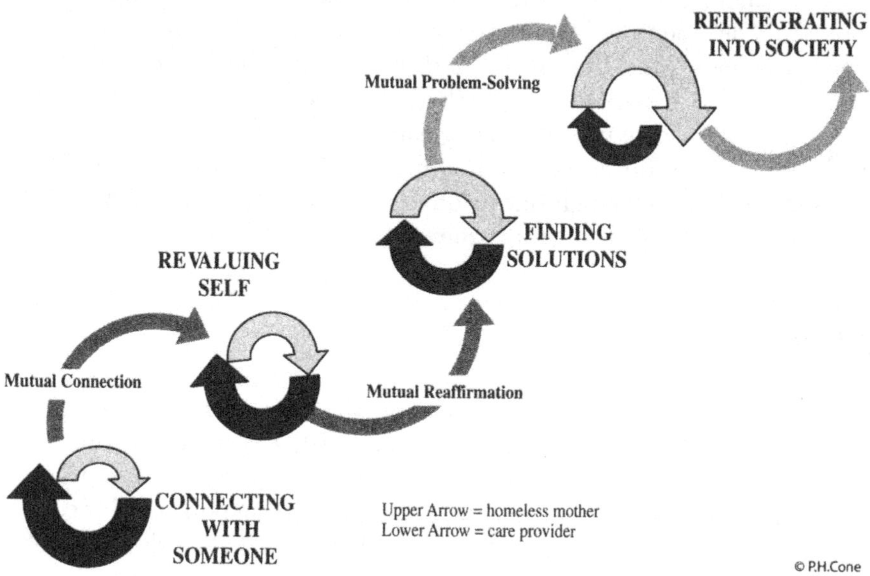

Figure 17.3 Mutuality: The key to Reconnecting.
Printed with permission from P. H. Cone.

One woman discussing the support of her new church family said, "I'll never worry again." This security helped with reintegration into society.

Reintegrating Into Society. Reinvestment in society was the outcome of mutually finding solutions to the challenges these mothers faced. This was only possible as mothers and care providers worked together and as mothers increased their engagement and investment into the process. Mutuality between the mother and the care provider continued to be a key factor in the move out of homelessness. For some, the journey was fairly swift; those who could easily envision having a home again had a more rapid trajectory out of homelessness than those who could not. The latter needed more hope instilled before they could see themselves as "homeful" rather than homeless, and sustained investment in the relationship by the provider was crucial. One mother embodied "homefulness" in a unique way.

> I knew I was finally free of the fear, free of the worry of becoming homeless again. I knew when I was shopping and I bought a plant. Because a plant means permanency, you know. It means you're gonna be there to water it and take care of it. It's a sign of stability. It's a sign that you're not goin' anywhere except to work. I knew then that we were okay!

While each mother had a different benchmark for seeing herself as "homeful," all identified a point at which they felt that they were no longer homeless, and they all felt a desire to "give back" in some way because of what had been given to them. Consistent and genuine caring on the part of the care provider, along with the investment of the mother, made a significant difference in their lives, and they were grateful. This attitude led them to reach out to others in need, mirroring the initial investment of care providers into their own lives.

DISCUSSION

Reconnection implies some level of mutuality. Over time, it becomes amplified, and the connection brings about positive results. Working effectively with disconnected individuals is possible when a readiness to change leads to a one-on-one connection with a caring person. This connection is the cutting point that moves the mother in the direction of reconnecting. A greater investment on the part of the care provider is evident in the early stages of the relationship, but the individual's investment in the process grows as the care provider nurtures it. With mutual investment, there is an opportunity for those who have lost dignity, respect, and a sense of self-worth to revalue self in a more positive light.

Woodward (1982) found that colostomy patients were able to revalue themselves when family and friends valued them. Respect for the individual's input throughout the problem-solving process increases dignity, which in turn influences the motivation to change. Mutually desired change moves the process toward success, especially when the disenfranchised person increases investment of time and energy toward that end. Establishment of a new social support network and the means to sustain it helps avoid repeat disconnection. Reinvestment into the lives of the needy is a clear sign of reconnection, restabilization, and reintegration into mainstream society.

Change as a Cutting Point Concept

Change literature reminds us that an individual must be ready for a change to actually occur, and the cutting point at which a person is ready to change direction is different for each. The decision to reconnect and to trust one person is the first step in the process of rebuilding trust in the society that marginalized the individual, so the importance of this step cannot be underestimated. Change can come very slowly for those who have been disconnected for a long time. A readiness to change cannot be forced, so care providers must be patient and consistent in their efforts to build trust and rapport with a disconnected individual. Change in perspective or attitude is a challenge, and being homeless makes looking at life differently and solving various problems more complex and challenging. The theory of Human Motivation (Maslow, 1943) points out that human beings are individually and societally motivated to act, so the mutuality of motivation on the part of both the mother and the care provider is important to the initial step of establishing a bond with one caring person.

Reconnection as a Concept

Reconnecting was the key to overcoming homelessness; it involved *becoming ready, connecting with someone, revaluing self, mutually finding solutions*, and *reintegrating into society*. What gave the homeless women energy to turn around was the sense that someone genuinely valued them. Their increasing investment in their journey out of homelessness was a direct result of reconnecting with the care provider (Miller, 1996). Short-term connections help with short-term problems such as food and shelter; long-term connections are important for the long process of reintegrating into society (Meadows-Oliver, 2005).

Many American families are fragmented or have fragile relationships. In a report on the increased vulnerability of homeless families, Page and Nooe (2002) explain that many women make choices on their personal views of what is best for them and their children, and often their perspectives are skewed. In any case, each mother indicated that the motivation for change relating to her child was a clear decision-making point in her life on the streets. This coincided with making a connection with a caring person who worked with her to overcome homelessness.

Social Support as a Concept

Social connections are important for restabilization after reconnection has begun. Networks must be developed and maintained to facilitate reconnecting. According to studies conducted by Jezewski (1995) and Lindsey (1997), being able to access a strong support system helps avoid renewed disconnection, and this support decreases the risk for repeated homelessness. Some support networks are available through various specifically focused support groups, such as drug abuse programs and programs for victims of domestic violence or the mentally ill (PATH, 2002).

People who do not fit these specific groups must find and build other networks and relationships through social, civic, and religious organizations (Letiecq, Anderson, & Koblinsky, 1996). Many homeless mothers developed and sustained social support networks through churches, providing a safety net for them. Others established connections with other mothers during their homeless experience or during the overcoming process (Cone, 2008). These networks needed to be maintained in order for those mothers to truly feel they had overcome homelessness. Some organizations have systems that help women problem-solve, such as job assistance or training (PATH, 2002). Staying connected through the process and afterwards helps individuals to feel that they are a valued member of society rather than a drain on societal resources (Jezewski, 1995). This facilitates the reintegration process.

In this study, those who reached out to homeless mothers were social workers, case managers, and volunteers from nonprofit organizations (Cone, 2006). Lindsey (1997) also found that genuinely caring trained professionals, particularly social workers, are of great assistance to mothers trying to get off the streets. Partnership with an organization that can subsidize initial housing costs or provide housing without preliminary fees is one way to meet this challenge (Hatton, 2001). An unstable and precarious state of finances is a major factor in repeat homelessness (Timmer, Eitzen, & Talley, 1994), so establishing and maintaining social support networks that can be accessed during times of crisis or sudden instability can serve as a buffer against that possibility. What makes the process possible is the mutuality between the mother and the care provider, both of whom are enriched by their mutual connection.

Mutuality as a Concept

Philosopher Charles Taylor reminds us that misrecognition practices are a major problem in our society today (1997), and that every human being has not only the right but also the need to be seen for the valuable person each one is. Many organizations do not recognize homeless mothers for the strong and courageous persons they are. Programs are often based on patriarchal or male-dominated thinking and planning that fail to meet the needs of homeless mothers (Whitehead, 2002). This exacerbates an already difficult situation. Another concern is that many care providers make plans without assessing the situation from the mother's perspective or asking the homeless mothers for their input (Miller, 1996). In addition to being an issue of loss of dignity, this lack of mutuality leads to poorly informed and therefore inadequate or ineffective programs (Averitt, 2003).

Becoming and staying connected has been found to be crucial in all aspects of overcoming homelessness. Through mutual connections, individuals can be assisted in figuring out solutions to the unique situation each one faces. Problem solving is a lifelong process that usually requires mutual social support, so the social networks these mothers establish are crucial to their long-term success in changing their situations and overcoming homelessness (Cone, 2008; Jezewski, 1995; Toohey, Shinn, & Weitzman, 2004). Mothers need to be given a voice in the problem-solving process. One caring person's ongoing investment in their lives produces energy in these mothers, enabling them to move forward and take increasing ownership of their journey out of homelessness. This causal effect amplifies as the mother's hope is renewed and she is able to envision a future with a home for herself and her child.

Causation as a Concept

The idea that investing energy can cause a positive response resulting in a change of direction is not new. It is the mutuality of this process that is of critical importance in causing the process of reconnecting to succeed. Mutuality was evident at each step, and the continual nurturing of the connection by both parties was crucial to success in overcoming homelessness. There needs to be a sense of mutual connection for the formerly disconnected person to move out of homelessness into reconnection with society. Mutuality then, is a key to Reconnecting and can be seen as causal in the process of overcoming adversity and being reintegrated into society. The theoretical code of amplifying causal loops emerged from the study of reconnecting to overcome homelessness. When there were mutual connections and an increasing investment of time and energy on the part of both the homeless mother and the care provider, the process moved forward toward the outcome of "homefulness."

CONCLUSION

Reconnection was discovered to be a theory of mutual connecting with increasing investment on the part of the mother and care provider. The cutting point occurred when the mother was able to accept the help of a genuinely caring person. The reconnecting process is possible through mutuality between the individual and the care provider. All participants went through the stages of this process, though the trajectory of each proceeded at a different pace. Every participant identified when and how helpful social connections were initiated. They described how mutuality was enhanced throughout the process, how creative solutions were discovered as mutual investment in the problem-solving process was amplified, and the point at which each one had a sense of overcoming adversity. While the investment of the care provider was far greater at the beginning of the process, the continued investment of the caring person encouraged a greater investment by the mother in an amplifying causal loop. By the end of the process, the individual was spending the greater amount of time and investing more energy than the provider. With this mutually amplifying causation, both parties were strengthened and enriched by the process.

According to Glaser (1978), a grounded theory is abstract of time, place, and people. The emergent theory of reconnecting can be applied to many situations and settings, particularly those following a crisis that results in disconnection. For example, soldiers who have had traumatic war experiences often come back home with a sense of disconnection from family, friends, and social networks. Their adjustment back to normal daily living, that is, their reintegration into society, is often very difficult. The use of this theory can help those working with such veterans to understand the disconnection, and with genuine kindness and caring, work to build a mutual connection with one caring person who can help them reconnect with family and society once again.

Through further analysis, the theory of Reconnecting has moved from a simple BSP to a substantive grounded theory integrated by two theoretical codes.

ACKNOWLEDGEMENTS

I would like to thank Dr. Catherine Waters, chair of my dissertation committee at UCSF, without whose assistance this study with Dr. Artinian as methodologist would not have been possible.

REFERENCES

Averitt, S. S. (2003). "Homelessness is not a choice!" The plight of homeless women with preschool children living in temporary shelters. *Journal of Family Nursing, 9*(1), 79–100.

Cone, P. (2006). *Reconnecting: A grounded theory study among formerly homeless mothers.* Unpublished doctoral dissertation, University of California at San Francisco.

Cone, P. (2008). Experiencing homelessness. In M. De Chesnay (Ed.), *Caring for the vulnerable* (2nd ed., ch. 20). Sudbury, MA: Jones & Bartlett.

Glaser, B. G. (1978). *Theoretical sensitivity.* Mill Valley, CA: Sociology Press.

Glaser, B. G. (1998). *Doing grounded theory: Issues and discussion.* Mill Valley, CA: Sociology Press

Glaser, B. G. (2001). *The grounded theory perspective: Conceptualization contrasted with description.* Mill Valley, CA: Sociology Press.

Glaser, B. G. (2005). *The grounded theory perspective: Theoretical coding.* Mill Valley, CA: Sociology Press.

Hatton, D. C. (2001). Homeless women's access to health services: A grounded theory of social network and managed care in the US. *Women & Health, 33*(3/4), 149.

Jezewski, M. A. (1995). Staying connected: The core of facilitating health care for homeless persons. *Public Health Nursing, 12*(3), 203–210.

Letiecq, B. L., Anderson, E. A., & Koblinsky, S. A. (1996). Social support of homeless and permanently housed low-income mothers with young children. *Family Relations, 45*(3), 265–272.

Lindsey, E. W. (1997). The process of restabilization for mother-headed homeless families: How social workers can help. *Journal of Family Social Work, 2*(3), 49–72.

Maslow, A. H. (1943). A theory of human motivation. *Psychological Review, 50*(4), 370–396.

Meadows-Oliver, M. (2005). Social support among homeless & housed mothers: An integrative review. *Journal of Psychosocial Nursing and Mental Health Services, 43*(2), 40–47.

Miller, S. (1996). Questioning, resisting, acquiescing, balancing: New mothers' career reentry strategies. *Health Care for Women International, 17,* 109–131.

National Coalition for the Homeless. (1999). The McKinney Act. *NCH Fact Sheet #18.* Washington, DC: National Coalition for the Homeless. Retrieved May 5, 2005, from www.nationalhomeless.org

National Coalition for the Homeless. (2004). Who is homeless? *NCH Fact Sheet #3.* Washington, DC: National Coalition for the Homeless. Retrieved June 11, 2004, from www.nationalhomeless.org/families

Netburn, M. (2005). *Press Release:* June 16, 2005. Los Angeles Homeless Services Authority. Retrieved June 17, 2005, from www.lahsa.org/pdfs/Current/Press%20 Release%20Final.pdf

Nunez, R. (2001). *Déjà vu: Family homelessness in New York City.* A report of The Institute of Children and Poverty and Homes for the Homeless. Retrieved August 10, 2005, from www.homesforthehomeless.com

Page, T., & Nooe, R. M. (2002). Life experiences and vulnerabilities of homeless women: A comparison of women unaccompanied versus accompanied by minor children, and correlates with children's emotional distress. *Journal of Social Distress and the Homeless, 11*(3), 215–231.

Projects for Assistance in the Transition from Homelessness. (2002). *Issue brief.* Washington, DC: Author (a branch of the Department of Mental Health Services). Retrieved May 5, 2005, from www.samhsa.gov/centers/cmhs/cmhs.html

Taylor, C. (1997). *Philosophical arguments.* Cambridge, MA: Harvard University Press.

Timmer, D. A., Eitzen, D. S., & Talley, K. D. (1994). *Paths to homelessness: Extreme poverty and the urban housing crisis.* Boulder, CO: Westview Press.

Toohey, S. M., Shinn, M., & Weitzman, B. C. (2004). Social networks and homelessness among women heads of household. *American Journal of Community Psychology, 33*(1–2), 7–20.

Urban Institute. (2000, February 1). *A new look at homelessness in America.* Retrieved May 5, 2005, from www.urban.org

Weingart Center. (2001, July). *Housing and poverty in Los Angeles. Just the facts.* Los Angeles: Institute for the Study of Homelessness and Poverty. Retrieved February 17, 2005, from www.weingart.org/institute

Whitehead, D. (2002). *Statistics on homelessness.* Washington, DC: National Coalition for the Homeless. Retrieved March 13, 2005, from www.nationalhomeless.org

Woodward, B. (1982). A descriptive study on the phenomenon of revaluing of self in colostomates. Unpublished master's thesis, California State University, Los Angeles.

18 Risking Involvement With Cancer Patients

BARBARA M. ARTINIAN

The helping relationship has been identified by Brammer (1988) as central to the practice of nursing. Its varying forms range from the minimal involvement of neutrality to the intense involvement of what nurses call a "special relationship." When patients experience a catastrophic illness such as cancer, a relationship with a nurse can be a major source of support. Although some practitioners question the ability of nurses to be therapeutic if they become too intimately involved with the patient and family (Donovan, 1981), such involvement may inspire the patient to maintain the will to live (Artinian, 1984).

THE STUDY

Aim

The purpose of this study was to explore and describe the process of how nurses form special relationships with cancer patients.

Adapted from Artinian, B. (1995). Risking involvement with cancer patients. Used with permission from *Western Journal of Nursing Research, 17*(3), 292–304. Sage Publications, Thousand Oaks, CA.

Method

Classical grounded theory methodology was used to collect and analyze the responses of the nursing personnel (Glaser, 1978, 1998, 2005).

Participants

Thirty-two nursing personnel who had worked for more than 6 months on cancer units participated in the project. Participants were recruited from a large public medical center and a private hospital with a large cancer unit, both of which were located in a Western state. Of these personnel, 11 were nursing attendants, 3 were licensed vocational nurses, and 18 were registered nurses. They ranged in age from 22 to 45, with a mean age of 29. Only one subject was male. All were involved in actual patient care and, therefore, had the opportunity to form relationships with patients. Because this was an exploratory study to describe the process of forming relationships, there was no attempt to limit the subjects to nursing personnel with the same level of skill or understanding.

Data Collection

In-depth interviews with the nurses were tape recorded and transcribed. Items were developed to explore relationships between nurses and cancer patients. For example, nurses were asked if they had ever developed a special relationship with a patient, how activities were different with that patient, and the meaning of their relationship. Additional questions were used to clarify or elaborate on the nurses' responses as the core variable emerged. These interviews were conducted with the subjects at their place of employment, in a quiet place such as a classroom or an office. Interviews ranged from 15 minutes to 2 hours in duration. The interviews varied widely in length because some nursing personnel spoke only long enough to explain that they had never formed a special relationship with a patient and why they considered a close relationship disadvantageous for them or the patient. The longer interviews were with those who had risked involvement, and they described in detail the many notable relationships they had formed. For the most part, participants reported accounts of their relationships with patients they had cared for in the past but not presently. Only one relationship involved a patient who was hospitalized at the time of the interview.

Data Analysis

Using constant comparative analysis, data were simultaneously collected and analyzed to identify the core process in the phenomenon of special relationships. Line-by-line analysis of the written transcripts and frequent listening to the audio tapes to capture the emotion-laden statements of the subjects led to the development of codes that described the behaviors and experiences of the subjects in their own words. These initial substantive codes were condensed into categories such as *initial attitude toward special relationships, selection criteria for special patient, activities typifying involvement,* and *strategies for resisting involvement* (Artinian, 1995). The properties of these categories were specified, and conceptual codes were generated by identifying the relationships among categories. The amplifying causal loops of practicing involvement and resisting involvement emerged from the data (Glaser, 2005).

Ethical Consideration

The study was approved by the institutional review boards of both hospitals. Nurses were interviewed after signing a consent form.

FINDINGS

Although the term *special relationship* was not defined for the subjects, their comments confirmed that they understood it to mean a relationship that went beyond the ordinary. By not being bound by a specific definition of the term, each subject was able to respond to it based on his or her own perception of its meaning and to describe examples of what he or she had observed. Nurses described their experiences in risking involvement in special relationships as either practicing involvement or resisting involvement. It was found that the main concern of the nurses in this study was to provide nurturing care to cancer patients. This concern was resolved by risking involvement when supportive relationships were in place to help the nurses resolve their grief when patients died. When supportive relationships were not available, nurses resolved their concern by providing deliberative affective neutral care rather than risking involvement with patients. In both cases nurturing care was provided to patients. The nurses' initial attitudes about caring for cancer patients, the supportive relationships available to the nurse, and the coping strategies they possessed set the stage for future relationships. Unresolved grief after a special relationship led to a conscious decision to reduce the risk of involvement, whereas the resolution of grief led to the decision to again risk involvement in special relationships. These processes are depicted in Figure 18.1.

Each experience made the nurse more certain that her decision had been correct and led to repeating the loop that gave her satisfaction or comfort. Of primary importance was the first experience of becoming involved. Even before beginning to care for cancer patients, many nurses had already decided that they were willing to risk involvement with their patients because they believed that was the only way to provide nurturing. One nurse stated, "I knew how I felt as far as my relationships with the patients and how I wanted to relate to them as a nurse . . . there is *no*

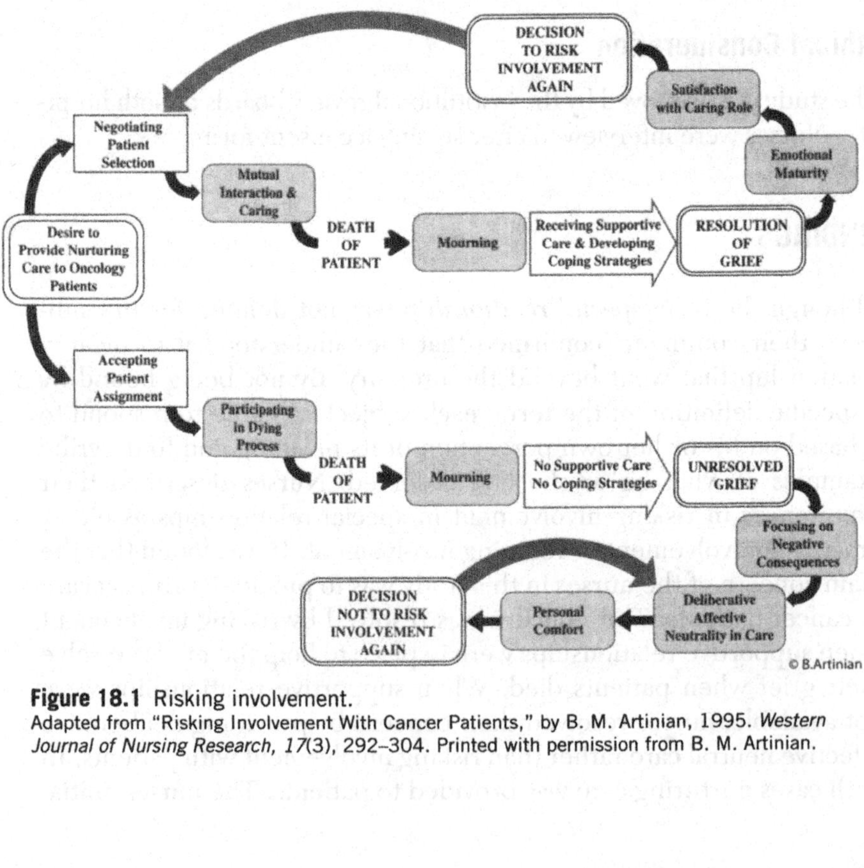

Figure 18.1 Risking involvement.
Adapted from "Risking Involvement With Cancer Patients," by B. M. Artinian, 1995. *Western Journal of Nursing Research, 17*(3), 292–304. Printed with permission from B. M. Artinian.

other way I could nurse." Other nurses believed that affective neutrality was the way to keep the nursing relationship objective, and they were drawn into special relationships over time without a conscious decision to do so. One nurse commented, "Before this happened, I wondered why other nurses got attached, but now I realize you can't help it. I resisted this for two years, and now I haven't done it on purpose." A nursing attendant said, "At first, I really couldn't see how they got attached to patients like that. Now I know. It happens."

During the first experience of involvement, the nurses were familiarized with the personal costs but also the benefits of having shared a life experience with another. Because they were no longer naïve about the experience, it would no longer happen outside of their awareness, and they could use deliberate strategies either to practice involvement in special relationships or to resist it.

Practicing Involvement

Selecting Involvement

Those nurses who chose to form special relationships did not involve themselves with every patient. They were selective, in that they entered into special relationships with some patients and not with others. The most important factor in selection was the personal attraction between nurse and patient, which was often instantaneous. Other factors that influenced the bonding process were the age of the patient, the vulnerability of the patient, similarity of life situation between patient and nurse, and mutuality when the patient showed concern for the nurse.

Nurses described the activities they used to get to know the patients. They said they laughed together and chatted, thus developing a friendship. They also learned about the special interests and needs of the patient.

Although nurses became attached to a patient for a variety of reasons, the concern they showed for a special patient was seen by the staff as beneficial to the patient and not disruptive to the unit. One nurse summarized the situation: "Somehow, everyone gets someone." Nurses were also very aware of the emotional consequences of forming attachments and did not believe that those who were not yet ready for such an involvement were giving inferior care.

Mutual Interaction and Caring

Minute Observation. When a special relationship was formed between a patient and staff nurse, the activities of the nurse changed. For example, she would scrutinize the written orders more closely:

- Maybe they ordered IM injections and I have to think twice. Wait a minute—the platelets are low, so you get the order changed.
- If it is someone that I am interested in, even if the day is heavy, I will go out of my way to check lab values or to read up on the progress notes.

Vigilant Protection. The nurse often knew the patient's wishes in terms of invasive procedures, and she was prepared to defend him or her from medical assault. One nurse guarded a female patient's right to die peacefully while being comforted by her husband. "I felt like I was a pillar outside of her room. Nobody did anything to her unless I knew about it. I knew everything that went on about her 24 hours a day. I was not going to have her hurt anymore."

She was successful in her goal to allow the patient to die peacefully. The husband would call her on the telephone and tell her what the physicians proposed to do for his wife's care, and the nurse would respond: "I'm not going to tell you what to do, but what I am going to say is that what J. has wanted from the beginning is just a nice death."

Special Consideration. Activities with special patients also took other forms, such as donating blood for patients, arranging special events, laughing with them, stopping to chat and make sure that they ate their lunch, or ensuring that patients understood the doctor's instructions. One nurse in the outpatient department arranged her work schedule so that one patient could have her chemotherapy early and get to work on time. Because the patient lived in her area, the nurse made two home visits to draw blood on her way to work.

Modification of Personal Schedules. A special relationship could also interfere with life plans. One nurse had planned to resign from a work situation but found that she could not do so because of her unwillingness to leave the patients with whom she had special relationships. Later, she deliberately decided against involvement so that she could change positions: "I think when I made my decision to leave, I also made the decision not to make a whole lot of new relationships." Another nurse felt guilty that she was on a short vacation when a special patient died even though the patient had urged her to go.

Participation in Death. Despite the personal impact, many nurses chose to be present at the time of patient death as a way of interacting with their patients. This involvement could also extend to their off-duty time. As one nurse described her behavior, "I used to call here all the time. I would get home and make dinner and I would call. And maybe I would call even two times a night—just to see how things were going." One head nurse summarized her staff's involvement in this way: "The people here really care about their patients, and they really care about each other. It's not a job. It's a life's work."

Consequence of Involvement: Mourning

Acceptance of Sadness. Those who experienced involvement with patients were certain to experience grief. A nurse said, "Every patient that you get attached to, you remember, and there is a certain sadness." One nurse said that during her first two years in cancer nursing, she had 10–15 special relationships and grieved at the death of each, to the extent that she was called "the cry baby." Her parents counseled her to change jobs, but she said, "I had a will within myself that I was going to fight this out and cope with and deal with it." This same willingness to continue involvement with cancer patients was expressed by another nurse: "We are confronted daily—many times a day, in some cases—with emotional depth that some people may never have to confront, or maybe just once or twice in their lifetime."

Physical Responses. Another nurse described the impact of her involvement with patients on her physical state. She recounted an interaction with a patient who had been on her unit off and on for four years who told her: "Your face is old." He thought she needed to leave this job and do something happy.

Nurses' grief sometimes resulted in a slowing of physical response that interfered with their ability to work. As one nurse said, "I mean I didn't do anything wrong. I didn't get things done."

Resolution of Grief

Supportive Relationships and Coping Strategies. Support was given both in the hospital setting and at home. For example, a charge nurse who had experienced special relationships with patients said that after a death of a patient with whom a nurse had a special relationship she allowed the nurse time to talk about it during coffee breaks and she also organized time to go out for a meal together. She also allowed the nurse to use her "comp" time to have days off so that she could mourn the loss and attend the funeral.

Nurses who had families described how they were helpful in resolving the nurses' grief. One nurse said that she would be sad at work, but while driving home she started thinking about her children, what to cook for them, and what they needed to do, and so was able to put her sadness out of her mind. Another nurse described the comfort her husband offered. She said that he was just a fireman and knew nothing about the hospital but that after the death of a special patient, he would rock her in a rocking chair until she felt better.

Maturity. One nurse compared her outlook on life with that of her sisters, who were close in age. She said that they were concerned about such little things as peeling wallpaper, but she had a larger perspective and was grateful and happy to be alive. When nurses were able to resolve their grief through supportive relationships and coping strategies, growth and maturity were positive consequences of entering the life experience of dying patients.

Satisfaction With Caring Role

These experiences led the nurses to decide to risk involvement again, and the process of patient selection and mutual interaction and caring recommenced in an amplifying casual loop. One nurse compared the experience of participating in the death of a patient with the experience of participating in the birth of a child. She felt privileged to be included; she had "unique and very touching and memorable" experiences that she would always carry with her.

Resisting Involvement

Decision Not to Risk Involvement

Because of the potential for negative consequences or unresolved grief following an experience of attachment, nurses often made a deliberate choice not to form special relationships with patients. "One day we had a patient die and I didn't even realize that it was bothering me until the end of the day. Then I thought—that is why I have been feeling crummy all day, and now I don't get real close to the patients."

A head nurse summarized the attitude of some of her staff: "You have got to be careful. It's the same old thing. Don't get too involved or you will get hurt. Don't get too involved—we are just going to lose them." Other nurses made the deliberate choice not to get involved with patients because they felt that involvement with some would decrease their job effectiveness. A charge nurse said,

> When you are in charge of everything, you can't give special care to one patient because emotions can cause you not to think about what's going on in the ward. You are upset and your body and mind are not working together. And since I couldn't function well, I thought I had better stop doing those things.

Other nurses described changes in their pattern of involvement:

> I used to start crying, but now—no. They need me and I am not going to get involved with them. . . . You can't get too attached because you know they are not going to be here for a long time. It kind of hurts and you know you had better back away now before they do pass away—you don't want to get attached because it really hurts.

Deliberative Affective Neutrality

Once the deliberate choice was made not to risk involvement, a number of strategies were used by nurses to control the extent of their involvement with patients.

Limiting Contacts. Perhaps the most commonly used strategy was to limit contact with the patient—to back off from relationships that could be painful. Nurses described their strategies to limit attachment:

- You see yourself—oh boy, here I go again. I'm getting too attached. I don't want that. I can have a patient two or three days in a row, but that is all.
- For some reason, yesterday I just wasn't able to deal with the closeness so I asked another nurse to give her treatment.
- I cut off patients eventually. Some of them just get to be too dependent. Then I have to get out.

Seeing All Patients as Equal. Another strategy used to control involvement was to see all patients as equal: "I try to balance it out—give everybody an equal amount of time so that everybody is going to have their chance."

Keep Patient in Patient Role. Another strategy was to see the patient as a patient and not as a friend: "I have to care for her as a patient, not as a girl friend." This attitude was in sharp contrast with the attitude of the involved nurse who said: "Your client relationship is kind of changed. You don't see them that much as a patient."

By concentrating on the patient as a patient and the job as a job, special attachments were avoided: "I am here and it is a job. I am here for 8 hours and I like to make the best of it. If a patient wants a certain nurse, that is her business."

Personal Comfort

The deliberate choice to provide affectively neutral care resolved the main concern of the nurses to provide nurturing care but not to experience the negative consequences of a special relationship. This provided personal comfort for them. By deciding not to risk involvement they were able to continue to provide care for cancer patients. This personal comfort reinforced their decision not to risk involvement and led to an amplifying casual loop in which their strategies to resist involvement continued to provide comfort to them.

Application to Nursing Settings

In GT, data collection and analysis are concurrent. Consequently, toward the end of the data collection period I was able to use the insights from this study in counseling a nurse. I interviewed a nurse who said he thought he was beginning to have a special relationship with a child. Knowing what the relationship could mean to him in terms of sorrow and satisfaction, I asked him about his family and friend support groups and outside interests and told him how important they were to nurses who chose to risk involvement.

DISCUSSION

The basic social process of Risking Involvement in special relationships that was studied in the research took the form of *resisting* or *practicing involvement*. These types of relationships are similar to those described by Morse (1991) who categorized relationships as clinical, therapeutic, connected, and over-involved. In the experience of nurses in this study, both resisting involvement and risking involvement were therapeutic for the patient. The process of resisting involvement could be called "clinical" and risking involvement, "connected." These findings were also consistent with findings of Ramos (1992), who identified three levels of relationships: the instrumental, the protective level with an emotional component, and the reciprocal relationship with resolved control issues. Nurses who risked involvement carried out protective activities and also experienced a reciprocal relationship with special patients. Nurses did not form special relationships with all patients, but only the ones they selected. However, one charge nurse commented that on her unit, "everyone had someone." The personal satisfaction the nurse received from the special relationships, knowing that she had met the needs of the dying patient and come to know a person at this point of life, supports the findings of Ramos (1992), who found that nurses perceived the most intense levels of attachment to be the most beneficial. The nurses' cognitive perception of their role, their capacity for establishing supportive relationships, and their use of healthy coping strategies influenced their ability to form special relationships. When they did enter into a special relationship, it was beneficial to the patient because the nurses acted in a concerned manner, as described by Benner (1989).

For novice nurses, the first experience of a special relationship could be immediate, because of their attitudes about caring for patients, or it could be delayed for a period of time or avoided entirely. When a special relationship did occur, it had the characteristics identified by Fosbinder (1991) of "going the extra mile." Fosbinder stated that both patients and nurses described the immediate rapport between them as "clicking," and this led to friendship and the willingness of the nurse to do extra things for the patient.

Experienced nurses who had practiced involvement in special relationships could decide to resist involvement because of changes in their life situations that made an involvement too costly, such as a change in support systems, or the taking on of additional responsibilities such as beginning graduate school. They would then begin to use the strategies of resisting involvement, even though it resulted in decreased satisfaction for them. Ramos (1992) also described how nurses could move between the levels of involvement.

CONCLUSION

An understanding of the strategies of *practicing involvement* and *resisting involvement* may be of value to nurses who desire to interact on an involved level but are uncertain about what the involvement would require of them. Further study needs to be done to describe an intermediate level of caregiving between affective neutrality and special relationships, such as the deliberative nursing practice described by Orlando (1961) or the role of concern as it informs nursing practice described by Benner (1989). In each of these forms of practice, the personhood of the patient is respected, but the nurse does not enter as completely into the life experiences of the patient. Further work needs to be done to elaborate the strategies used by nurses to provide this intermediate type of care.

REFERENCES

Artinian, B. (1984). Fostering hope in the bone marrow transplant child. *Maternal-Child Nursing Journal, 13,* 57–71.

Artinian, B. (1995). Risking involvement with cancer patients. *Western Journal of Nursing Research, 17*(3), 292–304.

Benner, P. (1989). *The primacy of caring.* Menlo Park, CA: Addison-Wesley.

Brammer, L. M. (1988). *The helping relationship* (4th ed.). Englewood Cliffs, NJ: Prentice Hall.

Donovan, M. (1981). Stress at work: Cancer nurses report. *Oncology Nursing Forum, 8*(2), 23–25.

Fosbinder, D. M. (1991). *Nursing care through the eyes of the patient.* San Diego, CA: University of San Diego.

Glaser, B. G. (1978). *Theoretical sensitivity: Advances in the methodology of grounded theory*. Mill Valley, CA: Sociology Press.

Glaser, B. G. (1998). *Doing grounded theory: Issues and discussions.* Mill Valley, CA: Sociology Press.

Glaser, B. G. (2005). *The grounded theory perspective III: Theoretical coding.* Mill Valley, CA: Sociology Press.

Morse, J. M. (1991). Negotiating commitment and involvement in the nurse-patient relationship. *Journal of Advanced Nursing, 16,* 455–468.

Orlando, I. (1961). *The dynamic nurse-patient relationship*. New York: Putnam.

Ramos, M. C. (1992). The nurse-patient relationship: Theme and variations. *Journal of Advanced Nursing, 17,* 496–506.

IV Role Theory

INTRODUCTION: BARBARA M. ARTINIAN

Interactions in terms of roles and positions have been explored for many years. The operational definition that I developed of role theory as a theoretical code is the reciprocal interaction between persons, which is organized into roles. It views behavior as the product of the interaction between self and roles.

This section presents two studies in which the emergent theoretical code related to role theory. Winter explored the organizational practices at a nursing home and identified many practices of care providers that helped to preserve the identity of patients who were entering a new role as a nursing home resident (see chapter 19, "Preserving Identity in a Nursing Home Setting"). For those experiencing a major role transition, it is helpful to recognize the change and modify behaviors to assist the person with this change.

In the second study, Hjälmhult studied the educational process for public health nursing, which in Norway occurs after the completion of baccalaureate education. The grounded theory of Conquering Operational Space emerged to resolve the participants' main concern of obtaining good learning experiences to become a public health nurse. The chapter presented here focuses on the first phase of her theory (see chapter 20, "Positioning in Operational Space: How to Become a Public Health Nurse in Norway"). The change of roles from seasoned nurse to novice public health nurse was a major hurdle in the participants' nursing career.

Understanding the challenges of role change can be very helpful to nurse educators, supervisors, students, nurses, and patients alike.

19 Preserving Identity in a Nursing Home Setting

VICTORIA WINTER
BARBARA M. ARTINIAN

Charlie, bless his heart, is actually interested in my story.
—*Water for Elephants* by Sara Gruen

The decision to surrender an elderly family member, be it a mother, or father, an aunt or uncle, or even a sibling to the care of others at a nursing home can be a time of crisis for a family. To admit to themselves that they can no longer care for this beloved member of the family, whose needs are beyond what they are capable of providing, fills families with feelings of guilt, helplessness, and failure. This task becomes even more arduous when the family member has become mentally incompetent, as in the case of Alzheimer's disease. How does one explain to this family member the decision to place him or her in a nursing home—especially a family member who is aggressive, or can no longer recognize son or daughter nor remember his or her own identity? Is there a good home, one that the family can trust and depend on to care for their loved one as they would if they could?

Once in a home, families need and seek to maintain a sense of attachment to their relative by engaged involvement to reduce their loss and create new ways of caring. The family becomes the reference group for the staff of a nursing home by affirming the staff's use of specialized knowledge of their family member as a basis for planning quality care. Seeing mother or father content and adjusted in a new environment, these families are eternally grateful for the care and concern that is shown.

One such facility that focuses on quality of life and quality of care is the Ararat Nursing Home in Mission Hills, California, an exemplary facility that has shown unprecedented success in the field of elder care. Under the leadership of Executive Nursing Director Margo Babikian, the facility has been chosen for a number of federal and state awards for excellence in nursing home care, including a zero deficiency evaluation from the California Department of Health Services for the past several years. This nonprofit skilled nursing provider, with 196 beds, has been providing compassionate care for seniors since its establishment in 1949.

The innovative Resident-Centered Care Model practiced at Ararat Nursing Home reflects a philosophical shift from mass care to individualized services. The organization of the home is based on the Intersystem Model (Artinian, 1997), which focuses on mutual decision making and development of a joint plan of care. Patient and caregiver are active participants in this process with collaboration needed along the continuum of care. The paradigm shift seen here is from an authoritarian relationship to a collaborative, supportive relationship that supports the resident's individuality as a dynamic entity.

THE STUDY

Aim

The purpose of the study was to identify organizational practices that are used by this facility to achieve quality patient care.

Method

Classical grounded theory methodology developed by Glaser and Strauss (1967) and in the later writings of Glaser (1978, 1992, 1993) was utilized for this study. The researchers used open-ended interviewing to explore the concerns of the nursing staff and their relationships with the residents, in particular the special relationships they formed with selected patients. The certified nursing assistants (CNA) were asked about their "adopted" residents, how they chose them, and what was special about their relationship. The questions served as a guide for the interview process. This study was done strictly from the viewpoint of the nurse.

Some of the questions used were: What new things did you learn during your orientation period? What things are done differently here at Ararat? What is most important to you when you work with a resident? Additional questions were used to clarify or amplify the nurses' responses as the core variables emerged.

Sample

Seven certified nursing assistants (CNAs) who work at the Ararat Nursing Home participated in this project on a voluntary basis. The nursing director and the head nurse assisted in recruiting the participants. As a group the subjects had worked at the Ararat home from 2 to 10 years. They ranged in age from 28 to 50 years of age, with a mean age of 38 years. The languages spoken by the subjects were varied and included English, Armenian, Turkish, Russian, Spanish, Italian, Arabic, and Farsi. All had immigrated to the United States from other countries such as Armenia and Russia. Previous occupations included nursing, medical student, epidemiologist, and hygienist. Only one subject was male.

All were CNAs who followed the innovative Resident-Centered Care Model utilized at the facility, which focuses on individualized service for each client and implementing state-of-the-art best practices. All were involved with actual patient care and as such had the opportunity to form relationships with the residents. One of the subjects was the senior team leader, another a team leader/charge nurse, and a third was a restorative CNA. Since this was an exploratory study, no attempt was made to limit the subjects to nursing personnel with the same level of skill or understanding.

Data Collection

In-depth interviews were conducted with the subjects at the facility in a quiet conference room off of the main dining area. Participant observation was also done in the common areas and in multidisciplinary conferences that were held every week at the facility. The interviews were tape recorded to provide clarity and detail to the data. They ranged in length from 30 minutes to 2 hours. The length of the interviews varied because some subjects had worked as a CNA for several years and had more experiences to share. Some were more open in describing their experiences with residents than were others. Subjects spoke of current residents as well as those they had cared for in the past, some of whom were deceased. The head nurse sat in on all of the interviews and helped to translate for those subjects that did not feel comfortable responding in English.

Data Analysis

Using constant comparative analysis, the data were simultaneously collected and analyzed to identify the core processes in the phenomenon under investigation in this study. The first author transcribed all of the interviews from the audiotapes. Line-by-line analysis of the written transcripts as well as frequent listening to the audiotapes, especially during transcription, helped to capture the powerful statements of the subjects that led to the development of the codes.

An expression heard frequently during the interviews was, "We are a family." During the initial analysis, it was thought that the core category was *family making,* but that proved to be inadequate because it did not integrate all categories. While reading the book *Water for Elephants* by Sara Gruen, the second author discovered the section that describes the conversation of an elderly nursing home resident with a young circus employee. Upon reading the comment by the elderly man, "Charlie, bless his heart, is actually interested in my story," she suddenly realized that the focus of the Ararat Home was to listen to the residents and incorporate that knowledge about them into the plan of care. From this realization the core category of Preserving Identity emerged. This category integrated all aspects of care provided by the nursing home.

Ethical Considerations

Approval for the study was obtained from the institutional review boards at the Ararat Nursing Home and Azusa Pacific University. The study was explained to all subjects and consent to participate was signed at that time. Data were given code numbers and kept confidential throughout the study.

FINDINGS

Self-identity is at the core of our being, our essence, our meaning in life. It is necessary to understand the danger to a sense of identity that occurs when a person enters a nursing home. When the core category of

Preserving Identity emerged, we turned to the literature on role theory to help us in structuring our data.

The organization of the Ararat Home provides the backdrop for preserving identity. Because each staff member is respected and appreciated as being part of the family, the entire team can work together to make the patient come first and be part of the family, thus preserving the identity of the resident. These practices will be discussed (see Figure 19.1).

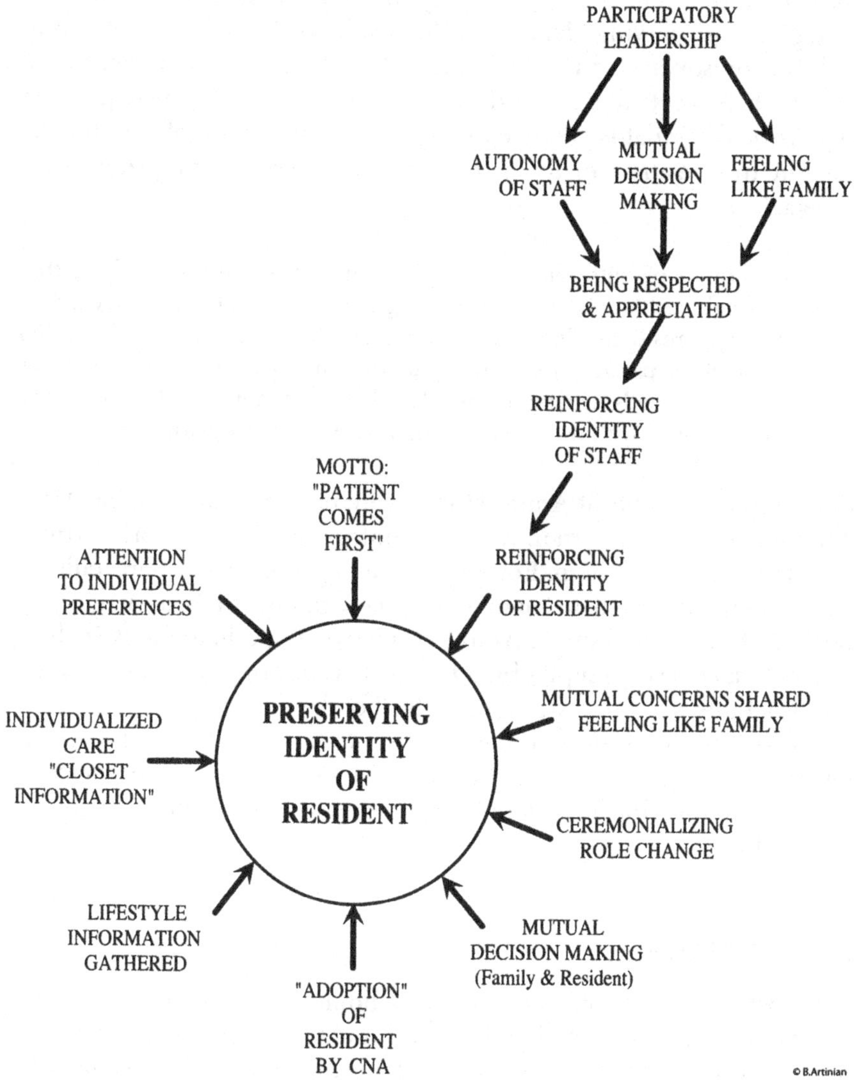

Figure 19.1 Preserving Identity in a nursing home setting.
Printed with permission from B. Artinian.

Motto Is "Patient Comes First"

The central focus of the care at Ararat is the individual resident. Each resident, each person, is treated as an individual with a life history that is significant, remembered, and cherished. The essence of that person is preserved from the time the staff first meets the patient at the front door in the lobby until the time of discharge or death. As expressed by one of the CNAs, "Patient is come first (sic). First patient care." This attitude then becomes the core strategy that acts as the basis for all other strategies in preserving identity for the residents. How does one accomplish this preservation? For the staff at Ararat, care of the patient is all done with respect, dignity, and compassion. "This is the first place (I have worked at) that is taking care of resident (sic). A lot of care for the resident from everyone. Even the supervisors are treating them with respect."

> Yes, there are big differences here. First thing I saw and I learned was that every single resident is different individual. There is individualized care for every single resident. There is no such thing like all are same. All of them are separate, separately assessed, separately. They teach me separately what this resident needs, what is his needs, what is his culture, what his ability and I have to be with them. This is the first thing that I learn at Ararat.

Many of the residents at Ararat Home were of Armenian descent. Most of these people were born in various countries around the world, Armenia being only one of them. For Armenians, a people in diaspora, culture is extremely important in maintaining their family, their heritage, and their ties to one another. At Ararat Home serving ethnic foods such as yogurt, feta cheese, and pita bread, as well as offering Armenian television programs, served to strengthen this bond.

Preserving Identity becomes a core category that has lasting qualities: abstract of time, place, and people (Glaser, 1993). The strategies to preserve identity for the residents experiencing a major role change will be described.

Ceremonializing

For most residents entering a nursing home, there is no ceremonial change. They are admitted and treated much like a patient entering a hospital, as if it were a temporary residence; they are only persons with a name and a diagnosis. At Ararat, at the time of admission, a place is prepared. Not just any room, but an environment that evokes the feelings of "home" for that person.

> I will start from the main entrance. Before the patient arrives I receive the paper that the patient is coming. The first thing I would like to make sure of is that the place he is coming to will be as his second home, if not first after a while. How do I do that? I orient the staff, all CNAs that the person is coming . . . to make sure the room will be in the best shape; and when the resident arrives, just as a friend in a very friendly manner but remaining professional, I will show him the place and try to make sure that he will not feel in a new place.

This rite of passage for residents becomes a change for the good, not a bad change.

Lifestyle Information Gathered

At admission there are two key forms that are filled out—the lifestyle and the "closet" information forms. With the help of the family and the patient, questions about their past lives are filled out as to vocation, hobbies, and spiritual preferences. If no family is available, every effort is made by the staff to contact family and relatives to obtain the most important details. The "closet" information is a summation of the lifestyle form that is posted inside the closet door in the patient's room. On this sheet is contained not only information on whether the resident is alert and oriented, can stand or walk, or has pain issues, but also what the resident loves. The resident may love to listen to the radio, watch TV, or go for walks in the garden. All these crucial details are noted so that nothing is lost. "They are becoming very attached to us and we love them—just love them as our own grandfathers and grandmothers. For myself, to have someone next to me, to have someone's attention, that is the most important thing that I will make sure they have."

"Adoption" of Resident by CNA

Most of the staff, though, already knows what is on the "closet" information sheet for each resident. Each staff member figuratively adopts several residents as a primary assignment. For some staff the resident they have adopted had a special need or concern. One CNA adopted a resident because of the language she spoke—Arabic. "Oh, with the resident I adopt, the first thing was her language. She speaks Arabic. Nobody understands but she also speaks Italian. I speak Italian. I try to talk to her. I know what she likes, what she wants and I help her."

Another CNA picked a resident who was also "very challenging":

> She loves me but sometimes she is fighting with her roommate, with the other residents, even with the CNAs sometimes. But with me I am going, "Oh, honey, I love you. Look how nice you look today. Look at your hair, your face. . . . When I adopt her someone asked me how can you get along with her? She is too much. I don't want to say nothing bad about her but so I am getting along with her.

Attention is given to every detail—nothing too small is overlooked. For these residents at Ararat the focus on helping each resident make the successful transition to a nursing home is done with much thought, attention to detail, and above all compassion for that individual person and his or her family. Many come to Ararat Home not talking, not smiling, or not walking. With personal attention these matters improve.

Individual Preferences

During a multidisciplinary conference, Margo, the executive nursing director, asked one resident about the things that she would wish for—food, activities, or hobbies. The resident replied that she enjoyed dogs, crocheting, and eating Armenian cheese as a snack. The team composed of the CNAs that care for her asked about the possibility of a small refrigerator for her room. This idca sparked much discussion about a trip with the resident to shop for the cheese and other favorite foods, the resident's responsibility to keep the refrigerator clean, and above all, a way to make the resident's place at Ararat more homelike. This discussion reinforced an earlier role for this woman of housekeeper, an important role in Armenian culture.

Mutual Concerns

Ararat exists as a community where mutual concerns are shared. At the time of the interviews the nursing director had recently had surgery and was away from the facility for 6 weeks. After her return, as the director walked the halls or stopped and spoke with residents in the dining hall,

all would ask how she was feeling and if she was doing well and not in any pain. This concern was also shown to other residents and the CNA staff. One resident who had to be moved to another wing to accommodate a broken arm was assigned to a different CNA team. The resident went to the nursing director's office to make a plea to either be moved back with her CNA or have the CNA moved to her wing. A compromise was reached and the resident was moved back.

Mutual Decision Making

All plans and decisions about residents at Ararat are made with input from the residents themselves and their families. This is especially apparent at the multidisciplinary meetings that are held every Wednesday. At each meeting approximately five residents are discussed. The CNAs that provide care for these residents are present along with the residents and their families or relatives. This is a time for the staff to discuss with each resident how he or she is adjusting to living at Ararat, his or her health and nutrition, whether pain is present, and the resident's potential for falls. Moreover, the residents' hopes and dreams are discussed. For many, their wishes to see family or relatives that are out of state are realized and plans made for travel. Families are encouraged to attend and give input. One son wanted to be sure someone was able to take his mother for a walk every day in the garden since he could only visit on the weekends. This daily walk became part of her plan of care.

If residents express issues such as difficulties adjusting to this new environment, the team is consulted for an answer. At times this consultation involves a root cause analysis to determine the factors involved. One woman was having trouble going to the dining room for meals. When asked, the resident said she was lonely. Her CNA also brought up the fact that this was the third nursing home this woman had entered in the past 6 weeks. Margo made arrangements to escort her to lunch in the dining room for the next week. Her CNA would sit with her for the other meals.

DISCUSSION

Moving into a new role is not always easy. A successful adjustment to the role of a nursing home resident is essential for what is to many a final transition in their lives. Over the course of a person's life progressive refinement of one's role gives a dynamic, developmental character to each individual, creating a unique identity (Davis, 1966). Preserving this identity is an essential part of this role change. One's identity along with past accomplishments are what we all hope we will be remembered for when we are gone—those things that our friends and family will speak of. For a nursing home resident to be remembered as the teacher, the violinist, or the grandmother with five sons is to be remembered for who she has been and still is.

One of the residents had been a concert violinist, so the staff obtained a violin for him to hold and carry. Even though he could no longer play, to have that instrument with him imparted a sense of comfort that was irreplaceable. A woman who had been a teacher was given a role in the Sunday morning program to teach about the scripture of the day. Again, this was a celebration of a life accomplishment for this woman.

New nursing home residents must constantly negotiate their new role between themselves, the staff, and their family. For this study, we looked at the negotiation between the residents and the certified nursing assistants. George Herbert Mead, in his seminal 1934 work *Mind, Self, and Society,* explored this notion of role negotiation. The learning of new roles is done in an interactive fashion; it is not meaningful to think of a role for one person alone, but for that person as an individual who is both cooperating and competing with others. This apparently self-contradictory mutual relationship between self and others is easily seen in encounters where there is considerable ambiguity, and is part of all social interactions. Each individual tries to define the situation or understand their role within it, choose a role that is advantageous or appealing, play that role, and persuade others to support it.

The nursing home resident's role is carried out in the context of each individual's orientation to the situation. Prior experiences with nursing homes will influence the perceptions of some. However, no person's behavior occurs in a random manner but is influenced by his or her own expectations and those of the other residents in the nursing home. At Ararat, all 196 residents are allowed to be people, not patients. As a consequence, each is seen not as a combination of medical issues, but as a real person.

Status and role represent conceptually the ideal patterns of behavior that are to be expected in given situations. Nursing home residents must assume that status of a patient in a nursing home. They are assigned rooms, with roommates usually not of their choosing, on a nursing unit with distinct meal times, visiting hours, and activities. Gone are their familiar surroundings, their freedom of choice for meals and foods, and their freedom to choose how to live out each hour of every day. Also gone is the choice to be placed in this situation, which for most nursing home residents is a decision made by others, family or otherwise. To adjust to this new situation is to accept the fact that they are now patients.

CONCLUSION

Relatives involved with a family member experiencing a major role transition need to know the rights and obligations of the role and the behavior changes that the transition entails. Those around the resident need to recognize this change of role and modify their behaviors in a corresponding fashion (Banton, 1965). The greater the change for the individual, the more others have to modify their behavior when the person is encountered in both the old and new roles. For the residents at Ararat, their time in the nursing home becomes a rite of passage to a new role in life, where it matters to all who they are and how they can best live their final days.

REFERENCES

Artinian, B. (1997). *The Intersystem Model: Integrating theory and practice*. Thousand Oaks, CA: Sage.

Banton, M. (1965). *Roles: An introduction to the study of social relations*. New York: Basic Books.

Davis, K. (1966). Status and related concepts. In B. J. Biddle and E. J. Thomas (Eds.), *Role theory: Concepts and research*. New York: Wiley.

Glaser, B. G. (1978). *Theoretical sensitivity*. Mill Valley, CA: Sociology Press.

Glaser, B. G. (1992). *Basics of grounded theory analysis*. Mill Valley, CA: Sociology Press.

Glaser, B. G. (1993). *Examples of grounded theory: A reader.* Mill Valley, CA: Sociology Press.

Glaser, B. G., & Strauss, A. L. (1967). *The discovery of grounded theory: Strategies for qualitative research.* Hawthorne, NY: Aldine de Gruyter.

Gruen, S. (2007). *Water for elephants.* Chapel Hill, NC: Workman.

Mead, G. H. (1934). *Mind, self and society.* Chicago: University of Chicago Press.

20

Positioning in Operational Space: How to Become a Public Health Nurse in Norway

ESTHER HJÄLMHULT

Caring for parents and babies is at the heart of public health nursing (PHN) in Norway. The shift from caring for people with health problems to caring for healthy people can be difficult. This study reports how Norwegian PHN students begin to see their new role. The concept *operational space* is used to explain how students had to move from focusing on illness and disease to a space of health and prevention. In the context of this study I define operational space as an actual zone or space required for professional agency, action, and conduct. *Positioning in operational space* is the first phase in a conquering process and is a process of obtaining learning experiences that students believe are relevant for their future practice. This knowledge could normalize the students' insecurity and contribute to confidence and improved learning experiences.

This study focused on PHN education. Unlike the parallel nursing role in the United States that is part of a baccalaureate program in nursing, PHN education in Norway is a postgraduate program requiring a BS in nursing and 1 year of full-time work as a registered nurse (Ministry of Education and Research, 2005). PHN education includes 10 weeks of practical training in districts within different rural or urban municipalities. Contracts between the University College and municipalities establish a framework for practice. Considerable administrative work is needed to provide sufficient placements. The typical clinic supervisor is a practicing PHN who receives minimal compensation and could be more or less enthusiastic about supervising a student. The faculty teacher has a peripheral facilitator role, meeting the student and supervisor two to three times during the student's placement. A PHN in Norway works with children and adolescents 0–20 years old and the focus of care is on health promotion and disease prevention. The services are provided at clinics run by Child Health Services and School Health Services, and are free of charge. These services are popular and are almost universally embraced.

THE STUDY

Aim

The purpose of this chapter is to describe the first phase of a generated grounded theory of Conquering Operational Space, which emerged from this study of PHN students in clinical practice.

Method

Grounded theory developed by Glaser and Strauss (1967) and Glaser (1978, 1998) was used for this design to explore the main concern of PHN students in clinical practice and how they acted to resolve this challenge.

Participants

I gathered data through 55 interviews with 21 PHN students and their 108 written weekly reports. I recruited participants in collaboration with the program director, who allowed me to enter the group. Forty-two PHN students, all women, received information and were invited to participate. Seventeen agreed, and four were recruited later to advance the emerging theory. They had nursing experience from different kinds of work in hospitals and communities and ranged in age from 26 to 43 years (average 36.5). Each participant was asked to complete a short weekly report with two questions: "Describe a situation from your practice in which you learned something this week," and "A challenge for me (professionally or emotionally) this week has been . . ." Because of increasing workload, students completed the reports fortnightly at the end of the study.

Data Collection and Analysis

I conducted the interviews in 2001–2002 and recorded, transcribed, and analyzed them continually. I arranged the interviews at the students' practical placement or in my office to avoid interruptions, and I tried to create a relaxed environment (Kvale, 1996). The weekly reports, with the two questions presented, served as an introduction for each interview, which lasted about one hour.

Substantive Coding

Data analysis comprised two activities: coding data, and memo writing about the coded data. Substantive codes involve (a) open coding in which all the transcripts are coded until a core category is identified that gathers and explains what happened, and (b) selective coding in which relevant categories are coded around the core category. In open coding I coded the transcripts manually line by line, constantly comparing them with previous coded transcripts. The focus was on the incidents—the meaning, action, and interaction—and was led by such questions as "What happens here?"

After I identified the main concern, the study progressed to identify patterns of behavior by which the students resolved this concern. The codes were grouped into broad categories. They moved from descriptive concepts such as *place oneself on the sideline* to broader concepts such as *role-seeking* and *dialogue-seeking.*

Theoretical Coding

Theoretical codes are abstract models that allow the researcher to talk about substantive categories and properties while thinking theoretically (Glaser, 2005). Theoretical codes conceptualize how the substantive codes may be related. After the core category was found, I tried different ways of correlating substantive codes to describe the identity transformation that was taking place in the students. Coding new interviews and rereading all the transcripts many times clarified which categories needed deeper understanding.

Ethical Considerations

My connection as a teacher at the university was clarified: I did not guide, follow up, or evaluate students. My research contract with the participants followed the ethical research guidelines related to confidentiality, possibility to withdraw without consequences, and my independent role as a researcher. Data obtained would not be given to the university or practice settings. (None of the participants dropped out.) Possible ethical implications would be managed with dialogue; however, some of the participants reported that the interviews had been valuable for them. I was informed that this study did not require approval from the Regional Ethical Board. The Norwegian Social Science Data Services was informed about the study.

FINDINGS

The students' main concern was identified as *how to obtain learning experiences to become a public health nurse.* They resolved this by the substantive grounded theory Conquering Operational Space, a basic social process consisting of three phases: *positioning, involving,* and *integrating into operational space.* The students directed their strategies within the student role, relations with the supervisor, and student activities. Each phase had its own conditions, strategies, and consequences. The full process is presented in my dissertation (Hjälmhult, 2007) and in an article (Hjälmhult, in press). This chapter explains the first phase.

Conditions About Positioning

Characteristic of the *positioning* phase is the experience of chaos and insecurity. This is related to loss of confidence and loss of identity as a nurse. The participants' nursing duties seemed to be inadequate. They were concerned about expectations, relations to supervisor, clients, and cooperating partners. They had to handle the insecurity of a new role in a new area, and strategies they used were important for how they obtained operational space. One student put it like this:

> In clinical practice they demand a lot of independence and initiative. This is my problem—and it concerns me and my identity that I, in a way, must change something in my head. . . . It may be related to confidence in my roles, that you have had a security and an identity as a nurse. You used to master what you do . . . and now the uncertainty and to be an adult and then a student is hard.

This illustrates the experience of role changing, a wavering nurse identity, and expectations of initiative taking. Students explained the difference between being a competent nurse whom everybody asks for advice and being a novice in a new professional area. Everything in practice seemed to be important. Questions they asked themselves were: What is the best way to start? How to engage? It was overwhelming when meeting children and adolescents, often as new target groups with needs, complicated family situations, and new procedures. The students' lack of knowledge and technical skills led to helplessness and confusion. They had no control over the situation. "I felt it was the same, whatever I could start with. I wanted them to tell me that tomorrow we have this and that, do you want this and this?"

Simultaneously, students expressed that they had expectations and were nervous about the pressure to succeed. Students said they needed to be alert and active, interested, and always in a good mood. They wanted to be clever and nice. They explained that they were afraid of being perceived as stupid or lazy by the supervisor:

"To be alert all the time, to be—and seem—to be very interested, and so I am too, but I think it is special. . . . I have performance anxiety; it is just what it is."

Strategies for Positioning in Operational Space

To overcome these feelings of inadequacy, students used the strategies of *role seeking, dialogue seeking,* and *occasionally participating.* The strategies became integrated, and, by degrees, the students glimpsed the operational space. They discovered "what it is about." See Figure 20.1 for a diagram of the first phase of the theory Conquering Operational Space.

Role Seeking

The students were engaged in finding their role. This included how to act as a student in relation to a supervisor and even to find a PHN role model. One student who had two supervisors said:

> The first two weeks I had only one supervisor—and that was very OK, even though I was a bit anxious about my student role—how it should be. It is even OK with two supervisors, but I have used a lot of energy in finding my role with the new one.

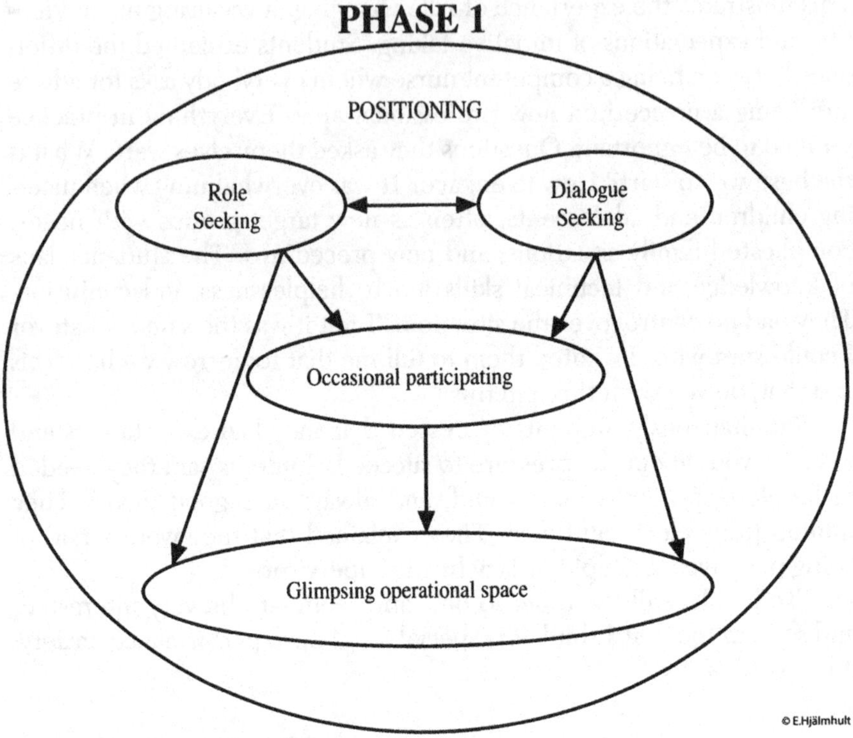

Figure 20.1 Positioning to conquer operational space.
Printed with permission from E. Hjälmhult.

Finding their role required engagement. The students wondered about their activity and how to access learning situations. Placing oneself on the sideline produced ambivalent feelings, but it gave the student the opportunity to observe without requiring participation. They wanted to let impressions sink in before acting. Their feelings were ambivalent because to be on the sideline might protect them from chaos, but it also rendered the students inactive and disengaged. From the sideline, the students sometimes observed poor practice but did not intervene because it was not easy to challenge a supervisor. One student described a group meeting that was not very successful because the leader did not intervene when there was teasing and bullying among the pupils. The student felt miserable and said, "Our oral agreement was not clear about my participation in the group meeting, and I did not feel it was natural to engage. I was on the sideline. I do not know the group or the leader."

When pursuing their role, examples showed how the participants kept a low profile and put up with situations where they actually wanted to respond but did not dare. They had a tactical approach to their activity. They said yes to some activities because they did not want to be discredited in the eyes of the supervisor. For example, they remained with the clients even when they wanted to leave the room to chart and work on care plans. Students felt that it could create a difficult situation if they wanted to withdraw to a silent place and write their notes. They felt that they were stealing away from the practice setting:

> I was frustrated by my student role. To sit down to note some cues as they arise—I experienced it as stealing away . . . then I am out of the practice setting. It was quite a dreadful dilemma; I did not know what to do. I talked with my teacher, and then to [my clinical] practice [supervisor]. It was much easier after being supported from school—it is really OK, you are really a student.

Dialogue Seeking

The students had to be active in seeking dialogue and good relations with the supervisor to secure a position in practice. Several students spontaneously expressed how satisfied they were with the dialogue, and one said:

> I think they are unbelievable, perhaps I have great luck; they are so positive and prepared. They know a lot, so I think that the seminar (for supervisors) was a good one. I experience that I am *wanted,* and even that they think it is nice that I am here.

It was a good feeling to be anticipated and welcomed. Being welcomed was a surprising situation for a lot of the students. Perhaps they had had opposite experiences from earlier situations in practice. Others were disappointed in the attitude of their assigned clinic, missed the encouraging dialogue with their supervisor, and felt rejected or depressed.

Students' motivations might be moderate rather than enthusiastic when they felt less welcomed. A clinic with personnel holding different attitudes and values from those of the student could make conversation a challenge. Sometimes motivated students could meet a less motivated supervisor, who perhaps felt pressure from having responsibility over a student. "They were drawing lots, who should have a student . . . because it is hard—they get tired of the students. . . . She had lost. Yes, I asked them if it was difficult to achieve a practical placement. It has been very strenuous to handle for me."

The students were seeking personal recognition. They wanted to be seen and listened to. In groups or individual consultations the clients were used to following the supervisor. Therefore students appreciated it when supervisors or even clients included them. The students felt vulnerable if a supervisor was absent or there were other hindrances in their learning situations.

In seeking learning experiences with supervisors, adverse elements may arise. Sometimes students missed out on situations if the dialogue was not open, and sometimes they were surprised at the relaxed dialogue. "It was no problem; I only had to say how I wanted to do it." The degree of honest, accepting dialogue with supervisors enhances or diminishes guidance for a PHN establishing operational space. Good dialogue with a supervisor was important for students who were positioning themselves to acquire essential learning experiences. It even formed a basis for participating in practice.

Occasionally Participating

Students' participation in this first phase was occasional, peripheral, and without obligation. The main activity was "to observe and to accompany" the supervisor everywhere, or to assist her, for example, talking with the clients in the waiting room. The students were afraid of missing activities and therefore missing learning opportunities.

Participating seemed to be voluntary, in contradiction to the next phase where participating was expected from both students and supervisor. To stay on the periphery had both advantages and limitations. One student put it like this:

> The first week, I think I was an inactive observer, but gradually got where it seemed to be easy and natural—it has been a lot of this in this practice. . . . Yes, because I do not need to be involved, I had a birds' eye view, seeing what was happening—without putting my foot in it or saying something wrong.

Sometimes the observer role touched and released overwhelming feelings of powerlessness. One student left the room to avoid a situation, while another stayed and asked questions. They had a "peripheral activity" and accessed learning situations through invitation or by taking initiative. By "observing and following" a supervisor in consultations and home visits and making scattered trials to participate, the operational space slowly took form. The advantage of observing an experienced supervisor was described as useful in this phase. To see, listen, and reflect gave insight. Characteristically, several students praised how the supervisor communicated with the clients. For example, they could describe how the PHN got contact with a four-year-old child and saw how she communicated: "She carried out all her investigations in a natural way by playing and talking, so that the child may show what she could do." The students realized that the communication and methods differed substantially from newborn to teenagers, parents and partners.

DISCUSSION

This study was conducted at an educational program for PHN students in Norway. Comparing the experiences of PHN students from other universities together with systematic observations provides further details on student experiences and how students act in practice.

The Student Role

Insecurity in the student role with a feeling of losing nurse identity was handled with three strategies of positioning, and continued until the student obtained an overall image of her role in the public health clinic situation. The three strategies that have been described are: *role-seeking, dialogue-seeking,* and *occasional participating*. They lead to a state of *glimpsing operational space.* The process of arriving at this glimpse varied in time and dimensions; it became an integrated part of the learning experiences and a vital basis for developing further competence. The students experienced ways of working out their role through reflection. This reflection contributed to shaping the outline of an operational space through cognitive impressions, attitudes, and emotions.

When they glimpsed their role as a PHN, they compared this glimpse with their own expectations from theory in PHN education and professional practice. These three following areas attracted attention for students at the end of positioning.

Meeting a New Paradigm

Here they saw that a PHN proceeds differently from a hospital nurse, because the focus in public health was on health promotion and disease prevention in ordinary family and community life rather than, "What is wrong with you?" Students felt that the work had a different mentality than in a hospital. "It is a new way of thinking—it is differently related to traditional nursing, because there the main focus is on disease."

Professional Secrecy

Students wondered about reading case records, making use of interdisciplinary cooperation, and interpreting confidentiality. How much could be said about schoolchildren or parents in a meeting with teachers, social workers, child welfare officers, or psychologists? The greatest challenge, however, was to *not* be allowed to tell parents when children or adolescents refused to give information or when parents refused to involve other professions.

PHN as a Public Person

Students even perceived that a PHN was a more public person than a hospital nurse. The PHNs had to balance their words and demonstrate skill, distinguishing between everyday knowledge and professional knowledge when seeing clients. The students admired the PHN for her overview and how she gained trust from the clients. The moment when the students understood what was going on, or glimpsed the operational space, marked a shift of perspective; they started recognizing and were able to move on into the next phase, *involving themselves in operational space.*

The Process of Positioning

Although the focus has been on Norwegian PHN students, research from other countries and professions show similar results concerning student insecurity, anxiety, and sense of chaos in practice (Bayer, 2001; Chapman & Orb, 2001; Charleston & Happell, 2005; Peyrovi, Yadavar-Nikravesh, Oskouie, & Berterö, 2005; Talvitie, Peltokallio, & Männistö, 2000).

Role Seeking

In clinical practice, Heggen (1995) describes how nursing students in their second year at a somatic hospital experienced insecurity, invisibility, and namelessness, being on the periphery of the social and practical community. They were striving to have a name, not just get referred to as "the student." The insecurity is identified by students as a part of their experiences in this study, but not the namelessness and feeling invisible, perhaps because they had already known what it was like to be a professional nurse, or because it happened that in their particular situations, they were appreciated.

To be placed on the sideline is to be on the periphery in practice. That position was not entirely negative; the student might feel like an outsider, but she did get an overview of what a PHN is. The temptation was for students to stay on the periphery instead of moving independently to accrue their own experiences. Bayer (2001) described the metaphorical "client room" through which students had to advance to be in a position to take advantage of learning situations. In Bayer's study, students had to comprehend the "client room," that is, to join the clinic situation at the respectful and submissive level of clients, before moving into the "pedagogical room," which meant to know how to approach the educators and comprehend the institutional rhythms and routines. PHN students often used the strategy of *tactically approaching* just to arrive in or stay in operating position. The question researchers are trying to answer is: Does the humble attitude of students work as a door opener to supervisors and communities, and paradoxically act as a way to conquer a position? My findings support an answer of "yes" to this question.

Positioning in operational space and finding her role in this way is vital to the student's learning process. This positioning effort is also described in a study of addiction nurses and their role development (Clancy, Oyefeso, & Ghodse, 2007). The study described the first of five stages to be the most distressing, with the core features being performance anxiety, feelings of being overwhelmed, and the absence of technical knowledge and skills. Failure to successfully navigate the first stage was likely to result in exit from the program. In my study, none of the PHN students dropped out even though two of them expressed wanting to change their local practical placement.

Dialogue Seeking

Some participants remained silent when they really wanted to contradict their supervisor. In a study of midwifery students (Davies & Atkinson, 1991), similar aspects are described. Midwifery students were ambivalent and insecure, polite, humble, and silent even if they knew their supervisors spoke incorrectly. They developed "studentmanship" in order to survive a hierarchical system, and focused on routine duties of nursing (temperature, pulse, respiration, and blood pressure). The authors in that study have questioned if the midwifery students would continue prioritizing submissiveness instead of developing more professional independence.

For PHN students, there are no routine nursing tasks like those the midwife students had, which could be one reason why the students in this study wavered or had a feeling of losing their identity as a nurse. Initially, we believed that they perceived that their nursing competence was insufficient. The client group was unknown to the students, and only a few had experiences working with children, adolescents, and their parents. Losing identity as a nurse is an underreported theme in the literature.

Another interesting issue is the value of contact with a supervisor for PHN students. They were seeking *personal* acceptance, in contrast to the *professional* acceptance that occurred in the next phase of this study. Although several students did feel integrated into routine practice, others strove to be included. It is suggested that they struggled with necessities of being a student, feeling uncomfortable when withdrawing to note cues, reflect on a situation, or prepare some activity. In the same manner, Heggen (1995) highlighted this problem, how students toned down their student role to be included in practice. They struggled to find the balance between school and practice, leading to self-restraint and subordination toward the supervisor in order to be accepted. Dialogue and good relations with supervisors are basic in practice and an important component in students' learning.

Some students had conflicts with their supervisor before they received a position in practice, and were at risk of being marginalized. This is in contrast with students who had a humble attitude and were rewarded with open doors (Mørck, 2003). On the other hand, there are examples of students who resisted their supervisor and nonetheless retained their position in the program.

In a literature review about effective supervision in medical clinical practice settings, Kilminster and Jolly (2001) concluded that the "supervisory relationship is probably the single most important factor for the effectiveness of supervision." They emphasize the necessity for clear feedback from supervisor to student and the importance of the students' control over, and input into, the supervisory process.

Occasional Participating

PHN students referred to being insecure about expectations from practice, and the need to be alert and acquisitive, so as not to be perceived as a lazy or inert person. Some of these aspects are discussed by Bayer (2001) concerning students from educational studies. He describes practice as "hidden curriculum," and specifies a number of invisible expectations of students in practice. One of them is to be engaged and to be active all the time. According to him, this "hidden pedagogy" controls the students. The findings in this study confirm that expectations or criteria for evaluation were hidden but effective in managing student learning. Other studies confirm the existence of supervisor attitudes that students should know their place, The hierarchical nature of the supervisory setup resulted in a sense of oppression and stood as a hindrance to autonomous practice (Begley, 2002; Currie, 1999).

The final main impression from my study is that students were in constant internal negotiation with themselves. They were always alert: to dare or not to dare was their concern. This parallels Chapman and Orb's study (2001) in that different types of students continually consider and negotiate finding an acceptable position in practice.

Positioning and Nervousness

Nervousness is recognized in other studies (Admi, 1997; Cusson & Viggiano, 2002; Löfmark & Wikblad, 2001). Several of the students were nervous in practice and sought clarity and good relations with their supervisor and others in the area. They balanced between subordination and understanding of the hidden curriculum, striving to be included in the community. To accomplish positioning in operational space, the students had to handle their roles, their cooperation with a supervisor, and their engagement in activities by choosing strategies in relation to these areas. The students' insecurity was related to the conditions they experienced, and to expectations from the supervisor or the clinical environment as well as from themselves.

Implications for Learning in Practice

The phase of *positioning in operational space* generated here illuminates PHN students' experiences in practice. It provides a framework for understanding the reasons why students act the way they do in clinical practice, and can be useful for PHN education, and even for practice. Supervisors can use this theory when planning and organizing student educational experiences. The notion of gaining insight into a wavering nursing identity may be a helpful construct to be managed during the students' education. Good relations and personal recognition are essential to student progress; they tip the balance of the students' energy flow toward having positive learning experiences.

CONCLUSION

Positioning in operational space, the first phase in a conquering process, is a way of obtaining learning experiences that students believe are relevant for their future practice. Educators should use this knowledge when preparing supervisors and students for learning in practice and to stimulate discussion focusing on positioning, relationship, and personal recognition. This knowledge could alleviate student insecurity and contribute to student confidence and improved learning experiences.

REFERENCES

Admi, H. (1997). Nursing students' stress during the initial clinical experience. *Journal of Nursing Education, 36*(7), 323–327.

Bayer, M. (2001). *Praktikkens skjulte læreplan* [The hidden curriculum in clinical practice]. Unpublished PhD dissertation, Danish University of Education, Copenhagen.

Begley, C. M. (2002). "Great fleas have little fleas": Irish student midwives' views of the hierarchy in midwifery. *Journal of Advanced Nursing, 38*(3), 310–317.

Chapman, R., & Orb, A. (2001). Coping strategies in clinical practice: The nursing students' lived experience. *Contemporary Nurse, 11*(1), 95–102.

Charleston, R., & Happell, B. (2005). Coping with uncertainty within the preceptorship experience: The perceptions of nursing students. *Journal of Psychiatric and Mental Health Nursing, 12*, 303–309.

Clancy, C., Oyefeso, A., & Ghodse, H. (2007). Role development and career stages in addiction nursing: An exploratory study. *Journal of Advanced Nursing,* 57(2), 161–171.

Currie, S. M. (1999). Aspect of the preparation of student midwives for autonomous practice. *Midwifery, 15*, 283–292.

Cusson, R. N., & Viggiano, N. M. (2002). Transition to the neonatal nurse practitioner role: Making the change from the side to the head of the bed. *Neonatal Network: The Journal of Neonatal Nursing, 21*(2), 21–28.

Davies, R. M., & Atkinson, P. (1991). Student of midwifery: "Doing the jobs" and other coping strategies. *Midwifery*, 7, 113–121.

Glaser, B. G. (1978). *Theoretical sensitivity: Advances in the methodology of grounded theory* (5th ed.). Mill Valley, CA: Sociology Press.

Glaser, B. G. (1998). *Doing grounded theory: Issues and discussions.* Mill Valley, CA: Sociology Press.

Glaser, B. G. (2005). *The grounded theory perspective III: Theoretical coding.* Mill Valley, CA: Sociology Press.

Glaser, B. G., & Strauss, A. L. (1967). *The discovery of grounded theory: Strategies for qualitative research.* New York: Aldine.

Heggen, K. (1995). *Sykehuset som "klasserom". Praksisopplæring i profesjonsutdanninger* [The hospital as a "classroom." Practical training in professional education]. Oslo, Norway: Universitetsforlaget,.

Hjälmhult, E. (2007). *Erobring av handlingsrom. Helsesøsterstudenters læring i praksis.* Unpublished PhD dissertation, The Norwegian University of Science and Technology, Trondheim.

Hjälmhult, E. (in press). Learning strategies of public health nursing: Conquering operational space. *Journal of Clinical Nursing.*

Kilminster, M., & Jolly, B. C. (2001). Effective supervision in clinical practice settings: A literature review. *Medical Education, 34*(10), 827–840.

Kvale, S. (1996). *Interviews: An introduction to qualitative research interviewing.* Thousand Oaks, CA: Sage.

Löfmark, A., & Wikblad, K. (2001). Facilitating and obstructing factors for development of learning in clinical practice: A student perspective. *Journal of Advanced Nursing 34*(1), 43–50.

Ministry of Education and Research. (2005). *Rammeplan og Forskrift for Helsesøsterutdanning* [National curriculum and regulation for public health nursing education]. Oslo, Norway: Author.

Mørck, L. L. (2003). *Læring og overskridelse av marginalisering. Studie af unge mænd med minoritetsbaggrund* [Learning and transcendence? of marginalizing: A study of young men with background from minorities]. Unpublished PhD dissertation, Århus Universitet, Denmark.

Peyrovi, H., Yadavar-Nikravesh, M., Oskouie, S. F., & Berterö, C. (2005). Iranian student nurses' experiences of clinical placement. *International Nursing Review, 52*(2), 134–141.

Talvitie, U., Peltokallio, L., & Männistö, P. (2000). Student teachers' view about their relationships with university supervisors, cooperating teachers and peer student teachers. *Scandinavian Journal of Educational Research, 44*(1), 79–88.

V Balancing

INTRODUCTION: BARBARA M. ARTINIAN

While some theoretical codes are used to indicate movement through a process, others emerge as the concept that keeps a phenomenon balanced. Balancing can be described as the action or actions to keep self or a situation on an even level between two extremes. Some balancing acts address inner conflicts and stressors while others are focused on activities.

Two studies illustrate the theoretical code of Balancing. In the first study, Giske found that patients undergoing diagnostic workups worked to keep themselves from experiencing extreme ranges of hope and despair while waiting for a diagnosis (see chapter 21, "Patterns of Balancing Between Hope and Despair in the Diagnostic Phase on a Gastroenterology Ward"). The activities of Preparative Waiting helped them balance the time during the diagnostic phase and the final interview when they would learn their definitive diagnosis.

In the second study, Artinian explored the balancing done by dialysis patients and their partners in order to achieve a successful marital relationship. The main focus was on the role expectations held by the spouses of dialysis patients (see chapter 22, "Bending Expectations by Spouses of Dialysis Patients: Balancing Between Alternatives"). Artinian found ways in which the spouses balanced marital decisions, marital responsibility for treatment regimen, and marital role performance. These individuals were balancing between alternatives in order to manage the problems they encountered while married to a person on dialysis.

Understanding experience of balancing is important to those who care for patients and their families who face chronic illnesses.

21 Patterns of Balancing Between Hope and Despair in the Diagnostic Phase on a Gastroenterology Ward

TOVE GISKE
BARBARA M. ARTINIAN

Most patients admitted to hospitals for diagnostic investigations go through a challenging time of waiting. The entire situation is filled with waiting: waiting for investigations and tests, preparing for and undergoing them, and finally waiting for results. They do not know what kind of disease they may have, what possible life changes are in store, or what treatment the disease may require. The time of waiting for a diagnosis is reported to be the most stressful time of the illness experience (Benedict, Williams, & Baron, 1994; Fridfinnsdottir, 1997; Lebel et al., 2003; Mishel, 1988, 1997; Neville, 2003; Poole, 1997; Poole & Lyne, 2000).

In this paper, we report the full analysis and development of the theory of Preparative Waiting, which has previously been published as a descriptive grounded theory (Giske & Gjengedal, 2007). The theory describes the experience of a group of gastroenterology patients going through the diagnostic phase. This paper shows how the theoretical code of *balancing between hope and despair* integrates the theory and how the theory is related to other research.

This chapter is a reprint of the article by T. Giske & B. Artinian. (2008). Patterns of "balancing between hope and despair" in the diagnostic phase: A grounded theory study of patients on a gastroenterology ward. *Journal of Advanced Nursing, 62*(1), 22–31. Reprinted by permission of Wiley-Blackwell Publishing Ltd, Oxford, UK.

After developing our substantive Preparative Waiting theory (PWT), we did a literature research to compare our findings with other research in the area. We found no papers reporting from the same patient group, or with as open an outcome of the investigation as in our group, which led us to widen our search for relevant literature. We found reports of investigations of breast abnormalities (Ambler et al., 1999; Benedict et al., 1994; Drageset & Lindstrøm, 2003, 2005; Fridfinnsdottir, 1997; Heskestad & Tjemsland, 1996; Lebel et al., 2003; Logan, Hackbusch-Pinto, & De Grasse, 2006; Poole & Lyne, 2000; Thorne, Harris, Hislop, & Vestrup 1999; Woodward & Webb, 2001). There were also studies of younger patients waiting for diagnosis in an acute ward (Sørlie, Torjuul, Ross, & Kihlgreen, 2006), studies related to waiting for liver transplantation (Jonsèn, Athlin, & Suhr, 2000), waiting for colon surgery (Moene, Bergbom, & Skott, 2006), waiting for diagnostic tests in chronic back pain (Rhodes, McPhillips-Tangum, Markham, & Klent, 2002), and waiting for surgery of knees and hips (Sjöling, Ågren, Olofsson, Hellzen, & Asplund, 2005).

Our substantive grounded theory (GT) of PWT was a process of balancing between *seeking and giving information, interpreting clues, handling existential threats,* and *seeking respite,* as illustrated in Figure 21.1. By comparing these research reports with our PWT, we found that most studies dealt with the emotional part of waiting and the need for information. To a lesser extent they dealt with existential aspects of waiting and how patients interpreted clues and sought respite. Just one study (Heskestad & Tjemsland, 1996) described all the aspects we identified in our study; however, the researchers did not organize them into higher-level concepts nor relate them to each other.

In GT, researchers search for theoretical codes that can conceptualize and integrate a substantive theory (Glaser, 1978, 2005). In our study, *balancing* emerged as such a theoretical code. In a study by Thulesius, Håkonsson, and Petersson (2003), the theoretical code of balancing described how health care professionals balanced the needs of end-of-life patients with available resources. They suggested that balancing is a fundamental process operating in all types of health care (p. 1371). Similar findings were reported in nursing literature. Irurita and Williams (2001) found that patients and nurses in acute care settings were in a reciprocal process of balancing and compromising to preserve the integrity of self and of others. In a GT study of AIDS/HIV patients, Kylmä, Vehviläinen-Julkunen, and Lähdevirta

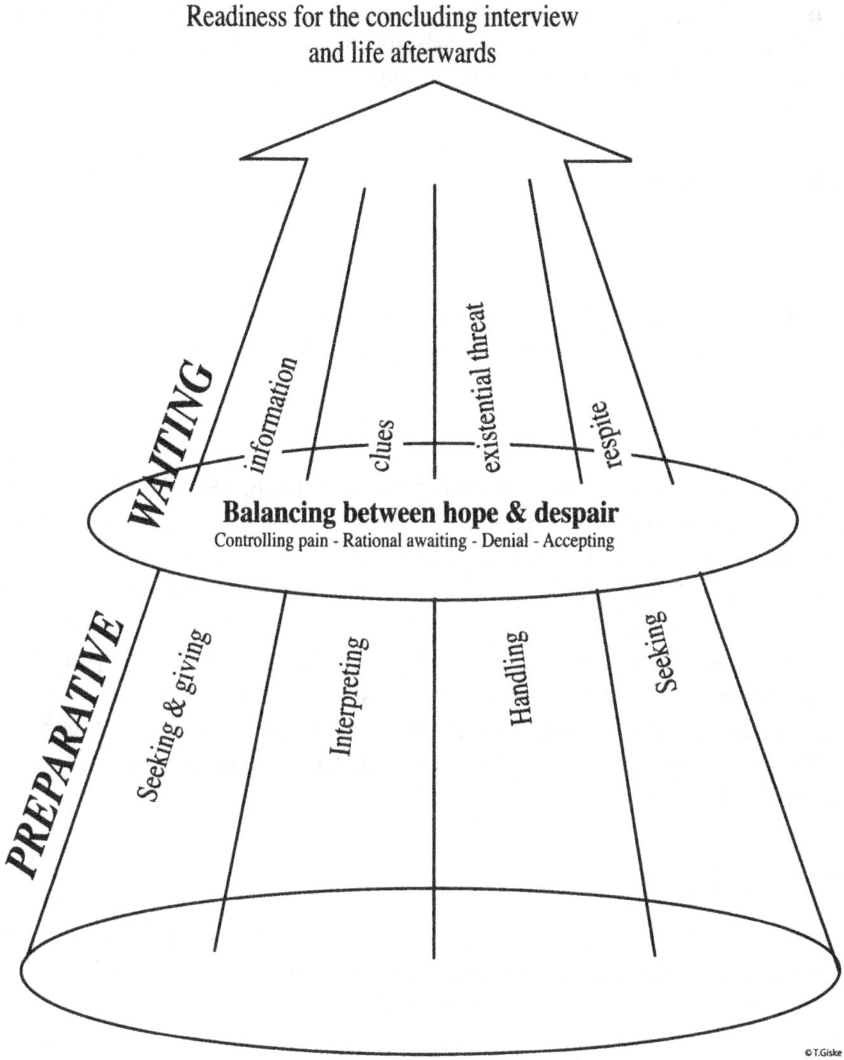

Figure 21.1 Model of Preparative Waiting theory.
Printed with permission from *Journal of Advanced Nursing* by T. Giske.

(2001) reported that patients balanced between hope, despair, and hopelessness in everyday life.

Against this background, this paper presents and discusses PWT from the perspective of how the different patterns we identified of balancing between hope and despair affected the ways participants sought information, interpreted clues, handled existential threat, and sought respite.

This use of the theoretical coding of balancing moved our analysis from the descriptive GT previously published (Giske & Gjengedal, 2007) to an integrated theory (Giske & Artinian, 2008).

THE RESEARCH

Aim

The aim of the study was to learn how patients going through the diagnostic phase experienced and handled their situation.

Method

Classical GT was chosen as method (Glaser, 1978, 1998, 2005). GT is well suited for studying complex and hidden processes (Morse, 2001). Full details of study methods appear in Giske and Artinian (2007), and a brief outline follows here. In GT, data collection and analyses are done concurrently. The data are first coded openly, later selectively according to the core concept, and finally theoretically. The purpose of theoretical coding is to relate the substantive codes to each other in such a way that the theory fits data, is relevant by letting the processes in the field emerge, and works to explain what is going on in the area studied (Glaser, 1978).

Participants

Eight women and seven men aged from 35 to 84 and admitted to a gastroenterology ward at a Norwegian University Hospital participated in the study. The age of 35 years and older was chosen because at this age most people are settled in the most important roles in their lives. When interviewed, their health problems had lasted from 1 day to 9 years. Participants were chosen in accordance with the development of the theory (theoretical sampling).

Data Collection and Analysis

Data collection (in-depth interviews) and analysis were done concurrently in 2002–2003. The 18 tape recorded and transcribed interviews (three patients were interviewed twice) were analyzed by open coding, moving on to selective coding when the participants' main concern was found to be, "How can patients prepare themselves for the concluding interview and future life?" and the core category of preparative waiting became clear. Memos were continuously written to aid the process of theoretical coding, which fitted the concepts to each other to constitute a dense and parsimonious GT.

In the analyzing process we developed many concepts. Two of the most distinct were *vulnerable dependency on staff and system* and *balance between hope and despair.* The first contained participants' experiences and strategies related to staff and being in the hospital environment. This category was eliminated because it described the condition of being a patient and had to be a condition for all categories. The second concept was early seen to be more guiding for the process than the other concept and we also identified four different patterns of how balancing was performed. As data analysis continued, balancing emerged as the theoretical code that integrated all the other categories.

Theoretical codes are abstract models allowing the researcher to talk about substantive categories and properties while thinking theoretically (Glaser, 2005, p. 3). Theoretical codes are flexible, and more than one may fit the same data. Glaser gives many examples of theoretical codes (Glaser, 1978, 1998, 2005), one of which is balancing. "Balancing is handling many variables at once in order to start an action, keep an action going or achieve a resolution. . . . Balancing is an abstract model that can be seen substantively or used as a substantive category" (Glaser, 2005, p. 29). Theoretical codes are "hard to understand in the beginning of research by the novice GT researcher" (p. 1). Therefore they are often ignored, left implicit, or just missed. A theoretical code is not necessary for a GT, but "a GT is best when they are used" because "a GT will appear more plausible, more relevant, and more enhanced when integrated and modelled by an emergent theoretical code" (p. 14). This became significant in our study. When the theoretical code of balancing emerged, it served to integrate the entire participants' experience. It also raised the PWT to a higher level, so that we could state hypotheses about relationships between patterns and categories.

Ethical Considerations

The study was approved by the region's Medical Ethics Committee. Participants were recruited to the study in collaboration with nurses on the ward, who prepared patients by giving oral and written information. The interviews started when participants had signed the consent form.

FINDINGS

Balancing: The Theoretical Code Integrating PWT

The theoretical code of balancing shows how participants in the diagnostic phase resolved their main concern by *seeking and giving information, interpreting clues, handling existential threat,* and *seeking respite.* Balancing was an intrinsic activity where participants moved between hope and despair. All participants had emotional boundaries concerning how deep into despair they could go before losing control, or how focused on hope they could be without losing track of reality. If they let despair and their worst fear become too strong, controlling and hiding how painful their situation was and how weak they actually felt became difficult. This moving between hope and despair influenced, for example, how they sought and processed information. The more hopeful they were, the more realistically they could appraise and process their situation. When they moved toward despair, they withdrew and were less able to process their situation. Different patterns of "balancing between hope and despair" emerged from the data. Patterns are behaviors patients engage in; they are strategies rather than labels, and so a person can use more than one pattern (Glaser, 2001). The four patterns identified were *controlling pain, rational awaiting, denial,* and *acceptance*.

Patterns of Balancing

Participants wondered what the truth might be about their situation, and they felt the *pain of uncertainty* about the future in large measure. To protect themselves, they controlled their thoughts related to future prospects: "I am nervous and tense, but I do not think my thoughts all the way through and finish." The pattern of *rational awaiting* was evident when a person focused on facts instead of hypothetical outcomes. Troublesome thoughts and feelings were not allowed to emerge as long as patients lacked accurate knowledge about their status. One man put it this way: "You cannot be anxious about things you don't know in the process, you must wait until you have a result. I keep it at a level that

I can handle." When the pattern of *denial* was recognized, participants focused on recovering from acute symptoms rather than brooding over possible underlying problems: "I have been ill for many weeks, and now I recover so fast. I haven't been thinking so much about how ill I am. What causes the enlarged liver I do not know, and I do not care so much about it either." The fourth pattern, *accepting*, was identified when participants had the confidence to openly seek information about what was at stake. The pain caused by fear of the future was combined with peace stemming from the belief that they would be able to cope. As illustrated in this quote, age, experience in life, and ability to reflect on former experiences were important conditions in this strategy: "I hope for a good outcome, but if not, I believe I will have no problem with facing it. I have some life experiences that will help me."

Seeking and Giving Information

The first concept of PWT was related to how participants sought and gave information. They sought information related to the content of their stay such as structure of the day, and how to prepare physically and mentally for investigations and their results. Such information gave them some emotional control and some possibilities of how to judge their situation. Participants saw it as the physicians' and nurses' responsibility to give the correct information to them in such a way that it was not misinterpreted. They also expressed a wish to have one main contact person in the medical team. The longer the patient had been waiting for a diagnosis, the more important it was that everything was done correctly to ensure accuracy of results. Participants also wanted to give the health care team information about how they experienced their symptoms so that physicians could be able to make the right judgment about their situation.

Participants themselves could be an obstacle to information exchange, because worry, fear, and their physical state limited their ability to process information. They sometimes heard only pieces of information, which made the overall meaning of what they were told unclear and led to misunderstanding. Some participants were afraid to ask questions or forgot what they had planned to ask the physician during ward rounds.

The more participants felt themselves to be on an even keel, the more they were able to process information and the better prepared they became. Information was best accepted when it was given in accordance with their patterns of balancing. Those using the pattern of *controlling pain* neither wanted too much information nor wanted to be involved in discussions about all outcomes with regard to care. One put it this way: "It's okay that they are worried [physicians] and wonder what this can be. For me it is better to get to know when they have something more specific to tell." Building trusting relationships with staff became a resource to lean on during their painful uncertainty. In contrast, poorly prepared ward rounds and new staff asking the same questions repeatedly drained them of hope and increased their despair.

Participants using the pattern of rational awaiting wanted information so that they could base their judgments on facts. Emotions related to different outcomes were kept on hold until the patients knew for sure what the outcome would be: "For me it is important to get a diagnosis, a serious one or a less serious one. I am concerned about the different alternatives, but I am waiting for the results to see how I can relate to it. I am a realist and this is how I am used to thinking."

Denial was seen when participants ignored signs of danger and overlooked negative possibilities. Some saw serious questions asked by physicians as impolite: "I have this itch, you see. When I was admitted, the physician pointed out that I had a problem with alcoholism. But there can be other reasons for this, [such] as kidney stones or a blocked blood vessel. One should be careful and not destroy people's self-esteem." With this pattern, the themes of an interview could change rapidly, jumping away from threatening topics only to return later and touch them briefly. Participants using the pattern of accepting sought information about their situation, and they were able to process it and relate to the emotions associated with the range of potential diagnostic outcomes.

Interpreting Clues

The second concept dealt with how patients interpreted clues. Participants remembered what had happened before they became ill, and they considered the changes in their body. Since they had different levels of medical knowledge and experience with illness and diseases, they interpreted bodily symptoms such as bleeding from the rectum, feeling lethargic, having a raised temperature, pain, diarrhea, enlarged liver, and weight loss differently. In addition to reflecting on their bodies, they paid attention to and considered how they were met in the hospital, what diagnostic interventions they went through, and what priority they were given. These internal considerations, together with interpretation of the interplay between themselves, staff, and the organization, were properties of the category of *interpreting clues* in our study.

The different patterns of balancing were related to how participants evaluated their situation. Participants using the controlling pain pattern were very sensitive to all clues, because they were vulnerable to feeling the distress of uncertainty. For self-protection, they did not allow themselves to consider fully the range of outcomes. Those using the rational awaiting pattern interpreted as many comprehensible clues as possible to try to make sense of their situation. Since emotions were put aside until the diagnosis and the prognosis were known, they hardly felt the emotional pain of considering the different scenarios: "They are reluctant to tell me something before they know, and this biopsy, that's what's decisive. It's obvious that it is considered to be a rather serious affair because it has been given top priority in this examination." Those using the pattern of denial turned their attention mainly towards positive signs, and compared their own situation with others that manage to live well despite diseases. When the pattern of accepting was seen, clues were considered and compared with knowledge and former experiences. One man shared his attempts at trying to make sense of his situation: "I have an ulcer in my duodenum that will not heal, and it's bleeding, and I have this increasing pain. You're thinking of cancer. . . . Today, the ultrasound showed a narrowing in the duodenum, and I am very tense about the result, if it's malignant or . . ."

Handling Existential Threat

The third concept was related to their experience of going through medical investigations and waiting for a diagnosis, which made participants consider possible outcomes of their illness. They were apprehensive about the future and what it might hold, questioning what might change for them and their loved ones. These concerns were intrinsic and often not expressed. Many outcomes were possible: It could be a serious and life-threatening disease leaving them with reduced lifespan, or it could be a chronic disease, a somewhat treatable problem easily fixed, or nothing at all. The possibility of more serious threats challenged them to reflect on what really gives meaning to life. Being admitted to the hospital added seriousness to the situation, and the smells, sounds, and sights of the hospital, staff, and fellow patients made it harder to hide from these thoughts.

To be in the diagnostic phase meant to be kept on hold in life and, even though they became more aware of life's meaning, this was not the time for making changes in such basic matters as outlook on life. For those having a Christian faith, a variety of images of God were found, which again influenced their way of seeking God in this hour of need. The way they experienced the existential threat was closely linked with the different patterns of balancing, as stated in the hypothesis that the more painful they felt the situation to be, the greater they felt the existential threat.

The pattern of controlling pain was used to protect themselves from dwelling too much on what they feared could be a serious outcome. For those believing in God, praying was a way of handling their distress: "I believe in God and the faith has become important to me. I pray; most of us pray when we are in some kind of need, I think. I say: God help me now"—she cries—"I cannot take any more, now I need help."

When the pattern of rational awaiting was seen, the handling of uncertainty for the future was dealt with by not considering the consequences of different outcomes before they had more facts about the situation. Their attitude was that nothing had changed before they had been given a diagnosis: "I'm a realist, and I think that will help me, because I'm not the type of person that can stand lulling myself about things. I'm impatient and want to get on with life." The nature of the denial pattern was to not to delve into threatening prognoses, which resulted in limited exploration as to what this could mean for the future. When acceptance was seen, participants discussed both the distress of an uncertain future and the trust related to the ability to handle their situation. This trust was built on former experiences of their own resources and available support of others: "There is a lot of uncertainty related to my future and what I can manage in relation to my family." He cries. "This is very painful for me. I have learned that life is not easy, but I have managed to be the strong one in the family, and my previous experiences have taught me how to cope."

Seeking Respite

The fourth concept was *seeking respite.* This dealt with stepping out of the constant tension of uncertainty, as when participants worked on balancing their hopes and despairs, making sense of their situation, handling worries for the future, and seeking an alternative mental state where their thoughts were concerned with things other than waiting. Respite granted rest and renewed strength: It offered a mental escape where they could disconnect from the smoldering tension of uncertainty, and it helped to "recharge the batteries," to prevent them from "exploding" or "becoming crazy," as participants expressed it.

Different conditions influenced the ability to find respite, such as where they slept—in the hospital, at the patients' hotel (nearby housing where patients could stay when health and the examination program permitted), or at home. How obedient or undemanding they were also made a difference. Conditions such as pain or nausea and preparations for investigations such as fasting also made it harder for participants to disconnect. In the hospital, respite was found through reading, listening to music, walking in the garden, and chatting with fellow patients.

Different patterns of balancing were also identified in ways of seeking respite. The more painfully patients experienced their situation, the more they felt the need for respite. When the pattern of controlling pain was seen, respite was sought to find a break from the pain caused by uncertainty. Such rest gave renewed strength to endure new investigations and prolonged waiting. One woman put it this way:

> When you can have leave and go home, I get more input from friends. I have the house and a dog—things that can occupy my thoughts. I need to recharge the batteries between the battles. When you are here, you are in bed and you see nurses, physicians, and fellow patients, and then all the smells. You do not get the chance to disconnect as easily here, even though I try.

For those using the pattern of rational awaiting, respite helped to kill time as they moved toward a conclusion. Respite was actively sought when denial was used; it offered a welcome break from bothersome threats in the back of their minds. The use of humor was tangible, and participants could keep themselves busy by following up on fellow patients' needs.

For those using the pattern of accepting, respite was also appreciated since it gave a welcome break from their work of dealing with uncertainty: "I'm doing a lot of thinking while I'm here. I read a book and listen to music to enter another world. I need to overcome a threshold to move away from what my head is full of."

Relationships Between the Categories

Table 21.1 summarizes how the theoretical code of balancing integrated the categories of PWT, and shows how different participants prepare themselves differently for getting a diagnosis.

Table 21.1

RELATIONSHIP BETWEEN THE DIFFERENT PATTERNS OF BALANCING BETWEEN HOPE AND DESPAIR AND THE OTHER CONCEPTS OF PREPARATIVE WAITING THEORY

PATTERNS OF BALANCING BETWEEN HOPE AND DESPAIR	SEEKING AND GIVING INFORMATION	INTERPRETING CLUES	HANDLING EXISTENTIAL THREAT	SEEKING RESPITE
Controlling pain				
Pain of uncertainty felt to a great extent	Wanting accurate information, not too much into discussion about different possibilities.	Work on making sense of all possible clues. Do not go into the worst scenarios.	Feel the existential threat to a great extent. Try to pull themselves back from going too much into it.	Seek respite since it gives a welcome break from the painful time of waiting that gives rest and renewed strength.
Rational awaiting				
Focused on facts and not on hypothetical outcomes	Focus on facts, not on hypothetical outcomes.	Work on clues to make the best estimate of their situation.	Nothing has changed. The existential threat is put on hold until knowledge and consequences about the situation are known.	Seek respite because it helps kill the time while waiting for the conclusion of the medical examination.
Denial				
Focused on improvements and overlooked signs of danger	Information is not actively sought. Recognize that something is wrong, and accept the need to know the result to be able to get help.	Focus on improvements and all positive signs in themselves. Compare themselves with others that got well or that manage to live well with disease.	Do to a limited extent go into this.	Seek respite actively since it offers a welcome rest from the bothersome threat of uncertainty.

(*Continued*)

Table 21.1

RELATIONSHIP BETWEEN THE DIFFERENT PATTERNS OF BALANCING BETWEEN HOPE AND DESPAIR AND THE OTHER CONCEPTS OF PREPARATIVE WAITING THEORY (*Continued*)

PATTERNS OF BALANCING BETWEEN HOPE AND DESPAIR	SEEKING AND GIVING INFORMATION	INTERPRETING CLUES	HANDLING EXISTENTIAL THREAT	SEEKING RESPITE
Accepting				
Uncertainty was bearable since there was confidence in enough resources available to cope with the situation	Seek and want accurate and adjusted information.	Work on making sense of all clues. Consider former experiences of coping with difficult life situations and compare them with the actual situation.	Experience the situation as less a threat since they find some rest in knowing there are resources available for them in relation to themselves, to significant others, and to God.	Need for less respite since the emotional pain of uncertainty is bearable.

Printed with permission from T. Giske.

DISCUSSION

In discussing the findings we must bear in mind that data from this study came from only one ethnic group and location. Understanding the theoretical code of balancing and how the patterns of controlling pain, rational awaiting, denial, and accepting relate the strategies of PWT to each other makes it easier to be sensitive to how different patients prepare themselves. But it will still be demanding for nurses to develop supportive interactions with patients. Patients' processes of preparing are dynamic, moving between hope and despair, levels of awareness, and more or less realistic appraisal of their situation (Giske & Gjengedal, 2007). A person can also move between different patterns, even though there was a tendency to use one pattern more than the other. This wavering between hope and fear is explicitly discussed by Benedict et al. (1994) and Heskestad &

Tjemsland (1996). Fridfinnsdottir (1997) identified three ways of coping, which she called denial, stoic acceptance, and selective attention. The first two ways are comparable to our patterns of denial and rational awaiting, and the last is best compared to the strategy of seeking respite. The different patterns made participants become prepared to various degrees; participants using mostly the pattern of accepting would be better prepared than those using mostly denial. This is in accordance with Drageset and Lindstrøm (2005), Fridfinnsdottir (1997), Heskestad and Tjemsland (1996), Poole and Lyne (2000), and Widerman (2004).

Patients using mainly the pattern of controlling pain go through a very harsh time, experiencing a great deal of emotional pain. Building of trusting and caring relationships, and continuous contact with a few key people, would offer these patients health care resources to lean on that would strengthen their hope and support them emotionally through the investigation process. Awareness of the existential pain these patients feel and their need to distance themselves from thinking about the worst-case scenarios should make staff aware of how they communicate potential possibilities along the process. To assist patients in reaching respite would be a way to help them gain a break from uncertainty-provoking anxiety. Such a break would give them renewed strength to endure the investigation process.

Patients mostly using the pattern of rational awaiting have limited conscious contact with emotions related to the uncertainty of their situation. They postpone emotional processing of their situation until they know the outcome. In relation to these patients, nurses need to consider to what degree they see it as helpful for patients to connect emotions to the cognitive preparation they go through. Newer theories of grieving after bereavement imply that it is possible to work thorough stressful situations without emotional catharsis (Guldin, 2007; Stroebe, Schut, & Stroebe, 2006). Accurate information is highly valued by these patients.

Patients using denial to a large extent tend to distort the judgment of their situation to protect themselves from the emotional threat of bad scenarios for the future. To the extent that nurses earn these patients' trust, they can strengthen patients' hope and thereby reduce the need for denial and other subconscious processes (Giske & Gjengedal, 2007). By demonstrating competence, continuity, and care, nurses can assist patients in a more realistic appraisal of their situation and thus help them to prepare more accurately for the concluding interview in which they receive the diagnosis, and for life afterwards.

Patients mainly using the pattern of accepting seem to be the ones who handle their situation best. These patients are able to appraise their situation realistically, trusting that there will be enough resources for them to cope with whatever the outcome might be. The situation of uncertainty and waiting is painful for these patients too, and a contact person, a well-coordinated investigation program, and continuity of physicians and nurses would make the situation more predictable for them and thereby ease their pain.

If we look at general implications of this study, one overall recommendation is to assign a knowledgeable and experienced nurse to each patient entering the hospital for diagnostic workups. Such a contact person could coordinate the investigation process and provide patients with accurate information and thereby reduce the pain of uncertainty. Information about hospital routines and details of procedures can improve patients' sense of control. Similar findings are reported by others (Ambler et al., 1999; Drageset & Lindstrøm, 2003; Lebel et al., 2003; Sjöling et al., 2005; Thorne et al., 1999; Woodward & Webb, 2001).

It is important for nurses and physicians to be aware of how patients feed clues into the process of making sense of their situation. Our participants tried to judge the seriousness of their symptoms by comparing their ongoing evaluation of the situation with knowledge and previous experiences in their own and others' lives. We found just one study that reported how patients tried to make sense of their bodily symptoms when no objective proof could be found (Rhodes et al., 2002). Participants in our study also paid attention to nonverbal clues in staff behavior and how staff appeared. Other studies report similar findings related to nonverbal signs from staff, such as facial expressions, gaze of the eye, tone of voice, and gestures (Heskestad & Tjemsland, 1996; Poole & Lyne, 2000; Thorne et al., 1999). Our participants also interpreted what investigations were done and the priority they were given, something also recognized by others (Poole & Lyne, 2000; Thorn et al., 1999). These findings show that patients invest time and personal interest in reducing uncertainty related to their case, and in doing so they take in as much information as they are capable of processing.

Handling existential threat was one of the main concepts of preparative waiting. The more participants felt the pain of uncertainty, the more they consciously dealt with the existential threat. Not knowing their diagnosis and prognosis challenged them to consider what was important in life. All participants pondered the image of God, even though some of them had a nonreligious worldview. The same results are reported in other Norwegian studies (Heskestad & Tjemsland, 1996; Mjølnerød, 1997; Ueland, 1997). Confronting one's own mortality is also reported in other studies to trigger awareness of spirituality (Logan et al., 2006; Sørlie et al., 2006), and being able to put one's life in God's hands through prayer helps coping (Benedict et al., 1994; Heskestad & Tjemsland, 1996; Lebel et al., 2003; Logan et al., 2006). For the participants who could do so, it is worth noting that praying gave confidence in a time of little control. Our study thus provides an integrated theory responding to Penrod's (2001) call for knowledge about how patients use mystical beliefs and practices in managing uncertainty.

The equivalent to our concept of "Seeking respite" was found in five other studies. Heskestad & Tjemsland (1996), Fridfinnsdottir (1997), and Logan et al. (2006) reported on diverted attention, where patients distracted their minds from thinking of investigations, possible cancer, or death. Benedict et al. (1994) called this phenomenon diversion, and Lebel et al. (2003) named it self-distraction. In acknowledging and respecting patients' individual use of and need for respite, nurses can assist them in regaining strength and enduring uncertainty in the diagnostic phase.

CONCLUSION

Our findings are important because they might assist nurses in further developing their role in relation to patients in the diagnostic phase. PWT outlines the complex and dynamic processes patients go through as they are preparing themselves variously for getting a diagnosis. In this process, nurses can be of invaluable support for patients and thereby strengthen their confidence and hope. Further research is needed to further clarify how different patterns of balancing influence patients' preparedness for the concluding interview. Further research related to how nurses can assist patients using mostly the balancing patterns of rational awaiting and denial is also needed.

REFERENCES

Ambler, N., Rumsey, N., Harcourt, D., Kahn, F., Cawthorn, S., & Barker, J. (1999). Specialist nurse counsellor interventions at the time of diagnosis of breast cancer: Comparing "advocacy" with a conventional approach. *Journal of Advanced Nursing, 29*(2), 445–453.

Benedict, S., Williams, R. D., & Baron, P. L. (1994). Recalled anxiety: From discovery to diagnosis of a benign breast mass. *Oncology Nursing Forum, 21*(10), 1723–1727.

Drageset, S., & Lindstrøm, T. C. (2003). The mental health of women with suspected breast cancer: The relationship between social support, anxiety, coping and defence in maintaining mental health. *Journal of Psychiatric and Mental Health Nursing, 10,* 401–409.

Drageset, S., & Lindstrøm, T. C. (2005). Coping with a possible breast cancer diagnosis: Demographic factors and social support. *Journal of Advanced Nursing, 51*(32), 217–226.

Fridfinnsdottir, E. B. (1997). Icelandic women's identifications of stressors and social support during the diagnostic phase of breast cancer. *Journal of Advanced Nursing, 25,* 526–531.

Giske, T., & Artinian, B. (2007). A personal experience of working with classical grounded theory: From beginner to experienced grounded theorist. *International Journal of Qualitative Methods, 6*(4), 68–80.

Giske, T., & Artinian, B. (2008). Patterns of balancing between hope and despair in the diagnostic phase: A grounded theory study of patients on a gastroenterology ward. *Journal of Advanced Nursing, 62*(1), 22–31.

Giske, T., & Gjengedal, E. (2007). "Preparative waiting" and coping theory with patients going through gastric diagnosis. *Journal of Advanced Nursing, 57*(1), 87–94

Glaser, B. G. (1978). *Theoretical sensitivity.* Mill Valley, CA: Sociology Press.

Glaser, B. G. (1998). *Doing grounded theory: Issues and discussions.* Mill Valley, CA: Sociology Press.

Glaser, B. G. (2001). *The grounded theory perspective: Conceptualization contrasting with description.* Mill Valley, CA: Sociology Press.

Glaser, B. G. (2005). *The grounded theory perspective III: Theoretical coding.* Mill Valley, CA: Sociology Press.

Guldin, M. B. (2007). *Sorg-reaksjoner—ny forståelse og behandling* [Reactions to bereavements—new understanding and treatment]. *Klinisk Sygepleje, 2,* 45–50.

Heskestad, S., & Tjemsland, L. (1996). *Du har kreft. En kvalitativ studie av kvinners akutte reaksjoner ved informasjon om brystkreftdiagnose.* [You have cancer. A qualitative study on women's immediate reactions to information about diagnosis of breast cancer.] *Tidsskrift for Norsk Lægeforening,* 9(116), 1067–1071.

Irurita, V. F., & Williams, A. M. (2001). Balancing and compromising: Nurses and patients preserving integrity of self and others. *International Journal of Nursing Studies, 38,* 579–589.

Jonsèn, E., Athlin, E., & Suhr, O. B. (2000). Waiting for a liver transplantation: the experience of patients with familial amyloidotic polyneuropathy. *Journal of Clinical Nursing, 9,* 63–70.

Kylmä, J., Vehviläinen-Julkunen, K., & Lähdevirta, J. (2001). Hope, despair and hopelessness in living with HIV/AIDS: A grounded theory study. *Journal of Advanced Nursing, 33*(6), 764–775.

Lebel, S., Jakubovits, G., Rosberger, Z., Loiselle, C., Sequin, C., & Cornaz, C. (2003). Waiting for a breast biopsy. Psychosocial consequences and coping strategies. *Journal of Psychosomatic Research, 55,* 437–443.

Logan, J., Hackbusch-Pinto, R., & De Grasse, C. E. (2006). Women undergoing breast diagnostics: The lived experience of spirituality. *Oncological Nursing Forum, 33*(1), 121–126.

Mishel, M. H. (1988). Uncertainty in illness. *Image: Journal of Nursing Scholarship, 20*(4), 225–232.

Mishel, M. H. (1997). Uncertainty in acute illness. In J. Fitzpatrick & J. Norbeck (Eds.), *Annual Review of Nursing Research* (*15*, pp. 57–80). New York: Springer Publishing.

Mjølnerød, H. (1997). *Pasientens åndelige/eksistensielle dimensjon slik den uttrykkes hos pasienter i livets sluttfase* [The spiritual and existential dimensions as expressed by patients in the terminal phase of life]. Publikasjonsserie nr. 32. Institutt for Sykepleievitenskap, Universitetet i Oslo, Norway

Moene, M., Bergbom, I., & Skott, C. (2006). Patients' existential situation prior to colorectal surgery. *Journal of Advanced Nursing, 54*(2), 199–207.

Morse, J. M. (2001). Situating grounded theory within qualitative inquiry. In R. S. Schreiber & P. N. Stern (Eds.), *Using grounded theory in nursing* (pp. 1–15). New York: Springer Publishing.

Neville, K. L. (2003). Uncertainty in illness: An integrative review. *Orthopedic Nursing,* 22(3), 206–214.

Penrod, J. (2001). Redefining the concept of uncertainty. *Journal of Advanced Nursing, 34*(2), 238–245.

Poole, K. (1997). The emergence of the "waiting game": A critical examination of the psychosocial issues in diagnosing breast cancer. *Journal of Advanced Nursing, 25,* 273–281.

Poole, K., & Lyne, P. A. (2000). The "cues" to diagnosis: Describing the monitoring activities of women undergoing diagnostic investigations for breast disease. *Journal of Advanced Nursing, 31*(4), 752–758.

Rhodes, L. A., McPhillips-Tangum, C. A., Markham, C., & Klent, R. (2002). The power of the visible: The meaning of diagnostic tests in chronic pain. In Sjöling, M., Ågren, Y., Olofsson, N., Hellzen, O., & Asplund, K. (2005). Waiting for surgery: Living on hold—a continuous struggle against a faceless system. *International Journal of Nursing Studies, 42,* 539–547.

Sørlie, V., Torjuul, K., Ross, A., & Kihlgreen, M. (2006). Satisfied patients are also vulnerable patients—narratives from an acute care ward. *Journal of Clinical Nursing, 15,* 1240–1246.

Stroebe, M., Schut, H., & Stroebe, W. (2006). Who benefits from disclosure? Exploration of attachment style differences in the effects of expressing emotions. *Clinical Psychological Review, 26,* 66–85.

Thorne, S. E., Harris, S. R., Hislop, T. G., & Vestrup, J. A. (1999). The experience of waiting for diagnosis after an abnormal mammogram. *The Breast Journal, 5*(1), 42–51.

Thulesius, H., Håkonsson, A., & Petersson, K. (2003). Balancing: A basic process in end-of-life cancer care. *Qualitative Health Research, 13*(10), 1353–1377.

Ueland, V. (1997). *Kommunikativ kompetanse. En beskrivelse av sykepleierens handlingsrettede kompetanse i å samtale om åndelige og eksistensielle spørsmål med kreftpasienter som har kort forventet levetid* [A description of the nursing careers' active directed level of skills in dialoguing the spiritual and existential questions with cancer patients with an expected short lifespan]. Publikasjonsserie nr. 28. Institutt for Sykepleievitenskap, Universitet i Oslo, Norway.

Widerman, E. (2004). Pathways to adult diagnosis of CF: The impact of pre-diagnosis experience on post-diagnosis responses and needs. *Patients Education and Counselling. 52,* 69–77.

Woodward, V., & Webb, C. (2001). Women's anxieties surrounding breast disorders: A systematic review of the literature. *Journal of Advanced Nursing, 33*(1), 29–41.

22

Bending Expectations by Spouses of Dialysis Patients: Balancing Between Alternatives

BARBARA M. ARTINIAN

The diagnosis of end-stage renal disease is an event that alters life in every dimension—physical, social, psychological, spiritual, and economic—and forces the person to evaluate life in terms of this new experience. There are a number of ways in which a dialysis patient can respond in terms of taking on new roles. Five dialysis roles have been described by Artinian (1983). The relationship among these roles are illustrated in Figure 22.1 and are:

- *undecided role,* in which the patient is not sure he or she really needs dialysis
- *waiting role,* in which all of life is put on hold in anticipation of a transplant
- *worker role,* in which the person needing dialysis continues to define self as normal and accepts the dialysis regimen to maintain optimal health
- *true dialysis patient role,* in which the dialysis patient centers life around dialysis
- *emancipated role,* in which a transplant or an ambulatory treatment frees the person from the demands of dialysis machines

The variability of response to the same disease situation suggests that individual characteristics of each dialysis patient are important in determining

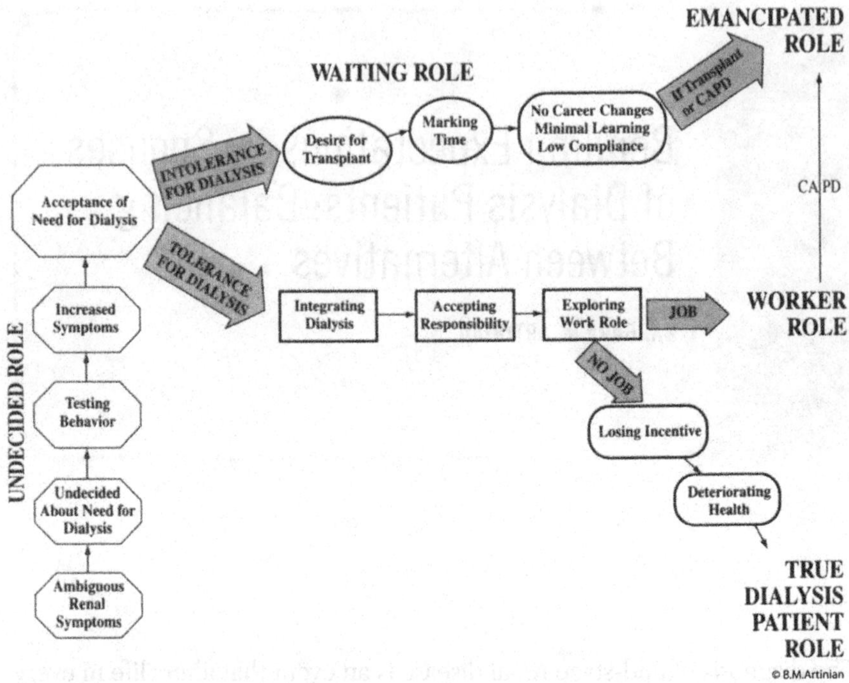

Figure 22.1 Careers of the dialysis patient.
From "Role Identities of the Dialysis Patient," by B. M. Artinian, 1983. *Nephrology Nurse, 5,* 10–14, with permission.

the response. One of the most important of these is the age at which the chronic illness occurs. For example, the experience of dialysis is qualitatively different for young adults than it is for mature adults who have already established themselves in the adult world before the onset of renal disease. Rather than pulling back from an established way of life, the young adult with end-stage renal disease must attempt to accomplish his or her developmental tasks while integrating the dialysis schedule into a school, work, and social schedule. The young adult must also attempt to court a partner and adjust to the give and take of marriage within the constraints imposed by the chronic illness. Since the majority of renal patients are mature adults rather than young adults, most of the studies about the experience of dialysis focus on that group (Baldree, Murphy, & Powers, 1982; Molumphy & Sporakowski, 1984).

The other important characteristic in determining response to the illness is the perspective each member brings to the situation (Antonovsky & Sourani, 1988). The role of the spouse in mediating the effect of chronic illness is important (Kerns & Turk, 1984). Therefore it is necessary to examine the expectations that both patient and spouse bring into the marriage to identify factors that either strengthen or weaken the marriage.

THE STUDY

Aim

The purpose of this study was to explore the marital role expectations held by the spouse of the dialysis patient and to understand how those expectations are met.

Method

Design

A qualitative approach that focused on understanding the main concern of the participants and how they resolved it was done using the constant comparative method for discovering grounded theory developed by Glaser (1978, 1998). This led to an understanding of how dialysis affects the experience of courtship and marriage for young adult couples when one member is a dialysis patient.

Sample

The sample consisted of a subset of 18 young adults in the worker role who were between the ages of 18 and 30 years. These were taken from a sample of 45 young adults. All subjects were maintained on hemodialysis, intermittent peritoneal dialysis, or continuous ambulatory peritoneal dialysis (CAPD). Of these participants, 8 were married at the time of the study, and 2 had been previously married but were divorced. All participants had been on dialysis for at least six months before being interviewed, so initial adjustment to the procedure had been accomplished. All the subjects had completed high school, and a number of them were enrolled in college on a part-time basis. Ten of the subjects had full-time employment.

Data Collection

Face-to-face interviews were conducted over a 2-year period in either the home setting or the dialysis unit, depending on the preference of the subjects. Most subjects were interviewed three times. Interviews ranged from 30 minutes to 2 hours and were all tape recorded. Open-ended questions were used to explore issues related to the young adult dialysis experience.

Data Analysis

Interviews were tape recorded and then transcribed for analysis. Names were changed in the transcripts to protect the subjects. Analysis at first focused on the strategies couples used to manage their domestic lives together as they integrated the demands of dialysis into their ordinary routines. The data-coding procedure followed the basic method outlined by Glaser (1978). Categories were developed and linked together to identify the main concern. The main concern that emerged was how to have a successful marital relationship. It was the expectation by the dialysis patient that the spouse would take into account the effects of the illness on the ability to carry out tasks. However, it was important to dialysis patients that they be expected to fulfill their roles as spouses. Through reflection on these divergent points of view, the basic social process (BSP) of Bending Expectations emerged. A BSP is a core category that has two or more clear, emergent stages that "differentiate and account for variations in the problematic pattern of behavior" (Glaser, 1978, p. 98).

Ethical Considerations

The study was approved by the Institutional Review Board of the University of California at San Francisco, and each of the six participating hospitals. Subjects were recruited by nurses at each dialysis unit. After an explanation of the study was given, an informed consent was signed. Patients were given pseudonyms to protect their identities in study transcriptions.

FINDINGS

Just as persons in authority learn to bend the rules to meet the exigencies of a particular situation while maintaining both the rules and the dignity of the person for whom the rules were bent, it was found that partners in enduring marriages learned to alter or to bend expectations to meet a particular situation while keeping intact the expectations for marital role performance that directed their lives together. This was a process of balancing between two alternatives (Glaser, 2005, p. 28). It was observed that were two types of interactions: when the healthy spouse expected no sharing of responsibilities by the spouse on dialysis, and when it was expected for the spouse on dialysis to always carry a full share of responsibility, making it impossible for the relationship to survive. Balancing between these two types of interaction was necessary to have a successful relationship.

By looking at the context in which bending expectations occurred, the conditions under which it occurred, and the consequences to the marriage of bending or failing to bend expectations, the theory was extended to include not only expectations about role performance but also expectations about mate selection and responsibility for physical care of the dialysis patient (Artinian, 1990). Although the process of bending expectations is an interactive one, it was the well spouse who was the most instrumental in carrying it out. The person on dialysis was forced to live with the effects of renal failure, but the well person had the option to leave and to establish a way of life independent of dialysis. The process of altering the normative expectations of Western society that state that partners be equally matched in physical attributes, be responsible for personal care, and share equally in the give and take of marital responsibilities took a long time. Three stages were identified: (a) bending expectations about who could be a marital partner, (b) bending expectations about involvement in the physical care of another young adult, and (c) bending expectations about marital role performance. Successful completion of each stage was necessary before the next could be attempted. The stages of the basic social process are diagrammed in a conceptual map (see Figure 22.2).

Stage 1. Bending Expectations About the Marital Decision: Balancing Between the Disability and Personal Characteristics

Presentation of self in the dating context is always problematic for the dialysis patient. Not to disclose the dialysis condition would be dishonest, but premature disclosure of too many details would be disastrous to the relationship. Some handled the problem initially by completely separating dialysis from the relationship. One patient said, "I don't want her to see it (the machine)—I don't think she is ready yet." Another said, "I don't let it get into our particular relationship."

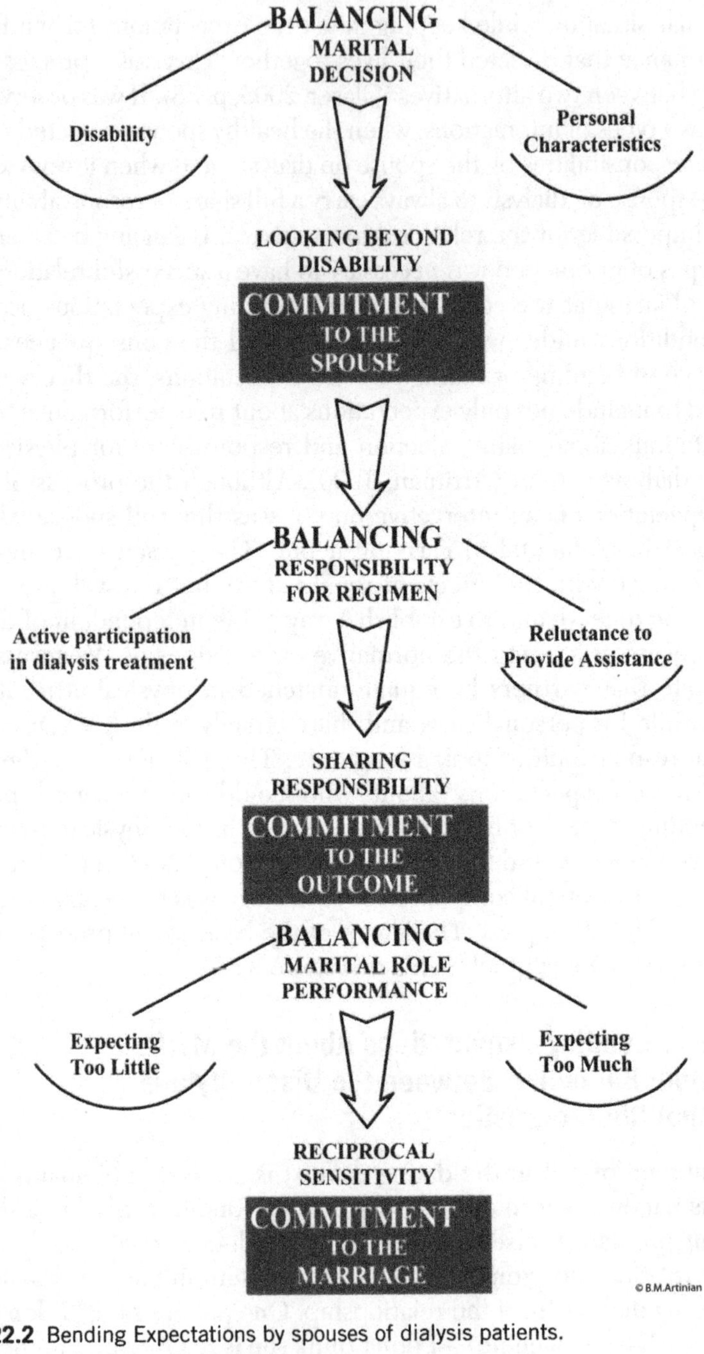

Figure 22.2 Bending Expectations by spouses of dialysis patients.
Printed with permission from B. M. Artinian.

Those who dated persons in the medical field considered themselves to be more fortunate because the person had some familiarity with medical procedures. In some cases when the date had a friend or relative in the medical profession, it made acceptance easier: "The girl I'm going out with now—she had a conception of what dialysis is—like a big heart-lung machine. But her father fortunately is a physician and explained the fundamentals, and she kind of accepted it."

In one case, family members tried to discourage the young couple:

> I was 17 when he got sick and had to wait until after I was 18 because my parents wouldn't sign for me to get married. My dad told me to get uninvolved. He didn't want me to see Bob anymore. He didn't want me to go to the hospital. I'd sneak off with the car and not bother to come back for a couple of days because he wouldn't let me go to the hospital. I'd never had any problems with my family before that, but as far as (my father) was concerned Bob was a bad problem and he didn't want me involved. So, we waited until I turned 18, then we got married. My dad's forgiven me, I think.

In addition to the negative comments from family members and friends, the patients' understanding of the effects of dialysis on normal living patterns also affected their approach to dating relationships. When I asked a 24-year-old if he was dating anyone, he said, "She's not old enough yet." When I asked if he had someone specific in mind, he said, "No, but in order to marry someone on dialysis she would have to be very mature. Since I think the husband should be older than the wife, she's not old enough yet." Another patient said, "It bothers me more than it bothers him—like you have a problem you are putting on someone else." She even suggested that couples should live together to see if the other person could put up with dialysis and with the scariness of it.

With all the problems inherent in looking forward to life together with a person who has a chronic illness, it is not surprising that relationships needed time to develop. One patient avoided telling his girlfriend about his dialysis until she had gotten to know him. When the time came to tell her, he said, "Actually it worked out well because it was at a time that she was ready to hear. We had been going together long enough that she wouldn't just run out the door, you know, and never call me again. So she handled it as well as she was able to."

Usually the decision to marry took a while to make. One couple dated three years before deciding to marry. In reflecting on the decision-making process, one patient said: "It took a lot for her to accept the fact that she was going to marry me. She saw dialysis a lot and saw what was going on. She's a hell of a lady." When the decision to marry had been made before the illness, the commitment to the person had already occurred. But in some cases it was challenged by the changed circumstances. In one case, however, the illness strengthened the commitment. The well spouse said:

> That's why we got married when we did. Originally we'd planned on waiting two more years to be married. I would have a chance to get out of school to see where I wanted to go, what I wanted to do. When they told us that Bob wasn't going to live very long, all I could figure was I'm going to have him for as long as I can and I think that's helped a lot—Bob's dialysis, and his treatment, and his progress.

This balancing between the realities of the disability and attraction to the person led to a commitment to the person and the decision to marry.

Stage 2. Bending Expectations About the Responsibility for Regimen: Balancing Between Active Participation in Treatment and Reluctance to Provide Assistance

When young adults marry, they expect that each will assume personal responsibility for self-care. When one of the young adults is a dialysis patient, this cannot be assumed. Most young couples rejected the alternative of hospital dialysis because it would cut into the hours they could be together. The amount of responsibility the partner was required to accept for the dialysis procedure depended on the type of dialysis used by the patient. The dialysis procedure is complex, but commitment to the person made the partners willing to learn it. After dating for three years, one man took off a month from work to go through the training for peritoneal dialysis with his fiancée so that she could dialyze at home when they were married.

Learning how to do one type of dialysis did not mean that the partner had learned all he or she needed to know. Changes in the medical trajectory or new advances in technology made new learning a part of the commitment. For example, when an infected peritoneal shunt sent the wife on dialysis back to the hospital for hemodialysis, her husband said. "It is hard having her gone three nights a week. If she had to go on hemodialysis permanently, I would train for it."

One couple on home intermittent peritoneal dialysis described their next project:

> We're going to learn CAPD for a vacation this summer so we can go camping. It will be the first time we've been able to . . . actually go. Before, we had the option of going and finding another unit, but you hear a lot of bad stories from patients who go and find units that are really not nice.

Another couple was getting ready to learn a new machine. They said: "We are getting a new machine that is portable. We are real excited about it because we will be able to go anywhere; it just needs three bags of saline."

After the training comes the actual stress of doing dialysis at home. Added to the stress from monitoring the machine is the stress of being busy. Someone has to set up the machine, clean it after use, and keep the treatment supplies stocked. If both partners had jobs or were students, this took considerable planning.

Sharing responsibility for the dialysis regimen sometimes required that the partners take on the role of assistor, as described by Strauss (1984). When an infected peritoneal shunt patient required hospitalization for hemodialysis and antibiotic therapy, the couple became collaborators. Both husband and wife were students enrolled in a nursing program. The wife described their strategy to keep her husband enrolled in a nursing program, since they had been told by school administrators that if he got sick enough to be put in the hospital, he would have to resign from the program. She said: "We never did tell his teachers at school about the infection. At six o'clock in the morning he took himself off the machine and I went downstairs to get the pass and checked him back in that afternoon for the rest of the four days. We have to work like a team."

Commitment to the Outcome

Although the dialysis procedure is the most visible part of the dialysis regimen, it is not the only part. However, it was observed that couples who worked together to carry out the procedure also worked together to manage the other parts. A wife monitored the medical care of her patient husband:

> I feel like the overseer of doctors. I know more about him than any of the doctors in the group. I watch his prescriptions and be sure [the doctors] know

> about him. I ask about everything. I have the determination to keep him as healthy and as well as he can be. He's learned a lot, and that has helped a lot in understanding and dealing with circumstances around his dialysis.

The balancing between taking responsibility for the regimen, either active participation in the dialysis treatment or reluctance to provide assistance to share responsibility, resulted in sharing responsibility or the decision to divorce.

When infants grow up in a family that shares this commitment to the outcome, they also become part of the vigilant protector system. A father who was on intermittent peritoneal dialysis four nights a week described the response of his 2-year-old daughter:

> The only people she'll let touch it are me, Steve, and Roberto. Roberto's the technician from the hospital; he used to come out with it. And Steve is the one who does maintenance. And I work on it, and anybody else—there was a guy who came out from Travenol who set up the new concentrate: "You don't touch my daddy's machine." Most of the time she doesn't think of it. What it is now, she thinks everybody, every daddy, is on the machine. She'll come up and we'll watch TV or we'll read because a lot of times I'll go on at 8 or 9 o'clock at night and it's before her bedtime so she'll bring her blanket in and a doll and her books or whatever she wants and she'll get up in bed with the tubing. As long as I don't yank it out of me or the machine, I can rough house with her and put her over my shoulder and play with her and stuff.

Not all couples experienced this shared commitment. One wife who went through the training to assist her husband on dialysis at home really wanted nothing to do with the machine. Her husband said:

> I know I'm responsible for it and I just do it. I'm not thrilled about it. I would like her to have more caring about the machine and me, but I understand her point of view, that she feels infringed upon—her time—so I just accept it. You would always like your spouse to be more caring about the machine. I don't love this, but it is something I have to do so I just do it.

For this couple there was no commitment to the outcome on the part of the wife. When I called six months after the first interview to schedule another interview, the wife informed me that her husband had suddenly requested a divorce just before the adoption of their child was to become final. She agreed to be interviewed and expressed her feelings about home dialysis:

> Why I let it in the house I don't know. I hated it from the day it came in. I despised it; I loathed it; and I resented it. Why I let it in is probably because, like anything else, you could get sick. You don't know. You're not raised to leave somebody because they get sick. That's not the way I was raised. And I guess I let it stay. It did give us certain flexibility that the hospital didn't, and probably the rest of it was guilt. I wanted it out, but I guess it was guilt.

Another dialysis patient described her husband's reluctance to participate in the treatment. She said that she was very independent and did everything herself. He just had to be there when she went on and came off. Therefore she said that she was very surprised when after several years he asked for a divorce, stating the he loved her but could not handle the stress anymore of worrying about her dying. She said, "It's obvious that I'm not dying, and he had never discussed his fears with me."

Stage 3. Bending Expectations About Marital Role Performance: Balancing Role Performance

Do Not Expect Too Little

Although it may initially seem that the dialysis procedure is the major problem facing the couple, once they work out ways to share responsibility for the procedure, they realize that life itself is the real challenge. A dialysis patient described how her spouse had helped her accomplish goals she did not think were possible when he pushed her to learn to ski. Another wife said, "I almost divorced my husband because he was babying me too much. But we had a long talk and now it is okay."

Do Not Expect Too Much

Although spouses can be very influential in helping the dialysis patient to achieve major goals, they must also be sensitive as to when to pull back. These couples would agree with Charlie Brown when he said, "The trouble with life is that it's so daily." For the dialysis patient to feel like a full partner in the marriage, there must be role obligations that he or she is expected to fulfill. In actuality, if temporary poor health prevents the obligations from being met, a helping hand is needed. A wife who was the dialysis patient explained it this way: "There are a lot of times I just don't feel good, and he has to be very understanding about that and it's just that I can't help it. Maybe I'm tired and the laundry doesn't get done right away. He has to be a lot more understanding of me than I of him."

Another wife described a happy resolution to the problem:

> I do it (shopping, banking, etc.), but when I don't feel good, he's pretty good about helping. I have to push him a little, but he . . . cleans around the house and does certain jobs, but he won't go shopping. The only time I can get him to, and I go too, is when I'm too tired to push the cart and load the groceries in.

When there is no willingness to change expectations about what the patient can do, it is not possible for the marriage to continue. One divorced patient who was again on hemodialysis after rejecting a transplant described how her husband responded to her medical problems:

> Not very well. It was just too much for him to accept. He didn't like me being sick all of the time and not being able to fulfill my household duties and wifely duties, and it just ended up failing. After I had my transplant he felt that I was capable of taking care of myself, and so he left.

Even when a patient is in good health most of the time, the fluctuations of a chronic illness need to be taken into account. A successful businessman said:

> Some days you just aren't going to feel on top of the world. But my wife just said, I'm sorry, I don't accept that. That was her way of dealing with it. I think that may have contributed to what happened (divorce). Technically you have a walking handicap, and yet when they see you walking around—in my case, playing racquetball, playing tennis—they look at you and say, this must be a piece of cake. They don't know that some days I don't feel good and some days my legs cramp so badly you can literally see the muscles. I don't tell people that because it is really none of their business.

RECIPROCAL SENSITIVITY

Because renal disease is a problem of such great magnitude, much of the couple's time and energy is focused on the patient. However, the well spouse also has needs that must be met. If the dialysis patient is not sensitive to these needs, much resentment can build up.

One wife resented the fact that her husband did not support her during the times she tried to become pregnant through artificial insemination:

> During the times when I was trying to become pregnant, going to the doctor, going for the insemination, he should have been there at the hospital because those were rough times when I should not have been left alone.

The well spouse can also experience health problems. One wife who was very conscientious about her husband's regimen said, "I've put so much weight on because of my thyroid. I don't have time to get the prescriptions filled. I'm not a good patient." But her husband gave no indication that he was concerned about her problem.

Following her husband's motorcycle accident that produced bruises but no broken bones, the wife who was the dialysis patient said:

> Of course he was hurting too, and he didn't have me to take care of him when he needed it, since I was dialyzing. He doesn't need (special care) that often, and I felt real guilty about (not being there for him). He just kind of felt neglected for a while plus always having a wife who is sick.

Commitment to the Marriage

When a couple learned to balance the demands of their marital role performance with reciprocal sensitivity as their relationship matured, the renal disease did not go away, but the dialysis regimen no longer dominated their thoughts. One well spouse said:

> There are periods of adjustment and acceptance. I think we are beyond those periods. We don't think about vacations we can't go on. This is the acceptance. We just plan ahead. If you had asked these same questions six months after she went on dialysis, the answer would have been much different. You learn a lot in those first years.

He talked about another patient who could only think of life in terms of a transplant and concluded, "She hasn't lived with dialysis long enough to find out it isn't so bad." What had appeared to be a major problem during the early days of dating and courtship now was seen as a constraint that needed to be worked out within the context of commitment to each other.

DISCUSSION

When one family member becomes chronically ill, all relationships within the family are profoundly affected. While some studies report negative consequences for the relationship (Halstrom & Schram, 1984; Peyrot, McMurray, & Hedges, 1988), others point to positive or neutral outcomes (Bowers & Kogan, 1984; Shapiro, 1983).

The analysis of the process of bending expectations by spouses of dialysis patients clearly indicates that it is a problematic process that takes time. At the beginning of each stage, the fact of dialysis dominated the relationship. But it gradually became less important as the personal characteristics of the dialysis patient emerged and the couple was able to balance between the disability and the person. This allowed the well spouse to initially look beyond the disability to the person, and it provided the well spouse the courage to enter the stage of actually assisting the patient with the dialysis regimen.

After the procedural part of the dialysis treatment had been mastered so that it was seen as routine, the couple was ready to work on the challenges of everyday living that confront any young couple. Their relationship was always under the constraint of uncertainty about the health of the dialysis patient. However, the gradual growth of commitment to the person and marriage that took place as societal expectations were replaced with expectations compatible with the facts of dialysis made it possible to work out solutions to problems that would have been impossible at first. For those who are able to balance the positive aspects of the dialysis experience against the negative ones, the outcome was commitment to the dialysis patient and the marriage.

CONCLUSION

There are young adults on dialysis who are trying to find a mate or who are trying to be successful at building a marriage with a well spouse. An understanding of the need to balance expectations can be of help to health care professionals who seek to provide support to these young people. The experiences of the subjects in our study may reflect the balancing problems experienced by other young adults on dialysis or by young adults with other chronic or handicapping conditions. Further research needs to be directed at analyzing the experience of other young adults who are balancing between alternatives in order to clarify this substantive theory of Balancing. In this way, a formal theory can be developed that could be used in working with any young adult patient with a chronic illness (Glaser, 2007).

ACKNOWLEDGMENT

This paper was supported in part by a National Institute of Health Grant, 5-T32-NU-07006–04, Research Training Program for Post-Doctoral Nurses.

REFERENCES

Antonovsky, A., & Sourani, T. (1988). Family sense of coherence and family adaptation. *Journal of Marriage &Family, 50,* 79–92.

Artinian, B. (1983). Role identities of the dialysis patient. *Nephrology Nurse, 5,* 10–14.

Artinian, B. (1990). Bending expectations for marital role performance of dialysis patients. *Family Community Health, 12*(4), 47–57.

Baldree, K. S., Murphy, S. P., & Powers, M. J. (1982). Stress identification and coping patterns in patients on hemodialysis. *Nursing Research, 31,* 107–112.

Glaser, B. G. (1978). *Theoretical sensitivity: Advances in the methodology of grounded theory*. Mill Valley, CA: Sociology Press.

Glaser, B. G. (1998). *Doing grounded theory: Issues and discussion.* Mill Valley, CA: Sociology Press

Glaser, B. G. (2005). *The grounded theory perspective III: Theoretical coding*. Mill Valley, CA: Sociology Press.

Glaser, B. G. (2007). *Doing formal theory.* In A. Bryant & K. Charmaz (Eds.), *The SAGE handbook of grounded theory* (pp. 97–111). Los Angeles: Sage.

Halstrom, J. L., & Schram, V. R. (1984). Chronic illness in couples: Selected characteristics, including wife's satisfaction with and perception of marital relationships. *Family Relations, 33,* 195–203.

Kerns, R., & Turk, D. (1984). Depression and chronic pain: The mediating role of the spouse. *Journal of Marriage & Family, 46,* 845–852.

Molumphy, S. D., & Sporakowski, M. J. (1984). The family stress of hemodialysis. *Family Relations, 33,* 33–39.

Peyrot, M., McMurray, J., & Hedges, R. (1988). Marital adjustment to adult diabetes: Interpersonal congruence and spouse satisfaction. *Journal of Marriage & Family, 50,* 363–376.

Shapiro, J. (1983). Family reactions and coping strategies in response to the physically ill or handicapped child: A review. *Social Science Medicine, 17,* 913–931.

Strauss, A. L. (1984). *Chronic illness and the quality of life.* (2nd ed.). St Louis: Mosby.

The Intervention Mode

INTRODUCTION: BARBARA M. ARTINIAN

PART IV

The purpose of the intervention mode is to test and modify an existing theory while improving clinical practice. When the relationships among the variables are adequately conceptualized, an intervention can be designed to improve practice and refine and extend the theory. In spite of the wide use of grounded theory methodology, few studies have been extended to affect clinical practice.

In order to use the findings of a grounded theory study, it is important to ascertain whether the intervention adequately represents the theory on which it was based. For example, in the study of risking involvement with cancer patients, certain conditions were identified that helped nurses resolve their grief following the death of a special patient, such as provision of time off following the death and supportive relationships at home and at work. In addition, engaging in outside activities that reduced the intensity of the experience was found to be helpful (see chapter 18, "Risking Involvement With Cancer Patients"). An experimental research design testing the effectiveness of a program that is designed to maximize these conditions with cancer nurses could be compared with a control group of cancer nurses for whom these conditions were minimal. A study of this type would evaluate the effectiveness of the program in resolving grief. Such a study would be different from one carried out in a quantitative mode because both the process of implementing the program and the program outcomes would be qualitatively analyzed using the same constant comparative methodology that has been used to generate the original theory (Artinian, 1988). In this way, the theory can be clarified and further developed.

In the absence of true experimental designs that could test and expand the grounded theory, the theory can be studied by an intervention in a clinical setting through an evaluation design. In his chapter in *The SAGE Handbook of Grounded Theory* (Bryant & Charmaz, 2007), Glaser (2007) explains, "grounded abstraction generates application" (p. 106).

The following section presents four interventions based on grounded theories presented in earlier sections. Giske has applied her understanding of preparative waiting theory (see chapter 21, "Patterns of Balancing Between Hope and Despair in the Diagnostic Phase on a Gastroenterology Ward") to developing an intervention that would increase nurse awareness of the problems experienced by patients in an ambiguous situation (see chapter 23, "An Intervention Study of Preparative Waiting Theory in a Hospital Unit"). Applying the theory of remodeling developed among MS patients (see chapter 14, "Remodeling the Course of Life: Moving On in a Changed Life"), Satinovic explores the use of the theory of remodeling the course of life among MS support groups to help people generate a good life with MS (see chapter 24, "An Intervention Program Using Remodeling the Course of Life Theory Among Persons With Multiple Sclerosis"). Hjälmhult works in educational research to discover if the use of her theory on positioning (see chapter 20, "Positioning in Operational Space: How to Become a Public Health Nurse in Norway") can be effective in helping PHN novices in a health care domain that is new to them to gain expertise more effectively (see chapter 25, "Implementing Conquering Operational Space Theory in Education Practice"). Cone has prepared research programs (see chapter 26, "Implementing Reconnecting Theory in Community Practice") to educate health care providers working with the homeless to modify care of homeless people based on the theory of reconnecting (see chapter 17, "Mutuality: Reconnecting to Overcome Homelessness"). Feedback from these programs can be used to modify and enhance the grounded theories under examination.

REFERENCES

Artinian, B. (1988). Qualitative modes of inquiry. *Western Journal of Nursing Research, 10*(2), 138–149.

Bryant, A., & Charmaz, K. (Eds.). (2007). *The SAGE handbook of grounded theory.* Los Angeles: Sage.

Glaser, B. G. (2007). *Doing formal theory.* In A. Bryant & K. Charmaz (Eds.), *The SAGE handbook of grounded theory* (pp. 97–111). Los Angeles: Sage.

23 An Intervention Study of Preparative Waiting Theory in a Hospital Unit

TOVE GISKE

The diagnostic phase has recently been researched more, both quantitatively (Drageset & Lindstrøm, 2005) and qualitatively (Leydon, Bynoe-Sutherland, & Coleman, 2002), especially in the area of breast cancer. All research points to this phase as the most stressful time owing to the amount of uncertainty patients and their families experience.

The grounded theory of Preparative Waiting (Giske & Artinian, 2008; see chapter 21, "Patterns of Balancing Between Hope and Despair in the Diagnostic Phase on a Gastroenterology Ward") presents the most well-developed theory of how the diagnostic phase is experienced by patients in hospital. The participants' main concern was found to be how they could prepare themselves for the conclusion of the investigations and life afterwards.

No reports were found describing systematic implementation of knowledge of patient experiences and processes in the diagnostic phase. Janice Morse, at a conference in 2008, discussed the lack of clinical changes coming out of qualitative research. She challenged us to move on and as researchers also to focus on how our findings can be implemented into practice and thereby make a difference in the clinical field. Grounded theory is especially fit for implementation as it focuses on the patient's main concern and how he or she acts to resolve it. The demand is for a grounded theory to be dense, with a few well-developed sensitive concepts with good grab, that fit the area of study, work to explain the processes going on, and show relevance by letting core problems and processes in the area emerge (Glaser, 1978, 1998). The focus on strategies participants use and how different conditions influence the process brings a grounded theory close to being put into practice and therefore makes it easy to develop into an intervention study.

The overall purpose for the study presented in this chapter is to improve practice for patients in the diagnostic phase coming to a medical unit in a Norwegian hospital and also to collect data to refine, modify, and extend the grounded theory of preparative waiting.

PREPARATIVE WAITING THEORY

The core category of the theory was named Preparative Waiting. The substantive Preparative Waiting theory explains how the participants handled their main concern. The theoretical code of *balancing between hope and despair* had four patterns: *controlling pain, rational awaiting, denial,* and *accepting* (see chapter 21, "Patterns of Balancing Between Hope and Despair in the Diagnostic Phase on a Gastroenterology Ward"). These patterns guided how participants balanced between the strategies they used to prepare for getting a diagnosis. Patients sought information related to the preparation for and the outcome of investigations to try to judge their situation. They wanted nurses and physicians, preferably one main contact person, to provide them with information and to follow them up during the stay. In the process of evaluating their case, they interpreted clues from their own bodies, diagnostic procedures, collaboration with staff, and priority given in the system. To be kept in uncertainty about the outcome of the investigation process and consequences for the future made them handle existential threats. It also made them consider what was important in life and assume more awareness of their view of life. They took care of themselves by seeking respite where they tried to keep themselves occupied with something other than the constant tension of uncertainty. This helped the waiting time to pass, and provided participants with renewed strength. All these activities are guided by the way they balanced between hope and despair. The movement between hope and despair made them get a taste of what they hoped and feared and thus prepared them to handle any outcome.

DESIGN

Method

Through data collection, analysis, and development of Preparative Waiting theory, patients had given me insight into how they prepared themselves for the concluding interview and life afterwards, as well as how different conditions eased or made the waiting time harder. In the implementation process, the action research design (Brown, 2001) was chosen since improved quality in the investigation process will need constant feedback from patients to help us keep focused on patients' point of view. Both qualitative and quantitative approaches will be used.

Aims

The aims of the project are specified in this way:

Specific aims related to patients

At the conclusion of this project, all patients will:

- Know who is their contact nurse or physician during the stay
- Have a good overview of the program of the day and the stay in hospital
- Be well informed about tests and investigations
- Receive information about tests and investigations, summing ups, and the final, diagnosis/conclusion as soon as possible
- Strengthen their ability to communicate with health care professionals

Specific aims related to nurses and physicians

At the conclusion of this project, all nurses and physicians will:

- Express good knowledge about their patients' diagnostic experience
- Identify conditions making it easier or harder for patients to go through the time of uncertainty and waiting
- Be motivated to follow up these patients in a thorough way
- Reflect continuously about what can ease the patient's investigative process, and what makes it harder

Specific aim for the system:

At the conclusion of this project, the health care team will:

- Develop a multidisciplinary care and treatment plan

Scientific aim for the researcher:

At the conclusion of this project, the nurse researcher will:

- Write a scientific article based on the project

Participants

This intervention study will collect data from patients, nurses, and physicians. After an initial contact with the unit, the head nurse, the nurse working with professional development, and I initiated discussion on the purpose and organization of the study. Physicians and nurses will be organized into groups on three nursing stations to promote optimal continuity in following up patients. It was decided that the implementation study should be limited to one group: the group that had the majority of admissions for gastrointestinal (GI) investigations. Four of the nurses and the two physicians working in this group were invited to take part in the study.

The inclusion for patients criteria are:

- All patients, aged 18 and above, are admitted to the defined group at the hospital unit for GI investigation.
- Patients must be mentally and psychologically capable of completing the questionnaire developed for the study.
- Patients must speak and understand Norwegian.
- Patients must be willing to give us feedback on the questionnaire.

Program Description and Implementation

Early in the planning process we had to make explicit who was responsible for what and how many should be directly involved in the project. After some discussion, we agreed to share responsibilities.

The director of research and development will:

- Finalize the purpose of the study
- Develop a questionnaire

- Send the application to the Norwegian Social Science Data Service and Regional Ethical Committee for final approval
- Teach, on a scheduled timetable and as needed, preparative waiting theory to the participating health care professionals
- Supervise all involved in the project through scheduled appointments and as needed
- Be first author of an article written for a research journal
- Supervise the development of the care and treatment plans for patients admitted to the selected unit for GI diagnostic workups

The head nurse at the unit will:

- Be a motivator for having the project carried out in the unit
- Organize the work so that the staff involved can take part in the project
- Keep in contact with director of research and development as needed
- Substitute for the nurse responsible for professional development as needed

The nurse responsible for professional development at the unit will:

- Participate in the process together with director of research and development and the head nurse in planning, implementing, and evaluating the project
- Manage study data of all participating patients for the duration of the project
- Participate in discussions and focus group interviews with the four appointed nurses
- Collaborate in developing the care and treatment plan for the study patients
- Be second author of an article written for a research journal

Four nurses appointed to be involved in the project will:

- Follow the study protocol as it relates to the nursing care of participating patients
- Participate in selected focus group interviews in the beginning, during, and at the end of the project
- Write weekly logs about their own experiences, including reflections about caring for these patients

- Distribute questionnaires to identified patients
- Specify what works/does not work for these patients and suggest reasons why
- Collaborate in developing the care and treatment plan for the study patients

Physicians working in this group at the unit will:

- Follow the study protocol as it relates to medical care of participating patients
- Prepare ahead of time for doctor's rounds
- Inform patients adequately and in a timely manner about the results of tests, diagnostic procedures, and the final diagnosis
- Collaborate in developing the care and treatment plan for the study patients

Nurses and physicians on the unit will be introduced to preparative waiting theory in the beginning of the research program so they gain insight into the patients' main concern in the diagnostic phase, which is how they (the patients) can prepare themselves for a diagnosis and what life will be afterwards. Also discussed will be how hospital conditions can promote or hamper patients' internal work, thereby making the waiting time easier or more difficult. Frequent feedback from the open comments in the patient questionnaires will be shared with the study personnel to assist in refining what works well in order to improve the patient experience, thus minimizing what is hard for them to endure.

The study team will review all information available about the routines of the day and brochures about actual tests and investigative procedures for this patient. When material is lacking, we will develop written material to support oral information. Patients will be informed about their rights, given an informational booklet, and encouraged to write down questions and concerns in preparation for the doctor's rounds. We will also prepare a folder presenting preparative waiting theory for patients so they can compare their own experience with the developed grounded theory.

Data Collection

Data will be collected from nurses and physicians involved in the study. The four nurses with a special responsibility to focus on the process will be asked to write regular logs, and they will take part in focus group interviews in the beginning of the study, after 2 months, and at the end of the study. The physicians working in this group will also take part in focus groups.

The patient questionnaire will be a 5-point Likert scale. Questions are developed from preparative waiting theory. Conditions reported to make the diagnostic workups easier or harder to go through are included, as well as patient experiences related to admission, information, investigations, doctor's rounds, contact person, how the diagnosis was conveyed, and how serious it was. All questions have an open space for comments in order to allow patients to convey their experiences and points of view throughout the process. Patients will also be invited to give suggestions for improvements and to share what has been important to them during the hospital stay. This feedback from patients can assist us in keeping up with what works well and help us see what needs further development in the hospital.

In 2006, a large study was carried out in Norway measuring patient satisfaction with hospital stays (PasOpp, 2006). Where relevant, questions from this research will be used to make later comparison possible.

The study will be started after approval of the regional ethical committee. Patients demonstrate consent to participate in the study by filling in the questionnaire and returning it to the unit in a sealed envelope. Anonymity and confidentiality will be kept by not asking for information that can identify patients.

Data Analysis

Data from the questionnaire will be analyzed by using statistical analysis software. The open comments will be analyzed according to grounded theory principles so that the theory can be refined, modified, and further extended as needed.

Data from nurses and physicians through focus groups and logs will also be analyzed according to grounded theory principles. These data offer health care professionals perspective on the diagnostic phase, and thereby make it possible to give an account of the complementary relationship upon which good care and follow-up depend.

CONCLUSION

The theory of Preparative Waiting explains how patients experience and work to prepare themselves as they go through the investigation process in the hospital. To live in uncertainty is most painful for these patients. Nurses and physicians are the key persons in the hospital, and the way they work and communicate with patients and organize the investigation process is very important for patients. Systematically implementing knowledge from preparative waiting theory on a hospital unit, and collecting data from patients, nurses, and physicians can be a fruitful way to improve quality of following up of these patients and further modify and extend Preparative Waiting theory.

REFERENCES

Brown, C. L. (2001). Action research. The method. In P. M. Munhall (Ed.), *Nursing research: A qualitative perspective* (3rd ed., pp. 209–243). London: Jones & Bartlett.

Drageset, S., & Lindstrøm, T. C. (2005). Coping with a possible breast cancer diagnosis: Demographic factors and social support. *Journal of Advanced Nursing, 51*(32), 217–226.

Giske, T., & Artinian, B. (2008). Patterns of "Balancing between hope and despair" in the diagnostic phase. A grounded theory study of patients at a gastric ward. *Journal of Advanced Nursing, 62*(1), 22–31.

Glaser, B. G. (1978). *Theoretical sensitivity.* Mill Valley, CA: Sociology Press.

Glaser, B. G. (1998). *Doing grounded theory: Issues and discussions.* Mill Valley, CA: Sociology Press.

Leydon, G. M., Bynoe-Sutherland, J., & Coleman, M. P. (2002). The journey towards a cancer diagnosis: The experiences of people with cancer, their family and careers. *European Journal of Cancer Care, 12*, 317–326.

Morse, J. (2008, May 19). Implementing qualitative research: Do we have a serious problem? Keynote address at the 5th Nordic Interdisciplinary Conference on Qualitative Methods in the Service of Health, Stavanger University, Stavanger, Norway.

PasOpp. (2006). *Pasienters erfaringer med døgnenheter ved somatiske sykehus: Resultater fra en nasjonal undersøkelse i 2006 [Adult patient experiences during medical inpatient care: Results from a national survey in 2006].* Nasjonalt kunnskapssenter for helsetjenesten [The Norwegian Knowledge Center for the Health Services]. Oslo, Norway. Retrieved May 17, 2009 from http://www.kunnskapssenteret.no/publikasjoner/1760.cms

24

An Intervention Program Using Remodeling the Course of Life Theory Among Persons With Multiple Sclerosis

MILKA SATINOVIC

A part of the substantive grounded theory on Remodeling the Course of Life (COL) as a means to generate a good life with multiple sclerosis (MS) is described in chapter 14, while the whole theory is described in a dissertation (Satinovic, 2008). The study was done to identify the main concern of persons living with multiple sclerosis and to discover how they resolved it. The main concern was found to be how to change in the course of life. This concern was resolved during a process consisting of four phases, in which the person with MS tries to remodel the course of life. The identified phases of the remodeling process are: *keeping up normal life, moving on in a changed life, doing the best possible in a changed life,* and *preventing illness from controlling life.* In this chapter, I present an intervention program based on Remodeling the Course of Life as well as an examination of the substantive grounded theory in nursing practice.

To facilitate my presentation, I make use of an approach to utilization of research described by Eastbrooks (1999). Eastbrooks delineates *indirect, direct,* and *persuasive* utilization. Indirect utilization of research can be done by teaching the theory to nurses and other health care providers, and encouraging them to use the principles when working with their patient populations. Direct utilization of research findings would be the direct use of the emergent theory with patients while extending and clarifying it through interviews, observations, and questionnaires. Persuasive research utilization denotes the use of findings in decision making about changing policies and practices of nursing care. This conceptualization by Eastbrooks will frame the discussion of how the theory of Remodeling the COL as a means to live a good life with MS can be used in nursing practice and how it can be extended to other fields of practice.

DESIGN

The study will use a Glaserian GT design to gain further information about Remodeling the Course of Life, its fit and relevance among patients with MS, and its application to other areas of practice.

Aim

The purpose of this study is twofold: (a) to improve practice in providing care to patients with multiple sclerosis; and (b) to gain further information about the substantive grounded theory on remodeling the course of life and its possible application to other domains.

Method

Grounded theory methodology will be used to guide data collection and data analysis. A questionnaire will guide interviews with MS patients, myalgic encephalopathy (ME) patients, personnel, and family members. Constant comparative analysis will compare the findings with the themes that emerged from the original GT study.

Participants

The research project has two parts with different participants in each. For phase 1 of the project, information from nurses working directly with MS patients is used for indirect utilization of the theory. This includes nurses who give care to patients with MS in a neurological department, MS–nurse specialists, and nurses working at rehabilitation units that serve patients with MS. For phase 2 the researcher will work directly with MS patients. Participants for this phase will include patients recently diagnosed with MS and referred by nurses working in the diagnostic center of the local hospital. Participants also include those recruited through the MS Society and the ME Society (supporting patients with chronic fatigue syndrome, or CFS).

PROGRAM DESCRIPTION

The two-part program is currently under way. Part one comprises the indirect and persuasive approaches and includes the education of nurses and other health care personnel who care for patients with multiple sclerosis. The second part is the implementation of the program among those who receive care, an examination of their perception of its fit and relevance, and an exploration of the theory's applicability to another group, namely those with chronic fatigue syndrome.

Indirect Use of Remodeling the Course of Life in Nursing Practice

Three different types of audiences could benefit from indirect use of research findings on how to live a good life with MS. I will first discuss my experience by presenting findings of the study at different levels of nursing education, at an MS society, and at an ME society (chronic fatigue).

Nursing Education and Practice

I have presented the developed theory of Remodeling the Course of Life at different levels of nursing education: bachelor, master, doctoral, and postdoctoral. The aim of the presentations to these audiences has been to offer a conceptualization of challenges that participants with MS experience in a Norwegian context when trying to live as good a life as possible. The conceptualization includes how they handle these challenges. The hypothesis is that by having the common conceptualization of the process of remodeling the course of life, health care personnel could meet people with MS where they are and understand what they worry about. For instance, when persons with MS are striving to accept the illness and to integrate it into the future course of life, it would be helpful if health care professionals in general and nurses in particular understand the depth and the gravity of this experience. Health care professionals can use the process of remodeling the course of life to become aware of a patient's situation, to promote and empower the patient to integrate the illness into his or her life, and to help the patient explore possibilities for a good life in spite of the illness.

Direct Use of Remodeling the Course of Life

Direct use of the theory of Remodeling the Course of Life is in effect when a program is presented to assist persons with MS to remodel the course of life in order to achieve as good a life as possible. At the same time, the researcher, when interviewing the patient, can test and evaluate the developed theory. I will discuss how one can start to develop a program of this kind.

Table 24.1 presents themes based on the stages in the theory of Remodeling the Course of Life. These themes were developed through in-depth analysis during the original study in which remodeling the COL emerged as a developing theory. The suggested themes will be used in two ways: (a) as an instrumental means to assess the process of remodeling or (b) as a means to facilitate dialogue with the patient.

An assessment questionnaire would test to what extent the theory of remodeling the course of life is able to give a patient and a nurse a picture of what is going on in a life with MS. At which stage in the process is the patient at present? How does the patient experience change and how does the change affect the life of the patient? What consequences are implied for the patient's life? These data can give us knowledge about differences between patient groups and make visible the patients who are at risk. The instrument will also be useful to help describe the process of remodeling in the group of people with different types of MS (progressive, relapsing-remitting, mild), and with differences in sex, age, and social situation.

Used as a means for a dialogue, the instrument can help the patient tell his or her unique story and develop awareness for the life situation and what is going on. It can help the person focus on what consequences the illness will have and how the focus changes as the illness progresses or goes into remission. The patient can give examples of shifts from one focus to another and describe the moving force for the change of focus. Using the themes from the instrument will help the patient see his or her choices as a process of generating a good life with MS. Such a process consists of both positive and negative fields of experience.

Table 24.1

INSTRUMENT BASED ON THE THEORY OF REMODELING THE COURSE OF LIFE
THEMES FOR DIALOGUE ON OR ASSESSMENT OF THE PROCESS OF REMODELING THE COURSE OF LIFE
Statement(s) for describing life with MS
Which are your challenges in life with an MS diagnosis right now?
Keeping up a normal life
1. Importance of living as you used to do before the diagnosis
2. Talking about your diagnosis with family members, workmates, neighbors
3. Energy used to keep up a normal life
4. Consequences of your way to tackle life with MS
Moving on in a changed life
5. Openness about the illness
6. Accepting MS as a part of life
7. Integrating the illness in life
8. Knowledge about changes in your body because of the illness
9. Strategies to strengthen your body, to generate energy, to improve your memory, to control your bladder function, to improve your quality of life
10. Competency to balance between the illness issues and life issues
Doing the best in a changed life
11. Value seeking
12. Fellowship
13. Activities that give you pleasure
14. Possibilities to use and develop your capabilities
15. Use of humor
Preventing the illness from controlling life
16. Obstacles when you try to live as good a life as possible
17. Encouragement in generating a good life
18. How much of your life is about illness
19. Hoping for the best

Printed with permission from M. Satinovic.

Persuasive Use of Remodeling the Course of Life

Persuasive use of the developed grounded theory means that it is used to persuade nurses and related health care personnel to improve current nursing practice among patients with MS at hospitals, coping centers, rehabilitation units, and nurse specialists. One other example of persuasive use of remodeling the life course is when it is used in policy making. The substantive theory of Remodeling the COL is developed from the patient perspective and as such it will differ from the perspective of health care personnel. Health care personnel who want to support persons with MS in their process of remodeling the COL will have to be familiar with the process and have the will and knowledge to implement the theory. Future courses will facilitate the development of competence of health care personnel by helping them understand the process of remodeling the COL, define its different phases, and help patients use its concepts to promote a good life with MS.

PROGRAM IMPLEMENTATION

The first phase of the training program has taken place, and the second is planned. The developed theory has been presented to health care personnel providing care to patients with multiple sclerosis and patients who receive care. Nurses at a neurological unit, home nurses, and nurses working at a rehabilitation unit have learned about the theory.

I have presented the developed theory at different levels of nursing education: bachelor's, master's, doctoral, and postdoctoral. The developed conceptual framework has also been presented to the MS societies at both national and local levels. The developed grounded theory of remodeling the course of life in order to live a good life with MS was also presented to a group of patients with chronic fatigue. Responses from the various groups are presented in the section on findings. The next step is to recruit participants for the direct use phase and to begin data collection and analysis.

Data Collection and Analysis

Phase 2 of the project requires meeting with patient groups and recruiting participants. I will use the instrument as an interview guide with patients, personnel, and family members of patients with MS. I will also conduct semistructured interviews with participants recruited from the ME Society. Observations, the interviews with participants, field notes, and memos will be included in data analysis.

The Glaserian GT method of constant comparative analysis will be used to analyze data. A comparison of findings from the MS group of participants and those from the ME group will indicate the fit and relevance of the theory of Remodeling the COL to patients suffering from chronic fatigue syndrome, thus validating and extending the theory.

FINDINGS

The first phase of the implementation project on indirect use of developed substantive theory has been completed, and a brief summary follows.

Nursing Education and Practice

The developed theory has been presented to students, researchers, and nurses working with patients with MS in settings such as hospitals, community, and nurse specialist. Those to whom the theory is presented immediately start to use it as a means to think and understand what is going on in the field. They tell new stories about its varying acceptance, or they describe cases where it has not been received and the consequent impact on patients, relatives, and health care personnel.

MS Societies

Patients with MS find training in Remodeling the Course of Life very useful. It gives them a framework to understand the process they have experienced more clearly and helps them articulate their life stories. They tell of hindrances to successful change in the course of life. They often raise issues such as the problems they encounter with reeducation, job reduction, and disability benefits, and how society is organized and functions when the health of an individual deteriorates.

Patients With Other Chronic Illnesses

The group of patients with chronic fatigue syndrome wondered if they could learn from the experience of patients with MS. Immediately after the presentation, I heard them comment, "This is the same process as we are going through" and "I am in the middle of this process," which indicates that the developed grounded theory of Remodeling the COL also reflects the experience of life with chronic fatigue syndrome. This immediate recognition is fascinating and suggests that the developed theory works and fits, and can be transferred to similar contexts where remodeling the COL is forced by chronic conditions.

These descriptions reveal (a) validation of the theory, as well as its relevance and modifiability, which are two of four criteria for assessing trustworthiness of the developed GT (Glaser, 1978), and (b) indirect use of the developed theory to understand what is going on in the field.

CONCLUSION

After presentations, persons with MS or their relatives often describe their own cases. These examples show that the concept of remodeling the COL as a process can be used indirectly by those involved to understand what is going on. The framework makes it possible to grasp why they act as they do, preview the consequences of different choices, and understand what prohibits or promotes the process of remodeling.

This research intervention uses the theory of Remodeling to describe the process of change in groups of persons who have different types of MS (progressive, relapsing-remitting, mild), and the theory applies across differences in sex, age, and social situation. These data can give us knowledge about differences between the groups and make visible patients at risk, such as patients who report that they are stuck somewhere in the process of remodeling. In the future, this knowledge can be used to develop programs and improve conditions in order to assist people with chronic and debilitating illnesses to generate a life that is as good as possible.

REFERENCES

Eastbrooks, C. A. (1999). The conceptual structure of research utilization. *Research in Nursing & Health*, 22(3), 203–216.

Glaser, B. G. (1978). *Theoretical sensitivity: Advances in the methodology of grounded theory*. Mill Valley, CA: Sociology Press.

Satinovic, M. (2008). *Omlegging av livskurs: en grunnleggende prosess i et godt liv med multippel sklerose*. Universitetet i Bergen, Bergen, Norway.

25 Implementing Conquering Operational Space Theory in Educational Practice

ESTHER HJÄLMHULT

Students' learning in clinical practice is important for many professions, but educational research in student clinical practice lacks empirical studies, particularly at the postgraduate level. Professionals to this day have too often been trapped in a tradition of abstract knowledge free from context, even in professional education, where theoretical knowledge is considered more important than knowledge developed by experience (Jensen, 1999). A study has been done to identify the main concern of how public health nursing students experienced situations in practice and how they resolved it (Hjälmhult, 2007, in press). The first phase of this theory is described in chapter 20 ("Positioning in Operational Space: How to Become a Public Health Nurse in Norway"). In this chapter, I will present an early phase of implementing the findings from the study into educational practice and start to briefly describe the theory.

THEORY OF CONQUERING OPERATIONAL SPACE

The grounded theory of Conquering Operational Space explains how public health nursing students resolve their main concern in clinical practice—how to gain access to learning experiences to become a public health nurse. This identified concern was resolved during a process consisting of three phases: *positioning, involving,* and *integrating into operational space.* Each of the phases has its own concepts, properties, and dimensions, which deal with the student role, relations with a supervisor, student activity, and the consequences of each phase. Through the complex and dynamic process, the students had to handle individual, social, and professional challenges simultaneously with feeling insecure and overwhelmed. They had to struggle toward obtaining independence, often by working against the system, handling the suspense of being in opposition to supervisors by daring to engage. In the period of clinical practice, the students aspired to define a sense of meaning, role, and function. As needed, they changed strategies along the way. The experience of successfully integrating into operational space demonstrated their attachment to their professional identity.

Aim

A grounded theory fits for implementation as it grabs what is important for the participants, and how they acted to resolve their main concern. The purpose of implementing findings from the theory of conquering operational space is to improve students' learning in clinical practice and to contribute to quality improvement within higher education and clinical practice. The aim is also to extend and modify this grounded theory and to investigate to what extent it fits in another area.

DESIGN

The first step in using and developing the conquering theory has been dissemination of the findings in different ways and areas to the people who are responsible for facilitating the learning process. There are at least three partners involved in the learning process: students during postgraduate education, nursing educators, and clinical supervisors. One researcher question has been: Will a common understanding of awareness of the conquering theory among all partners increase the quality of students' learning process?

Educators must define their focus and agenda in order to prepare both students and their supervisors in professional practice. To make a difference in practice requires that the generated theory should be constantly taught and integrated both in theory and practice. This idea corresponds to Coomarasamy & Khan (2004), who in a systematic review observed that clinically integrated teaching improves knowledge, skills, attitudes, and behavior, in contrast to seeing only knowledge improvement from classroom teaching. Therefore, evidence-based practice should be integrated into clinical practice to achieve desired improvements with substantial outcomes. "Situated learning" also develops in practice. In this theory, social interaction is a critical component and students become involved in "community of practice" (Lave & Wenger, 1991; Wenger, 1999).

When I have presented the findings of our study of conquering operational space to public health nursing students at the end of their programs, they have immediately recognized common experiences from their own internships, experienced an "aha," and understood some of their experiences in a new way. The framework of concepts made sense. Students recommended that they be informed about the conquering operational space theory *before* clinical practice.

Based on this suggestion, students new to the program are now introduced to the theory in their clinical orientation prior to their clinical experience. Some students who had been taught about conquering operational space before their placement reported more control in their practice and clearer sense of meaning to what happened with them. The feeling of insecurity and stress was more accepted and normalized, and the conceptual framework became a means to understand what had occurred in the field. Therefore, it can be valuable to systematically implement knowledge from conquering theory and systematically evaluate student feedback. This study result harmonizes with the criteria that a grounded theory should fit, be relevant, be modifiable, and work for those involved (Glaser, 1978, 1998).

Method

Both quantitative and qualitative methods will be used in our future study. The quantitative part of the study will use a questionnaire, which will be administered to the two groups of students at the end of their practical studies. The qualitative section of the study contains the open-ended questions at the end of the questionnaire and focus group interviews.

Participants

This study collects data from public health nursing (PHN) students and student midwives. Based on feedback already received, I have chosen student midwives as a comparative group. It is interesting to compare the PHN and midwife students. Norwegian midwifery education as well as public health nursing education is a postgraduate program requiring a bachelor of science in nursing and at least one year of full-time work as a registered nurse. Each student group in our study consists of 40 students and all are invited to participate. PHN students have two clinical periods (total 10 weeks) and student midwives four (total 40 weeks). Participation in the study will depend upon availability and willingness to participate.

Program Description and Implementation

The generated theory has identified that PHN students had to conquer their operational space in practical placements and distinguish how different conditions facilitated or hindered the learning process. In my meetings with the directors of the two programs, we have discussed how to organize a study, and I have permission to meet each of the two student groups in their classrooms. Two weeks before their first practical period the students will be informed verbally and in writing about the investigation and invited to participate. Supervisors will be given a 1-to-2-day seminar by the teachers at University College prior to students' clinical placements. Students participate to some extent in these seminars. The first day, I will introduce the theory of conquering operational space for supervisors, stimulate discussions and comments around the theory, and discuss their role in the learning process for students. They will also be informed about the study, the aims, and the student questionnaire.

Data Collection

Data will be collected by means of a self-administered questionnaire using questions developed from the theory of conquering operational space. A pilot study from public health nursing students at another University College will be carried out and necessary changes made. The structure of the questionnaire is a five-point Likert scale and covers student experiences related to positioning, involving, and integrating into operational space with a special focus on student role, dialogue, and participating, as well as reported conditions. Questions will provide the opportunity to share what has been important to them during the learning process in clinical practice. The questionnaire will be administered at the end of the students' practicum. The students at the university college are familiar with an electronic learning management system, "It's Learning," and the questionnaire is accessible via this system. The Regional Ethical Board does not require approval for this study. The Norwegian Social Science Data Services will be informed before the study begins.

Further data collection will continue after analyzing the questionnaires from the different practice periods. This will be accomplished by conducting focus groups from each program in order to gain deeper insight into students' experiences in practical periods. I will be the moderator for the groups with a teacher as co-moderator.

Data Analyses

Data from the questionnaires will be analyzed statistically using appropriate software, and grounded theory principles will be used in analyzing the open questions and data from focus groups (Glaser, 1978, 1998, 2005). The findings from different sources in this way can refine, extend, and modify the theory.

CONCLUSION

Conquering Operational Space explains how students experienced the learning process and acted to obtain learning experiences in their clinical practice. The students' role is vulnerable, and by gaining support from supervisors the ability to conquer the required operational space is increased. Close cooperation between University College professors and clinical supervisors is necessary in professional education; educators have a key role in preparing students and, to a degree, the supervisors for practical placement. By systematically implementing knowledge from the theory of conquering operational space and collecting data from students, the learning process of students will be improved and a contribution made to quality improvement within higher education. To gain a better picture of the whole process, a complementary study should be conducted to focus on the clinical supervisors' main concerns working with students in practice and thus generate a theory that presents the supervisors' point of view on the students' learning process. In this way, the two generated theories can shed light on each other and together drive the learning process forward.

REFERENCES

Coomarasamy, A., & Khan, K. S. (2004). What is the evidence that postgraduate teaching in evidence based medicine changes anything? A systematic review. *British Medical Journal, 329,* 1017–1021.

Glaser, B. G. (1978). *Theoretical sensitivity: Advances in the methodology of grounded theory*. Mill Valley, CA: Sociology Press.

Glaser, B. G. (1998). *Doing grounded theory: Issues and discussions.* Mill Valley, CA: Sociology Press.

Glaser, B. G. (2005). *The grounded theory perspective III: Theoretical coding*. Mill Valley, CA: Sociology Press.

Hjälmhult, E. (2007). *Erobring av handlingsrom. Helsesøsterstudenters læring i praksis.* PhD dissertation. The Norwegian University of Science and Technology (NTNU), Trondheim, Norway.

Hjälmhult, E. (in press). Learning strategies of public health nursing students: conquering operational space. *Journal of Clinical Nursing.*

Jensen, K. (1999). *Mellom tradisjon og fornyelse* [Between tradition and renewal]. In K. Nielsen & S. Kvale (Eds.), *Mesterlære: Læring som Sosial Praksis* [Master/apprentice: learning as community of practice]. Oslo: Notam.

Lave, J., & Wenger, E. (1991). *Situated learning: Legitimate peripheral participation.* Cambridge, MA: Cambridge University Press.

Wenger, E. (1999). *Communities of practice: Learning, meaning, and identity*. Cambridge, MA: Cambridge University Press.

26

Implementing Reconnecting Theory in Community Practice

PAMELA H. CONE

American policies that make life even more difficult for the poor and disenfranchised of our nation need to be revised (Whitehead, 2002). Programs of lasting assistance need to be developed (Institute for Children and Poverty [ICP], 2008). The current sociopolitical environment causes a sense of separateness from the larger society and a loss of personal and family stability for homeless families. The prevailing negative attitude of society toward the homeless starts the demoralization process and increases the sense of helplessness and marginalization that homeless mothers experience. Even those services that are supposed to help people who have limited financial resources are fraught with such difficulties as poor accessibilty, attitudinal barriers, and complex procedures and paperwork that often end up causing humiliation (Whitehead, 2002).

In today's already fragmented, disconnected society, those who do not fit the social patterns or common understandings of families and mothers are disempowered (Averitt, 2003). Findings from a study based on the perspective of formerly homeless mothers were used to develop a theory-based program to assist homeless mothers in overcoming their homeless situation. The initial study was conceived with the long-term goal of informing the practice of those who serve the homeless. This chapter discusses the implementation of a theory-based program for care providers who work with the homeless.

DISCUSSION OF RECONNECTING THEORY

The basic social process (BSP) of Reconnecting to Overcome Homelessness emerged through a Glaserian GT study among formerly homeless mothers (Cone, 2006). The stories of the 30 participants were further analyzed to reveal a cutting point in the theory of reconnecting. The theoretical code of *amplifying causal loops* emerged to explain the relationships of the concepts to each other and the movement of the process toward its outcome of reintegrating into society (see chapter 17, "Mutuality: Reconnecting to Overcome Homelessness").

Reconnecting has two stages, each with several steps. The stage of *moving out* includes becoming ready and connecting with someone. A cutting point of the decision to make a stable connection separates the first and second stages. The stage of *overcoming* includes revaluing self, mutually solving problems, and reintegrating into society. Mutuality is a key concept in the process, and the relationship between variables is an amplifying causal loop that increases as the care provider invests time, energy, and caring into the life of the homeless mother and helps her to reconnect with society. The intervention described here focuses on reconnecting as a means to overcome adversity and the research proposes to examine the effectiveness of the theory in program planning and implementation.

INTERVENTION MODE

Aim

The purpose of the study is to improve practice in providing care and protocols of assistance programs for homeless mothers and to test and extend the theory of Reconnecting (see chapter 17, "Mutuality: Reconnecting to Overcome Homelessness").

Design

This intervention study is based on the basic social process of Reconnecting to Overcome Homelessness that emerged from a Glaserian GT design for qualitative research (Glaser, 1998). This research is proposed as a type of political activism advocating involvement in policy making at the local, state, and national levels. At the local level, the East San Gabriel Valley Coalition for Health Care for the Homeless (ESGVC-HCH) will be provided with the protocol and the board requested to use it in giving in-service training for their personnel. They, in turn, will pass on the protocol to the case managers and social workers from the state who work with the homeless at their sites.

At the national level, the theory of Reconnecting will be displayed in a poster format at a national Health Care for the Homeless (HCH) conference for leaders who work with the homeless. Attendees will be invited to fill out a survey assessing the fit and relevance of the poster information to their own work with homeless people. They will be asked to apply the intervention program in their HCH programs. They will also be asked to reassess the program later on using a questionnaire to send back to the researcher that will be attached to the original survey.

Participant

For the local ESGVC-HCH, participants will include the board and on-site leaders who will be invited to participate in the study by applying the new protocol in preparation of the HCH Winter Cold Weather Shelter program in December 2009 and then to evaluate its effectiveness in March 2010 using a survey questionnaire. In addition, a convenience sample will be used to recruit participants at a major conference on homelessness by the National Center for Health Care of the Homeless in Washington, DC, and invite them to participate in the study to test the theory of reconnecting.

PROGRAM DESCRIPTION

The two stages and five steps of the reconnecting process are used as the framework for application to practice (see Figure 17.1). A brief explanation of the theoretical framework underpinning the protocol will be attached to the research questionnaire. Those who work with homeless mothers through various agencies will be given strategies based on the findings from each stage. The protocol is a new approach that is simple and cost-effective, though it is time-intensive (see Table 26.1). Its use will require a change of attitude and focus, both on the part of program administrators and care providers.

Table 26.1

PROGRAM FOR THE PHENOMENON OF EXPERIENCING HOMELESSNESS

PROGRAM PLAN

Reconnecting
to overcome homelessness

Moving on

1. *Becoming ready*
   - Encourage personnel to make contact over and over and not give up
   - Teach personnel to be supportive when the homeless hit bottom
   - Train personnel to identify cues for the readiness to change
2. *Connecting with someone:*
   - Develop the personnel for making caring connections that will bring hope to homeless mothers
   - Utilize only genuinely caring personnel in street and shelter work areas
   - Train personnel to build rapport and trust in order to solidify connections

Overcoming

3. *Revaluing self*
   - Train personnel to assist in the values clarification process
   - Provide counseling that will assist with revaluing self and establishing a new belief in self-worth
   - Encourage personnel to instill a sense of love and belonging in the mothers
4. *Mutually solving problems*
   - Train personnel in the mutuality needed for true collaboration with mothers
   - Mutually cooperate to find solutions for financial instability and home establishment
   - Demonstrate respect for the mother's ideas and choices through the technique of active listening
   - Brainstorm with the mother and encourage the mother to express her dreams and goals as well as strategies for reaching them
5. *Reintegrating into society*
   - Sustain long-term one-on-one connections
   - Build and solidify accessible support networks

(*Continued*)

Table 26.1

PROGRAM FOR THE PHENOMENON OF EXPERIENCING HOMELESSNESS (*Continued*)

- Assist in finding jobs and homes where social support is accessible
- Encourage mothers to maintain social connections and strengthen networks
- Identify and support activities the mothers choose that indicate a desire to give back to society

Context: Formerly homeless motherhood

Conditions: Reconnecting with someone, self, and society

Outcome: Homeful and reintegrated into society

Printed with permission from P. Cone.

Data Collection

Initial data will be collected in June 2009, when a colleague and I will present a poster at the National Health Care for the Homeless conference in Washington, DC. These data will be gathered from conference attendees, who will be asked to answer a short survey with questions relating to the poster presenting two stages and five steps of the reconnecting theory. They will be asked about the fit and relevance of the findings from the study on reconnecting to overcome homelessness. Those who agree to participate in the long-term project will also be given the handout with a clear description of the intervention and the protocol itself (see Table 26.2), and they will be asked to use the intervention in their work with the homeless. A self-addressed stamped envelope with an attached questionnaire will provide a means for sending a program evaluation to the researchers after implementation.

For the local portion of the study, I will attend ESGVC-HCH planning meetings and provide the same packet of materials to coalition leaders. Initial responses to the survey will be gathered and a request to use the long-term intervention with follow-up evaluation of the program will be made. In this way, both a specific local site and a group of scattered national sites will be included in data collection.

Table 26.2

PROGRAM HANDOUT ON RECONNECTING TO OVERCOME HOMELESSNESS

The process of *Reconnecting* demonstrates clearly the importance of genuine caring and concern on the part of care providers and a one-on-one connection with homeless mothers to facilitate the processes of *moving on* and *overcoming homelessness*. It begins with establishment of mutual connections, requires mutual problem solving, and only succeeds with the establishment of long-term social networks. The process is cost-effective but time-intensive.

The choice of workers who have a genuine desire to help homeless mothers move out of homelessness is important. Personnel should keep on offering themselves as mentors until they see indicators of the homeless mother's readiness to change. Establishing a mutual connection is the key to empowering these women to envision "homefulness" and to take the first step toward getting into a home of their own. Care providers must respect the way each mother manages her mothering and her trajectory out of homelessness. Training on how to apply values clarification with the homeless that will assist in changing their perspective on themselves from worthless to valuable human beings is crucial. Caring connections must be established and maintained, requiring interdependence and mutuality, in order for effective problem solving to occur.

Developing and maintaining support networks requires mutuality as well. Caregivers must learn how and where to access a wide variety of resources, taking into account the accessibility of resources in the long term, in order to avoid instability and the risk for repeat homelessness. Maintenance of social networks and support is crucial for long-term success; restabilization precedes reintegration into society.

Printed with permission from P. Cone.

Data Analysis

Upon collecting initial survey answers, the Glaserian GT method of constant comparative analysis will be used for open coding of answers to discover themes and categories. Reflective memos will record my thoughts and analysis. With the availability of a large pool of possible participants, saturation may occur at one national conference and one local organization. If necessary, I will continue data collection at other conferences and sites.

I anticipate that findings from this study will shed light on the emergent theory of reconnecting, and give insight into its fit, relevance, and workability in the care of the homeless. Evaluation of the theory-based intervention will reveal more clearly the most effective strategies for helping single female-headed homeless families to get off the streets into stable housing as rapidly as possible. Future testing of the theory will take place among another sample of people disconnected by adversity.

CONCLUSION

Programs with some success include programs such as PATH (Programs for Assistance in Transition from Homelessness) administered by SAMHSA (Substance Abuse & Mental Health Service Administration), a branch of the U.S. Department of Health and Human Services, and "Homes for the Homeless" in New York City (ICP, 1998, 2008). What these programs have in common is their focus on a broad range of services. However, what they lack is an extended network to support families until the time these families self-identify as ready to be independent. The services also lack a focus on establishing and sustaining a support network for these vulnerable families, so with increasing numbers of newly homeless, these programs are actually failing to meet the need (ICP, 2008). Programs for homeless families need to be flexible and multifaceted and should be promoted by genuinely caring individuals. They need to be based on mutuality and the continuing input of the families they serve. In addition, they need to encourage establishment of mutual support networks that "mend the torn fabric" of societal connections for these families (Letiecq, Anderson, & Koblinsky, 1996).

"Give a man fish, you feed him for a day; teach a man to fish, you feed him for a lifetime" is an old adage that, while couched in gender-based terms to which feminists might object, holds true for the situation of homeless mothers today. In light of this study, one could add "Connect him/her to a fishing village, and you provide a support for his/her family." Family homelessness can be overcome, as these formerly homeless mothers have demonstrated. It is up to society's leaders, such as health care providers, to work with homeless families to help them to avoid becoming another homeless statistic by reintegration into mainstream society.

REFERENCES

Averitt, S. S. (2003). "Homelessness is not a choice!" The plight of homeless women with preschool children living in temporary shelters. *Journal of Family Nursing*, 9(1), 79–100.

Cone, P. (2006). Reconnecting: A grounded theory study among formerly homeless mothers. Unpublished PhD dissertation, University of California at San Francisco.

Glaser, B. (1998). *Doing grounded theory: Issues and discussion.* Mill Valley, CA: Sociology Press.

Institute for Children and Poverty. (1998). *Ten cities: A snapshot of family homelessness across America, 1997–1998.* Institute For Children and Poverty, in cooperation with Homes for the Homeless. Retrieved on June 21, 2005, from www.homesforthehomeless.com

Institute for Children and Poverty. (2008). *Failure at the four-year mark, 1998–2008.* Institute for Children and Poverty, in cooperation with Homes for the Homeless. Retrieved June 21, 2005, from www.homesforthehomeless.com

Letiecq, B. L., Anderson, E. A., & Koblinsky, S. A. (1996). Social support of homeless and permanently housed low-income mothers with young children. *Family Relations, 45*(3), 265–272.

Whitehead, D. (2002). *Statistics on homelessness.* Washington, DC: National Coalition for the Homeless. Retrieved on March 13, 2004, from www.nationalhomeless.org

Index

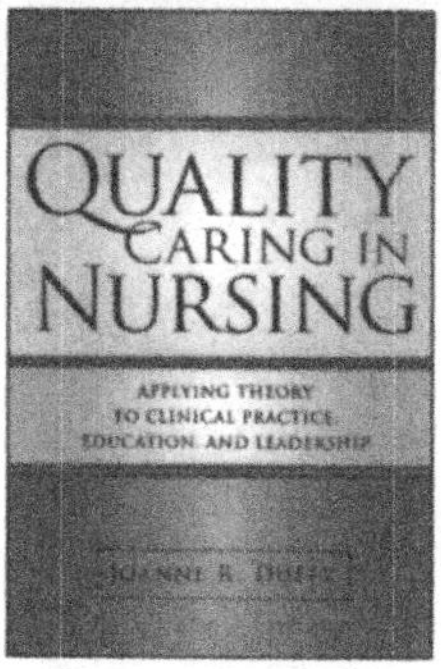
QUALITY
CARING IN
NURSING

Made in the USA
Monee, IL
13 September 2026

62977348R00216